Medical Myths, Lies, and Half-Truths: What We Think We Know May Be Hurting Us

Steven Novella, M.D.

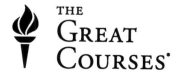

THE
GREAT
COURSES

PUBLISHED BY:

THE GREAT COURSES
Corporate Headquarters
4840 Westfields Boulevard, Suite 500
Chantilly, Virginia 20151-2299
Phone: 1-800-832-2412
Fax: 703-378-3819
www.thegreatcourses.com

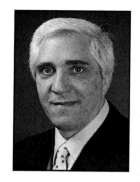

Steven Novella, M.D.

Academic Neurologist
Yale School of Medicine

Professor Steven Novella is an Academic Neurologist at Yale School of Medicine. He is active in medical education at every level of experience, including patients, the public, medical students, and continuing education for medical professionals. He also performs clinical research in his specialty area, including publications on amyotrophic lateral sclerosis, myasthenia gravis, and neuropathy.

Dr. Novella received his M.D. from Georgetown University and went on to complete residency training in neurology at Yale School of Medicine. He is also trained in the subspecialty of neuromuscular disorders, which continues to be a focus of his practice. Although he treats all types of neurological disorders, he specializes in diseases of nerves and muscles.

Dr. Novella is the president and cofounder of the New England Skeptical Society, a nonprofit educational organization dedicated to promoting the public understanding of science. He is also the host and producer of their popular weekly science podcast, *The Skeptics' Guide to the Universe*. This award-winning science show (2009 winner of the People's Choice podcast award in the education category) explores the latest science discoveries, the presentation of science in the mainstream media, public understanding and attitudes toward science, philosophy of science, and critical thinking.

Dr. Novella was appointed in 2009 as a fellow of the Committee for Skeptical Inquiry, an international organization dedicated to the promotion of science and reason; he writes a monthly column for their publication, the *Skeptical Inquirer*. Dr. Novella maintains a personal blog, the award-winning *NeuroLogica Blog*, which is considered one of the top neuroscience blogs. On *NeuroLogica Blog*, he covers news and issues in neuroscience but also general science, scientific skepticism, philosophy of science, critical thinking, and the intersection of science with the media and society.

Dr. Novella is also the founder and senior editor of *Science-Based Medicine*—a group medical and health blog with contributions from dozens of physicians and scientists. *Science-Based Medicine* is dedicated to promoting the highest standards of both basic and clinical science in medical practice. This prolific health blog is geared toward both the general public and health professionals. *Science-Based Medicine* is recognized as a top health blog and is increasingly influential in the ongoing discussion of the role of science in medicine. ∎

Table of Contents

Table of Contents

Table of Contents

SUPPLEMENTAL MATERIAL

Disclaimer

This series of lectures is intended to increase your ability to recognize medical misinformation and make use of reliable, evidence-based information when making health-related choices. These lectures are not designed for use as medical references to diagnose, treat, or prevent medical illnesses or trauma. Neither The Great Courses nor Dr. Steven Novella is responsible for your use of this educational material or its consequences. If you have questions about the diagnosis, treatment, or prevention of a medical condition or illness, you should consult a qualified physician. ■

Medical Myths, Lies, and Half-Truths:
What We Think We Know May Be Hurting Us

Scope:

True or false: Eight glasses of water a day are mandatory for staying hydrated. Vitamin C protects you from catching a cold. Frequent snacking is the quickest way to bust your diet. Natural foods are always better for you.

You hear advice like this all the time. But what do these would-be nuggets of medical wisdom have in common? They're all myths, half-truths, and misconceptions—pieces of information so familiar that we take them for granted without considering the scientific truth about them.

In today's information age, when supposedly accurate medical advice and diagnoses can be found online with the click of a computer mouse, medical myths are all around us. Using them to make decisions about your health—whether it's how to treat the symptoms of the common cold or how to care for a child or aging relative—can be harmful, even deadly.

Because you are ultimately responsible for your own health, it's critical to understand the accuracy of medical information—to break down the growing body of misinformation and discover the truth about everyday health and well-being. These 24 lectures are an empowering learning experience that will give you evidence-based guidelines for good health, will enhance your ability to be better informed about common medical myths, and will strengthen your skills at assessing the scientific truth behind medical information and advice. ■

Medical Knowledge versus Misinformation
Lecture 1

There are hundreds of cancer cures promoted on the Internet. There are all kinds of concoctions and unusual or bizarre treatments that will sell themselves because of claims that there's a conspiracy of silence in the medical community—that the government and physicians are all in on it for some reason. But, at the end of the day, what they're trying to do is sell you on a myth of the hidden or secret cancer cure.

We are all responsible for our own health and health care and for that of our children. Yes, there are healing professionals who are there to help, advise, and perform technical procedures—like surgery—that we can't do ourselves. But, ultimately, we make our own decisions. We live in the age of information, where we can simply go on the Internet and get access to all the information that professionals have access to. Being armed with accurate information can help us make the best health decisions for ourselves and our families. But the flip side is that being confused by myths and misinformation can be dangerous—sometimes even deadly.

On the Internet and elsewhere, there are rumors, urban legends, and myths that are spread as fact. There are many ideological groups spreading misinformation to promote their particular worldview. There are also plenty of people who are trying to separate you from your money by making false or misleading marketing claims or using hype rather than real information to promote a product.

The best source of reliable information is still health-care professionals. Your physicians are there primarily to advise you. Don't be afraid to ask questions: When you have a visit with a physician or other health-care professional, come prepared. If you are going to do some research on your own, do it before you go in, and bring your specific questions. Bring a friend or family member, because the more people that are in the room hearing the information, the more you will remember. Also, don't be shy about seeking second opinions; it's pretty much par for the course these days.

There are other trusted sources besides health-care professionals. If you are wading through the information on the Internet, stick to trusted sources like known universities—Yale, Harvard, the Mayo Clinic, or Johns Hopkins. There are also many research institutions like the National Institutes of Health, the National Cancer Institute, and the Muscular Dystrophy Association. There are professional organizations for every specialty, like the American Academy of Pediatrics and the American Academy of Neurology. There are also patient or disease advocacy groups like the Multiple Sclerosis Society.

But there are also a lot of posers. Anyone can create a snazzy website and make it seem like they're an impressive organization. Therefore, here are some red flags to look out for:

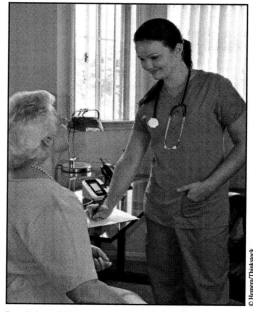

Don't be afraid to ask questions of your health-care providers.

Beware of so-called institutes or organizations that seem to be doing nothing more than promoting a single individual. Beware of sites that seem to be trying to sell you something; they are probably distorting information to make that sale. Also, beware of outliers. If you're visiting various sites that all seem to have one opinion, but Bob's Institute of Syndrome X has a completely different opinion, it's probably Bob's Institute that you should be wary of. There are also well-meaning but misguided patient and disease-oriented groups. There are groups that honestly want to do what's best for patients, sufferers, and society, but they don't have a culture of science.

Finally, there is no substitute for just thinking critically. At the end of the day, you have to think for yourself. Here are some more tips for reading information on the Internet: (1) If something sounds too good to be true, it probably is. If someone's promising you the cure for cancer, you should be a little wary of that. (2) Don't trust testimonials. They are just anecdotes, and as we say, the plural of anecdote is anecdotes, not data. Sites use testimonials to support their claims because they don't have the scientific evidence to back them up. (3) Look for contrary information and opinions. If someone is trying to sell you a product, treatment, or therapy, specifically go out of your way to see what the critics of this are saying. (4) Finally, is there published, peer-reviewed evidence? That's the ultimate currency of medical information. Having a peer-reviewed article is not a guarantee that the results will hold up over time or that they're accurate, but it's at least a good starting point. To search for this research yourself, go to the website PubMed.org.

The best source of reliable information is still health-care professionals.

Over the next 23 lectures, we're going to go on a journey together through many medical facts and myths. I will also discuss many controversial topics. Some of these topics may touch very close to home on beliefs that you have, and I ask you to listen with an open mind. My job is to go through the scientific literature, to try to make sense of the science as we understand it today. Sometimes that may lead to conclusions that are not necessarily popular or that are controversial. I also try to separate out real controversies within the scientific community itself from false controversies—ones where the scientific community is generally on the same page, but there are still public opinions that are contrary. I'll also try to make clear when I'm giving you my own opinion or interpretation that may not be the definitive answer on a particular problem. ■

Suggested Reading

Note: Additional references for most lectures are listed at the end of the Bibliography.

Bausell, *Snake Oil Science*.

Centers for Disease Control (website).

Ernst and Singh, *Trick or Treatment*.

Mayo Clinic Online Reference.

Sagan, *The Demon-Haunted World*.

Sampson and Vaughn, *Science Meets Alternative Medicine*.

Science-Based Medicine (blog).

Questions to Consider

1. How do we know which treatments are safe and effective for which conditions?

2. What role do you think informed consumers should play in their own health care?

Medical Knowledge versus Misinformation
Lecture 1—Transcript

Hi, I'm Dr. Steven Novella, an academic physician and neurologist. The reason why I spent my career in academia is because I love teaching—teaching students, patients, my fellow physicians, and the public. It's why I contribute to several science blogs, why I produce a science podcast, and why I'm really excited about teaching this course on medical myths.

To give you some idea of the types of questions that we encounter, let me tell you about a patient who came to me with a very serious illness—a fatal illness in fact. He wanted to know if he should fly to China to spend $20,000 plus all the expenses involved for a risky and experimental stem-cell treatment that they read about on the Internet. That person needed serious information.

I also get many questions from friends, family, and acquaintances. For example, new parents want to know if they should vaccinate their children to protect them from disease. Should they worry about all those risks they've been hearing about and reading about on the Internet? Then there are the more simple questions like, should you really wait an hour after eating before going swimming?

We're all ultimately responsible for our own health and healthcare and for that of our children. Yes, there are healing professionals, like myself, who are there to help, advise, give you information, and perform technical procedures—like surgery—that you can't do yourself. But, ultimately, we make our healthcare decisions for ourselves. We also live our lives day to day not under the care of a professional, but making decisions that affect our health.

We live in the age of information where everyone can be their own expert. This is because you can simply go on the Internet and get access to all the information that professionals have access to. Being armed with accurate information can help us make the best health decisions for ourselves and our families. But, the flip side is that being confused by myths and misinformation can be dangerous, sometimes even deadly. Sometimes even physicians are still harboring medical myths and could learn to correct it and hear the truth.

There is a tremendous amount of healthcare information on the Internet. In fact, two-thirds of adults in a recent Pew poll said that they go on the Internet specifically to search for healthcare information. It is one of the most common types of information that is available on the Internet. There's so much, in fact, that people are overwhelmed with too much information. It can be bewildering to sort through all the various conflicting sources and claims.

On the Internet and elsewhere, there are rumors, there are urban legends, there are myths that are spread as fact, sometimes even seeming authoritative. There are many ideological groups that are spreading misinformation because they want to promote their particular worldview. And there are plenty of people who are trying to separate you from your money by making false or misleading marketing claims or using hype in order to promote a product rather than real information. Of course, there are lazy and sometimes sensationalistic journalists who are promoting it all.

Still the single most reliable source of reliable information is healthcare professionals. Don't be afraid to use those resources. Your physicians are there primarily to advise you. Don't be afraid to ask questions. Some other tips on making the most of that resource—when you do have a visit with a physician or other healthcare professional, come prepared. If you are going to do some research on your own, do it before you go in and go in with specific questions. Physicians basically expect that these days and it's part of the interaction. Bring a friend or family member because the more people that are in the room hearing the information, the more you will remember and take home. That's clear.

Don't be afraid to ask for more time if you feel you need it, even if that requires making another appointment. The most important part of the interaction with the physician and a patient is the educational component—make sure you get that out of it. Also, don't neglect your wellness visits. This is part of the reason why you want to go to a physician even when you're well—so they can update you on things you should be doing to stay healthy. For most healthy adults, an annual visit is fine. Of course, if you have a chronic illness you may want to visit more frequently. Also, don't be shy about seeking or asking for second opinions. It's pretty much par for the course these days and you shouldn't shy away from it.

Other than your physician, there are other trusted sources as well. If you are wading through the information on the Internet, you need to have some rules of thumb to figure out what sources are likely to be reliable and which ones you should avoid. Trusted sources include known universities—my own institution of Yale, Harvard, the Mayo Clinic, or Johns Hopkins. Those old and trusted names are good sources of reliable information.

There are also many research institutions like the National Institutes of Health, the National Cancer Institute, and the Muscular Dystrophy Association. There are professional organizations like the American Academy of Pediatrics and the American Academy of Neurology. Pretty much, there's one for every specialty that there is. There are many patient or disease advocacy groups like the Multiple Sclerosis Society.

But, there are also a lot of posers. Anyone can create a snazzy website and make it seem like they're an impressive organization. Therefore, here are some red flags to look out for. Beware of so-called institutes or organizations that seem to be doing nothing more than promoting a single individual. Anyone, again, could name themselves an institute. Beware of sources that seem to ultimately be trying to sell you something; probably they're going to be distorting the information to make that sale.

And beware of outliers. By which, I mean, if you're visiting various sites that all seem to be giving one opinion, and Bob's Institute of Syndrome X has a completely different opinion, it's probably Bob's Institute that you should be wary of—not all of the other tried and true institutions. This is especially true if they're claiming that they're being persecuted or they're the victim of some kind of conspiracy of silence. These are just ways in order to distract you from the fact that they're giving you a rather unusual opinion.

Other types of misinformation include marketing—again, as I said, promoting an ideology. But, there's also well meaning but misguided patient and disease oriented groups. There are groups that do honestly want to just do what's best for patients, sufferers, and society, but they don't have a culture of science. They're not dedicated to accurate information. Thus, they can easily form an echo chamber of misinformation. You have to be wary of that as well.

Finally, there is no substitute for just thinking critically. At the end of the day, you have to think for yourself. Again, here are some rules of thumb that should set off your critical thinking filters when you're reading information on the Internet. One, if something sounds too good to be true, it probably is. Beware of hype that seems way out there. If someone's promising you the cure for cancer, you should be a little wary of that. Also, don't trust testimonials because they're just anecdotes. As we say, the plural of anecdote is anecdotes, not data. The reason why sites are using testimonials to support their claims is because they don't have the scientific evidence that reliably backs them up.

Also, look for contrary information and opinions. If you're reading someone trying to sell you some product, treatment, or therapy, specifically go out of your way to see what the critics of this are saying. What does the other side believe? See which side sounds more credible. Also, if there is one, see what the consensus is. Are most sites that are reliable promoting one point of view as opposed to an outlying point of view?

Finally, is there published, peer-reviewed evidence? That's the ultimate currency of medical information. Having a peer-reviewed article is not a guarantee that the results will hold up over time or that they're accurate, but it's at least a good starting point. Don't believe conspiracy theories. Again, they're there to distract from the actual evidence. Don't trust friend-of-a-friend urban legends. Make sure that the sources are all verifiable.

I mentioned that peer-reviewed published scientific medical research is the most reliable kind of evidence out there, but that breaks down into different kinds of evidence as well. It's important to understand that because the wrong kind of evidence can be used to support the wrong kind of claims. For example, there's basic science research. That's what's done in test tubes and Petri dishes to try to understand the basic mechanisms of how cells work and how things function. But, they can't be used to make ultimate clinical claims about what's safe and effective. Biology is still just too complex for us to extrapolate from basic science knowledge. But, it does help point the way towards clinical research.

When the basic science looks promising, then we do animal research because there's no substitute for looking at something in a complex biological model. Again, animal models of disease and animal research cannot be used to see what happens in people because people aren't rats and guinea pigs. But, it does help set us up to do more safe and effective clinical research.

Clinical research is what we base clinical claims on. That breaks down into a few types as well. There's observational research and experimental research. With observational research, we're just looking at what's happening out there in the real world. We're looking for correlations. We can't control all the variables so when we find a correlation we can't know what the cause and effect is. But, if we see a correlation holding up, no matter how we look at it—for example, smoking cigarettes correlates with various types of lung cancer in observational studies—we can still come to reliable conclusions.

But, the best kind of clinical evidence is experimental evidence where we actually have subjects that we experiment on. This is because we can control all of the variables and we can isolate the variable that we're interested in. Does this treatment work for a specific disease? But, then again, there are preliminary clinical trials with small numbers of patients that are usually unblinded or just minimally blinded. There again, they're just to see if this is a promising treatment when we actually give it to people.

All of this leads to the most reliable kind of information for clinical claims. That is definitive, large, double-blind, placebo-controlled studies where as many variables as possible are controlled. There's large numbers where you can get statistical significance. Even then we like to see a consensus of multiple such trials before we really close the door on any specific question. If you want to look at some of this research for yourself, I suggest you go to a website called PubMed.org. That's where I go when I want to look at the actual published literature.

Now that we've set the stage for how to think about information and how to sort through all of this, I'm going to give you a few examples. I'll start with some simple, easy bites, just a few common medical myths. Then, we'll see what the information really is about them.

I'm going to start with hiccups. A hiccup is an involuntary spasm of the diaphragm that causes the abrupt inhalation of air followed by a sudden glotic closure, causing the typical hiccup sound. Normally, hiccups are intermittent. They occur at random for a short period of time. Most of us have encountered them. When they're brief and intermittent, they don't cause a problem. They may be embarrassing if nothing else. They can be caused by eating a large meal, laughing, drinking too much alcohol, emotional stress, or even just stretching.

There are plenty of folk hiccup treatments out there. The most common ones are holding one's breath, breathing into a bag, being startled, swallowing sugar, the Valsalva maneuver—which is basically holding your breath and then bearing down like you're having a bowel movement, like this—or trying to hiccup. Do any of these home remedies for hiccups work? There's no evidence to support any of them. They really are just folk remedies without any evidence behind them.

There are even some amusing and bizarre folk remedies that have been proposed for hiccups. This includes stroking your earlobe, repeating to yourself "I am not a fish," flatulence, saying the word "pineapple," drinking vinegar, and my favorite, jumping out of an airplane. I'd like to see that one in a double-blind trial.

There are, however, interestingly, hiccup treatments that actually work. But, these are not ones that you're going to get at home. There are several medications that we use to treat what we call intractable or persistent hiccups which can actually become a serious problem. These medications include gabapentin, Thorazine, and baclofen. In extreme cases, we can even implant a vagal nerve stimulator or a phrenic nerve pacer to actually override the hiccups by controlling the nerves.

Let's go from the hiccup to the sneeze. The sneeze is an involuntary explosive expulsion of air from the nose and mouth. It's triggered by irritants on the nasal or oral mucosa, by bright lights, allergies, and respiratory infections. It serves a protective function. It expels irritants and germs from our upper respiratory system. What happens if you hold the sneeze in?

I've heard lots of stories about all the horrible things that can happen to you when you hold a sneeze in, such as your eyes popping out. But, in honesty, none of those things are going to happen. There's no real danger to holding in a sneeze although you probably shouldn't do that. You should let this sneeze serve its function—to expel irritants and germs. Although, if you do have to sneeze, you should do it into a tissue or your elbow so you don't spread those germs around.

There are, however, real risks to sneezing because sneezing is a fairly violent and explosive event. It can very rarely—and I want to emphasize this, very rarely—lead to some medical complications. These include an arterial dissection, which is a tear in one of the arteries leading up your neck—very dangerous and can lead to a stroke—retinal damage from the sudden pressure; fainting from that Valsalva maneuver I spoke about which you can do when you sneeze. It could drop your pressure; you get less blood flow to your brain and you can pass out. It can cause headaches by a similar mechanism and also can dislodge a clot from your legs and cause a venous embolism. But, don't worry, those are all really rare side effects.

What about swallowing gum? Parents always tell their children, don't swallow the gum, it's dangerous. Many of you have probably heard that, if you swallow gum, it will stay in your intestines for up to seven years. Gum is made from resin. It is not digestible, so you won't break it down and digest it. However, it doesn't stay in your intestines. Your intestines have what we call peristalsis—they move things through. The gum will pass through your intestines with the normal passage of time. You will expel it on your next trip to the bathroom.

There are some potential risks, though, to swallowing large amounts of gum over a short period of time—something that really only a child might do. It can, in fact, cause an obstruction, especially if you eat it with other bulky items, like fiber, for example. It may actually get stuck so much in your intestine that it will cause a blockage that could be potentially serious, even requiring surgery. Therefore, it is the standard recommendation that kids under five are not allowed to chew gum because they may think that they're supposed to swallow it just like candy. Also, a minor point is that gum does contain a lot of sugar, so sugarless gum is better for your teeth and your health.

What about hangovers? Here are the symptoms of a typical hangover: dehydration, fatigue, fever, nausea, vomiting, headache, diarrhea, flatulence, sensitivity to light and sound, trouble sleeping, and difficulty concentrating. It doesn't sound very pleasant. It's no surprise that people have been seeking cures for hangovers for many years.

What causes all those horrible symptoms? First is dehydration. Alcohol inhibits what we call the anti-diuretic hormone. In other words, alcohol makes you pee, makes you lose water. There are also impurities in alcohol such as other types of alcohol—other than ethyl alcohol—zinc, and so-called congeners, which are other substances in there that give the alcohol its flavor. In fact, darker liquors have more of these congeners in them. It is not a myth and it is, in fact, true that darker liquors may therefore cause a worse hangover for that reason.

Also, the ethanol—which is the alcohol that we drink—is metabolized in the body to acetaldehyde. Acetaldehyde is a nasty chemical that is 30 times more toxic than alcohol itself. To a large degree, it's the acetaldehyde that causes the hangover. Also, drinking may impair the liver's ability to regulate blood sugar. Therefore, the hangover may also go along with hypoglycemia or low blood sugar.

What are the real cures for hangover? There's really only one tried and true treatment. That's what we call tincture of time. It simply takes time to metabolize the acetaldehyde into acetic acid. Nothing is going to take a hangover completely away until that has had time to occur. You can also treat some of the symptoms. For example, if you're dehydrated, you can treat that with hydration, drinking a lot of fluid. That may improve the headache and fatigue. Also, alcohol irritates the stomach and may cause nausea. Therefore, milk or other foods that are settling may settle the stomach and relieve those symptoms. Also, if you're hypoglycemic, you can eat food, especially carbohydrates. That may make you feel a little bit better as well.

But, that's pretty much it. Time and those symptomatic treatments are the cure for hangovers. But, there are a lot of folk remedies. For example, there's caffeine, so-called hair of the dog, drinking more alcohol, all sorts of potions and concoctions, hot showers, and exercise. Unfortunately, none of those home remedies have any effect. They simply don't work.

There are some not-at-home remedies, however, that may help. If you find yourself or someone finds themselves in an emergency room because of a severe hangover, then you may get treated with oxygen or certain medications that help deal with the metabolic effects. This includes tolfenamic acid, chlormethiazole, and acetylcysteine.

Let's get back to that question I asked at the beginning of this talk—should you wait an hour after eating before you go swimming? This one's been around for a long time, since at least the 1960s. It's based on a somewhat plausible notion—the idea that, when you eat a large meal, your blood gets diverted to the digestive tract and away from your muscles. Therefore, if you then try to engage in activity, your muscles won't be getting enough blood flow and they will tend to cramp up. If you're swimming when your muscles get a large cramp, that could be very dangerous and you could drown. That's the source of that urban legend.

However, it turns out that, while some blood is diverted to the digestive system from the muscles, it's not enough to cause any problems with muscle function. There's plenty of blood flow to go around and there is no correlation with eating and cramping. There simply is nothing to that myth and, of course, there's nothing about the magical number of one hour. Really, the only risk from eating a large meal and then engaging in strenuous activity is that it may be uncomfortable. But, it's not a medical problem.

Over the next 23 lectures, we're going to go on a journey together through many medical facts and myths. I will also discuss many controversial topics.

Some of these topics may touch very close to home on beliefs that you have and I ask you just to listen with an open mind.

My job is to go through the scientific literature, to try to make sense of the science as we understand it today. Sometimes that may lead to conclusions that are not necessarily popular or that are controversial. I also try to separate out real controversies, controversies within the scientific community itself, from false controversies—ones where the scientific community is pretty much all on the same page with a specific conclusion, but there are still public opinions which are contrary to that scientific consensus. I'll try to make it clear also when I'm giving you my own opinion or my own interpretation that may not be the definitive final answer on any particular problem.

We started in this lecture with some fun, mini-medical myths. We're going to be running the whole gamut including some very in-detail and very serious misinformation and mythology. For example, let's get back to that patient that I spoke about at the beginning of the lecture. He wanted to know if they should travel to China in order to get experimental stem-cell therapy for his terminal illness. That's a really serious question. He wanted to know if he should mortgage his house and get money from his friends, family, and co-workers in order to do this.

Unfortunately, he was following a trail of misinformation. It was a trail that was laid there specifically to lure people who are desperate and looking for information with the latest hype in order to essentially take them of tens of thousands of dollars. I've even seen cases of people spending over a hundred thousand dollars seeking these stem-cell therapies.

At the present time, in the spring of 2010, there are no legitimate stem-cell therapies for sale that are out there. Therefore, if you see anyone claiming to cure anything with stem-cells, it's probably marketing hype and probably a scam. Stem cells are a legitimate avenue of research. It's a very exciting and very sexy potential treatment where we could actually replace dead, diseased, or dying cells with healthy new cells. We're certainly hoping that it will potentially treat many things, like Parkinson's disease and Alzheimer's disease.

But, it's not at the level of human use yet. We're basically making the transition from animal research to the earliest human research with stem-cell therapy. The only stem cells that should be given to people at this point in time for these types of therapies should be done in the context of a legitimate and ethical experimental protocol, not in some clinic in China or Mexico. But, that information is on the Internet. It is there in order to provide misinformation to lure you in.

There are many other equally serious issues. For example, there are hundreds of cancer cures promoted on the Internet. There are all kinds of concoctions and unusual or bizarre treatments that will sell themselves because of claims that there's a conspiracy of silence in the medical community—that the government and physicians are all in on it for some reason. But, at the end of the day, what they're trying to do is sell you on a myth of the hidden or secret cancer cure. These are very serious because they are attempting to lure patients away from proven therapies, therapies which may even have the potential for a cure in some cases for some types of cancer. In others, it may just extend the duration and quality of life.

But, if you forego proven therapy for the false hope of a cure that you read on the Internet, that is one of the good examples of the dangers of medical misinformation. There are many other types of treatments as well. There's chelation therapy, for example. This has been around since the 1950s. Chelation therapy is a legitimate treatment for heavy metal poisoning. But, there is a subculture of even physicians who are promoting chelation therapy for heart disease and other indications, for autism, for things that have nothing to do with heavy metal poisoning and for which the evidence shows it doesn't work.

In a perfect world, chelation therapy for heart disease would've been abandoned 50 years ago, but the subculture persists. Now they're using the Internet in order to spread their alternate view, essentially a big medical myth. Some are true believers; some I think are just trying to market it to the public. That's another thing to be wary of, these subcultures that could have all the trappings of legitimate scientific institutions. That's another good example of why you have to go with the consensus of opinion. If you have one institute that is saying one thing, but all the other scientific institutes, universities, and professional organizations are saying something else, that should give you pause.

In my own specialty of neurology, I frequently encounter a claim that a treatment called patterning or psychomotor patterning could actually cure children of serious neurological disorders like mental retardation, Down's syndrome, or things like that. I have had many parents ask me. Sometimes it's my patients, sometimes it's just my friends or neighbors that ask, should they go to this institute, dedicate a large chunk of their lives and a lot of resources of time, emotion, and money to this therapy—because they want to do everything for their child.

I certainly understand that they want to do that, however, the scientific evidence settled this question in the 1970s. It was an interesting idea; it just didn't work out. It doesn't work and now we understand why it doesn't work. The underlying theories didn't really pan out. But, some of these disproven therapies that should be discarded—and were discarded by science—live on. They live on in myth. They live on on the Internet because people became dedicated and too invested in these notions to give them up. They couldn't go beyond the scientific evidence.

These are the kinds of issues, the range of issues, that I'm going to be talking about over the next 23 lectures. Some are fun and easy medical myths. A lot are very serious and involved medical situations dealing with serious diseases, sometimes life threatening. Other times, it's just how to live an optimal, healthful life. I'll be talking about weight control and dieting, which is very fraught with medical myths. I'll talk about things like hypnosis and all kinds of mythology around vaccines, pregnancy, and many other topics. I'm looking forward to discussing all of those issues with you over the next 23 lectures.

Myths about Water and Hydration
Lecture 2

So-called juicy foods like fruit contain a great deal of water, maybe 60%–70%. There are some surprising foods, like a cooked hamburger, that have 40%–50% water.

About 65% of the adult body by weight is made up of water. We all need water to survive, yet there are many misconceptions and much false information out there about this most basic element of life. How much water should we drink every day? If you are dehydrated, should you drink beverages with caffeine in them? Are expensive water purifiers really worth it?

The primary mechanism by which we maintain our hydration is thirst. Thirst is a powerful emotion that motivates us to eat and drink. Thirst actually serves two functions. First, it regulates the concentration of salt and other electrolytes in our blood—a property of the blood and tissues called osmolality. Also, it regulates the overall volume of water in our bodies. The other primary mechanism by which our bodies regulate our own fluid is urination. Many people ask how useful urine color is in determining our overall state of hydration. It turns out that it's actually a pretty good rough marker.

Another way our body loses water is through sweating. Sweating primarily is a mechanism to regulate body temperature, but it involves excreting saline from our sweat glands. In hot and dry environments or with physical activity, sweating can be a significant source of water loss. This may dramatically increase the amount of fluid we need to drink in order to replace what we lose through sweat.

One of the big myths of water is how much water we should drink every day. Typically, you'll hear that you need to drink eight 8-ounce glasses of water per day. This myth probably originates from the Food and Nutrition Board, which calculated the average water needs of an average adult with average activity and environment and came up with the figure of 64 to 80 ounces per day. However, in that same report, they also noted that most people get 20% of their fluid intake from food. Thus, even if you need 64 or 80 ounces, you don't have to drink it all as water, and you don't have to go out of your way to count up how many glasses of water you're drinking.

What about thirst myths? I've often heard that by the time you're thirsty, it's too late—you are already dehydrated. When you think about it, that doesn't really make much sense, because thirst has evolved over millions of years to be a mechanism to tightly regulate how much fluid we need in our body. It wouldn't work well if you didn't become thirsty until after it was too late. In general, you can rely on your thirst. You will become thirsty long before you are actually dehydrated. Thirst works, and you don't have to force fluid when you don't feel like drinking.

The diuretic effect of caffeine is actually very mild, and the fluid in most caffeinated beverages will more than compensate for this effect.

What about the myth that caffeinated drinks do not hydrate and in fact will make your hydration worse? This is based on a kernel of truth, as many myths are. Caffeine is a weak diuretic; therefore, if you drink a lot of caffeine, it could plausibly make you lose fluid. However, the diuretic effect of caffeine is actually very mild, and the fluid in most caffeinated beverages will more than compensate for this effect. If you're out on a hot summer day and all you have is a caffeinated beverage to drink, go ahead and drink it. It will still hydrate you.

What about special situations in which we need to pay more attention to our hydration? In hot weather, we sweat more to cool ourselves off, and we therefore lose more fluid. Whenever you're in a warm or hot environment, make sure you have access to fluid so that you can hydrate continuously. Fortunately, our bodies also acclimate to a hot situation by holding onto more fluid. Athletes often push human endurance to its limits, and water is no exception. Athletes can lose as much as 2 liters of sweat per hour. That means they may need to drink 12 liters of fluid in a day in order to just maintain their hydration.

However, there's a cautionary downside to this as well. Aggressively hydrating, even with sports drinks that contain electrolytes, can actually worsen the dilution of electrolytes. The only way to really maintain your osmolality when you're drinking that much fluid is to eat salty snacks. When you push the body to its limits with extremes of athletic endurance, you overwhelm the regulatory systems. You have to be careful about how much you drink, what you drink, and that you eat.

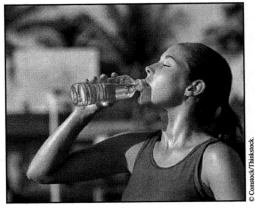

© Comstock/Thinkstock.

In a warm environment or with physical exertion, make sure you hydrate continuously.

There are a few questions that frequently come up with respect to water. One is bottled water—is there an advantage to it? Interestingly, bottled water costs about 1900 times as much as tap water. But bottled water, if you look at it statistically, is no better than tap water. It's no more healthy, and in taste tests, it hasn't been shown to taste any better. Bottled water, overall, is basically a scam.

What about water purifiers, which you install in your home to filter out organisms, impurities, or heavy metals from your water? Most modern industrialized countries have agencies, like the Environmental Protection Agency in the United States, that closely monitor and regulate water. Currently, there are no major safety issues with tap water in the United States or other industrialized countries. If you have any concerns, you can look up these agencies' reports on the quality of the water in your area. The legitimate use for water purifiers is to increase the taste of water. There, you can just follow your own taste. If your tap water tastes fine to you, then don't worry about it. If it doesn't taste right, you may want to get a water purifier—even though it won't necessarily be more healthful. ■

Suggested Reading

Segal, "Body Fluids."

Questions to Consider

1. How does the body maintain its delicate balance of water and electrolytes?

2. Are some sources of water better for hydration than others?

Myths about Water and Hydration
Lecture 2—Transcript

This lecture is all about water, something that we all need to know about. For example, let me tell you about the time I was hiking during a hot summer when I was feeling thirsty. A friend of mine who was hiking with me warned me against drinking the carbonated and caffeinated beverage that I had. They told me that the caffeinated beverage would not rehydrate me and, in fact, it would make me more dehydrated.

Another time, I was visiting the Mt. Wilson Observatory. It's a beautiful telescope 10,000 feet on the top of Mt. Wilson. Despite the fact that I was drinking on a regular basis and thought I was doing well to keep hydrated, I became fairly dehydrated fairly quickly. Also, I have many patients that have to be concerned with their hydration. For example, I have migraine patients who may get a migraine if they become dehydrated. Many have noted to me that they get dehydrated if they take a jet ride. They're curious as to why that might happen.

About 65 percent of the adult body is comprised of water by weight. That's a lot. Water is the elixir of life. We all need it to survive. It's not surprising, therefore, that psychologically, it represents to us the very notion of purity and health. We all need to protect our precious bodily fluids. Even in cool temperatures, a person can only survive for only about ten days without fresh water.

Yet, there are many misconceptions and much false information out there about this most basic element of all life. How much water should we drink every day? If you are dehydrated, should you drink drinks with caffeine in them? Are expensive water purifiers really worth it?

Where do we get our water from? Of course, we get water from drinking fresh water and pretty much any fluid that we drink will be mostly water and will rehydrate us or keep us hydrated. But, interestingly, about 20 percent of the water that we get comes from the food that we eat. That's an average number, 20 percent. There's actually a lot of variability in how much water there is in food. So-called juicy foods like fruit contain a great deal of water;

they may be 60 to 90 percent water. There are some surprising foods, like a cooked hamburger, that have 40 to 50 percent water in it.

Of course, very dry foods will have less water. Depending on the kind of foods that you eat, you'll get different amounts of water from your food. But, again, about 20 percent of your water intake comes from the food you eat rather than fluids that you're drinking. In other animals, interestingly, they may get more water from their food. Koala bears, in fact, rarely drink water at all. They don't have to drink water. They can get 100 percent of their fluid from the eucalyptus leaves that they eat. Of course, sea creatures get all of their water from what they eat because they live in salt water; they have no access to fresh water.

The primary mechanism biologically by which we maintain our hydration is thirst. Thirst is a powerful emotion that motivates us to eat and drink. When we feel as if we are thirsty, our body is telling us that we need fluid. That motivates us to engage in the proper behavior. This actually is in fact a very fine tuned system of self-regulation. Generally speaking, you don't have to think too much about how much water is in your body. You just follow your thirst and let your body do the rest.

Thirst actually serves two functions. First, it regulates the concentration of salt and other electrolytes in our blood. That is a property of the blood and tissues called osmolality. It's basically a technical term for concentration in the blood. Also, it regulates the overall volume of water in our bodies.

Since thirst and other mechanisms that I'll mention are regulating both osmolality and fluid volume, it's interesting to understand how the two things interact. By and large, they go hand and hand. When you're on the dry side, when you're dehydrated, your fluid volume will be lower and your osmolality will be increased at the same time. Therefore, drinking fresh water or most of the sources of fluid that we would drink will correct both a high osmolality and dehydration. There's no problem. But, generally speaking, most of the time the osmolality gets the priority.

Actually, our bodies have evolved to very carefully and closely regulate osmolality within a fairly narrow range. This is because it has the priority in terms of the mechanisms of regulating these two things. However, the more dehydrated we get and the lower our fluid volume becomes, the more that fluid volume takes priority. If you are severely dehydrated, overall fluid volume takes absolute priority. All of your body mechanisms will shift into a mode where they are conserving water at all costs.

The other primary mechanism—other than thirst—by which our bodies regulate our own fluid is micturition. This is just a fancy word for urination. Our kidneys and our genitourinary system are the primary mechanism by which our bodies will regulate water volume and concentration. Simply put, our kidneys will flush our blood. Basically, the blood filters through the kidneys. The kidneys, moment to moment, are sensing the amount of overall concentration in the blood. They're also receiving hormonal signals from other parts of the body like the heart and the brain, which are telling the kidneys what the overall fluid volume in the body is. Then the kidneys will concentrate the urine based upon all these signals. They will also adjust the concentration of many specific components—not just the overall concentration, but the individual concentrations of sodium, potassium, calcium, and chloride, for example.

One question that comes up is how useful is urine color in determining our overall state of hydration? Is that a myth that you can rely upon, the color of your urine? It turns out that it's actually a pretty good rough marker—although there are a few caveats. When your urine becomes more concentrated, it will go from a pale, pale yellow at the dilute end to a darker yellow, then amber, and even a brownish color at the maximally concentrated end.

For example, you may notice that your first urine in the morning—you haven't had anything to eat or drink for eight plus hours—is usually pretty dark. But, if you drink a lot of fluid during the day, it may become very, very pale yellow. That's your kidneys doing their job, varying the concentration of urine depending on how much fluid there is in your body. If you want to get an idea about your overall state of hydration, you can simply look at your urine although you probably should use the average color over several urinations.

Here come the caveats now. For example, there are certain things that you can eat, which can also change the color of your urine. There are certain vitamins; there are certain food coloring dyes that may alter the specific color of your urine. That may throw you off a little bit. But, generally speaking, it's a good reliable indicator. We do more in terms of our fluid status than just drink and urinate although those are the two primary mechanisms by which we regulate our osmolality and overall fluid volume.

There are other ways in which our body loses water, for example, sweating. Sweating primarily is a mechanism to regulate body temperature, not body fluid. However, it does involve excreting saline, salty water, from our sweat glands. That water then evaporates and that evaporation takes heat away from our skin and that cools off our bodies. In hot and dry environments or with physical activity, sweating, however, can be a significant source of water loss. Therefore, it may dramatically increase the amount of fluid we need to drink in order to replace what we lose through sweat.

When we're dehydrated, again as I said, the more dehydrated we become the more all of our bodily fluid mechanisms shift into conserving fluid. The amount that you sweat will progressively decrease the more dehydrated you become. If you stop sweating, not because you're cool, but because you're dehydrated, then you lose a very important mechanism of regulating your temperature. This can lead to heat stroke. In fact, that's the most common cause of heat stroke—dehydration combined with the hot temperature.

As I said, sweat is not just water; it's salty water. You've probably tasted sweat, it tastes salty. We're losing salt, sodium chloride, and other electrolytes in the sweat as well. Those too need to be replaced. Therefore, drinking just water is not going to be sufficient.

Another thing that we do every day that causes us to lose water is breathe. With every breath you take—as the Police song goes—we lose water. Water is lost through evaporation. When we have patients in the hospital and we are carefully regulating their fluid input and output in order to monitor the function of their organs—like their kidney, heart, and lungs—we can calculate everything we put into the body and everything that comes out of the body.

But, there's what we call insensible water loss. Insensible water loss is what we can't measure, but it's happening nonetheless and we just estimate that. In a hospital environment, an average person will lose a couple hundred cc's of water just from evaporation through breathing. However, the drier the environment, the more water you will lose through breathing. This could become very significant. Here, dryness is probably more of a factor than the heat itself.

In fact, mountain climbers learn that, when they are at a high altitude, the air becomes not only thinner, but typically much drier. Even though there may be snow on the ground and it can be very cold, the dryness can cause a tremendous increase in the insensible water loss through breathing. In fact, that's what happened to me when I was on the top of Mt. Wilson. It was cool. I wasn't really engaged in any strenuous activity, but at 10,000 feet, it was very dry. I lost a lot of fluid much more quickly than I usually do.

One of the big myths of water is, How much water should we drink every day? Typically, what you'll hear is that you need to drink eight 8 ounce glasses of water per day. But, is that really what you need to drink? Do you have to go out of your way and count up how many glasses of water you drink? This myth probably originates from the Food and Nutrition Board who calculated the average water needs of an average adult with average activity and environment. They came up with the figure of 64 to 80 ounces per day; eight times eight ounces is 64. That's probably where the eight by eight myth came from.

However, in that same report, they also noted that, on average, most people are also going to be getting 20 percent of their fluid intake, of their water intake, from the food that they eat—and the rest from fluids. Thus, even if you need 64 or even up to 80 ounces, 20 percent of that is coming from your food so you don't have to drink it all as water. Also, it's interesting to note that most people just going about their day without paying any attention to how much they're drinking are going to be getting more than the 64 to 80 ounces of fluid. Again, you don't have to go out of your way to count up how many glasses of water that you're drinking.

What about thirst? I've often heard that, by the time you're thirsty, it's already too late—you are already dehydrated and therefore you have to consciously hydrate yourself and not just rely upon thirst. When you think about it, that doesn't really make that much sense overall because thirst has evolved over millions of years to be a mechanism to tightly regulate how much fluid we need in our body. It really wouldn't work very well if you didn't become thirsty until after it was too late. That would be like the gas gauge on your car only telling you when you've already run out of gas.

In general, you can rely upon your thirst. You will become thirsty long before you are actually dehydrated. Again, the systems have evolved to very tightly regulate our fluid intake. The bottom line is trust your thirst. Thirst works and you don't have to force fluid even when you don't feel like drinking.

I mentioned before that that friend of mine had heard that caffeinated drinks do not hydrate and in fact will make your hydration worse. They'll dehydrate you. This is based on a kernel of truth like many myths are. Many myths are often based upon that little kernel of truth. Caffeine is a weak diuretic. A diuretic is something that stimulates your kidneys to excrete more fluid, to dilute the urine, and to waste water. Yes, caffeine is a slight diuretic. Therefore, if you drink a lot of caffeine, it could plausibly make you lose fluid. However, when you dig down a little bit deeper, it turns out that the diuretic effect of caffeine is actually very mild.

Also, frequent caffeine drinkers will become tolerant to that effect. They don't get the diuretic effect from caffeine after a while. After even just a few weeks of regular caffeine use, it no longer has that effect on your body. Also, the fluid that is contained in most caffeinated beverages will more than compensate for this mild diuretic effect. If you're out on a hot summer day and all you have is a caffeinated cola or other beverage to drink, go ahead and drink it. It will still hydrate you.

What I've been talking about up to this point mostly is usual environmental conditions as most people go about their day to day life under most circumstances. However, there are special situations in which we do need to pay a little bit more attention to our hydration—and where dehydration can occur so quickly that if you don't have ready access to fluid, you may become dehydrated.

The first to talk about is hot weather. This one I think is the one that would make most sense and that most people would think about. As I said, the hotter it is, the more we sweat in order to cool ourselves off and the more fluid we will therefore lose. We also will lose more fluid through the insensible loss, the evaporation from breathing. Therefore, whenever you're going to be in a warm or hot environment, you need to make sure that you have access to fluid so that you can continuously hydrate yourself.

Dehydration results from just not having access to fluid for a period of time. Fortunately, our bodies also do what's called acclimate. They acclimate to a hot situation by adjusting. Our bodies will naturally hold on to more fluid. We will lose less water and salt through our sweat as we spend more and more time in a hot climate. This also means that, when you are traveling from a cool environment to a hot environment—you're taking a vacation in the tropics, you're not acclimated to the heat—you can become dehydrated even quicker. Also, that first really hot day in the spring when the thermometer climbs above 90 and people are outside, they don't realize that, after a long winter and a cool spring, they're not acclimated to the heat. Therefore, you have to be especially cautious at those times.

Athletes often push human endurance to its limits and water is no exception. Athletes can lose as much as two liters of sweat per hour—two liters! That means they may need to drink 12 liters of fluid in a day in order to just maintain their hydration. That's a situation where, if you're not going out of your way to steadily drink, you can easily become dehydrated.

However, there's a cautionary downside to this as well. Aggressively hydrating, even with sports drinks that contain electrolytes, can actually worsen the dilution of electrolytes or the loss of electrolytes from the blood. Remember how I spoke about osmolality and fluid concentration and fluid volume? If you're struggling to maintain your fluid volume, you can actually dilute out and reduce the osmolality in your blood. That could actually even get to dangerous levels. Most people think that if you drink a sports drink that has electrolytes in it this won't happen. It puts back what your body is missing, as the advertisements say. However, while they are much better than straight water, they're still what we call hypotonic, meaning they have less salt than electrolytes. There's much less than what's in your blood. Therefore, it will still tend to dilute out the electrolytes in your blood when you have to drink gallons and gallons or liters and liters of this fluid.

The only way to really maintain your osmolality when you're drinking that much fluid is to eat especially salty snacks. When you push the body to its limits with extremes of athletic endurance, you overwhelm the regulatory systems. You do have to be careful about how much you drink, what kind of fluid you're drinking, and you do need to eat.

I had spoken about high altitudes and my trip to Mt. Wilson. There are other situations—other than being at a world famous telescope—where you might be at a high altitude. Probably the most common situation in which the average person finds themselves at a high altitude is when they're flying in a jet to go somewhere. At 6000 feet, just from the thinning of the atmosphere, water loss through breathing is double normal. You will lose water at twice the rate. This becomes progressively more of a factor as you get higher and higher in altitude. At 10,000 feet, where I was at Mt. Wilson, it's triple. You lose it at three times the rate.

Jet cabins are partially pressurized. If you're flying 39,000 feet, you're not feeling the pressures that are outside the airplane at 39,000 feet. You would pass out. That's why they instruct you about how to breathe through those breathing masks. But, if you're in a Boeing 747 at 39,000 feet the cabin is pressurized to about 6900 feet of pressure. Again, you're at a little bit more than double the rate of insensible loss through breathing in the cabin.

Also, jets like to keep their cabins dry. It's better for the equipment and everything inside the airplane. Now you're in a dry and low pressure environment where water loss can be much more rapid than you think and you're used to. Also, you're confined to your seat so access to water may be limited. The stewardesses or stewards may be slow in bringing you water. Therefore, it's actually recommended that you have some kind of fluid with you when you're going to be taking an especially long flight in order to make sure that you don't become dehydrated.

There are many medical conditions in which fluid management becomes more complicated. Again, what I've been discussing up to now is your average healthy adult or healthy person. But, there are many medical conditions where we have to pay particular attention to fluid status. I already mentioned that, in the hospital when patients are sick, we may count up every cc, every milliliter of fluid and very, very carefully manage it.

Let me give you some examples of some medical conditions where fluid management is more in point and where the regular mechanisms of thirst and micturition may not be adequate. For example, if the kidneys themselves are not working with kidney insufficiency or kidney failure, the kidneys may not be able to keep up with their demands and put out enough fluid. You might need to restrict your fluid intake in order not to overwhelm the kidneys' ability to deal with the fluid.

In heart failure, the heart can't pump enough blood to the kidneys. The fluid starts to get backed up in the heart and backed up in the lungs. Again, the only real treatment for that is fluid restriction—or doctors may prescribe artificial diuretics that will sort of coach the kidney into getting rid of more fluid.

There're also kidney stones. If you've ever had them, you'll know it's one of the most painful medical conditions that there is. These are usually formed from calcium oxalate or calcium phosphate. They are sharp, little crystals that get stuck in either the ureter, the tube that connects the kidney to the bladder, or the urethra, the tube that drains the urine from the bladder. That could be extremely painful. You have this small, little, delicate tube with this sharp, knifelike crystal inside that has to work its way all the way down this long tube—it's very, very painful.

If you are at risk for developing kidney stones—because you have a family history, a particular metabolic situation that can lead to increased risk of kidney stones, or you're on certain medications that increase the risk of kidney stones—you may have to pay particular attention to your hydration. It may not be enough to just listen to your thirst. You may actually need to keep an eye on your urine. We tell patients to look at your urine. It should always be pale yellow. Force a little bit more fluid than you would naturally drink just from thirst in order to keep your urine very dilute. That will minimize and reduce the risk of developing those painful kidney stones.

Diarrhea or dysentery is actually a serious medical condition. Throughout most of human history, this has been a very significant cause of death. In fact, before the modern age, most soldiers who die in an army campaign don't die of their wounds—they die of things like dysentery. What happens is that an infection in the intestines will cause the bowels to stop absorbing water from the food and fluid that we eat and drink. But, even worse than that—even worse than the fact that it's not absorbing fluid—it actually can secrete fluid into the intestines. This then, of course, comes out the other end as diarrhea.

In fact, a severe case of dysentery can cause somebody to secrete and lose 10 or 12 liters of fluid every day just through the intestines. Imagine losing that much fluid and not being able to replace it by drinking, by absorbing it. It's no wonder that people become rapidly dehydrated and die from this condition. In fact, only modern medicine really can save people from death from dysentery. In essence, we have to give them intravenous fluid. We have to bypass the intestines until they have a chance to heal. We have to replace all the lost fluid with intravenous fluid—usually saline—something that's close to what the blood is. This gives people time and keeps them alive in order for the infection or whatever is causing the dysentery to have a chance to work itself out.

Migraines are another medical situation where hydration becomes important. I'm a neurologist; I treat migraines every day. It's one of the most common situations that I see. Migraines can be triggered by dehydration. Often, migraineurs have to be especially careful not to get caught behind the eight ball, as we say. Don't let yourself be stuck without access to the fluid. I don't force them to drink a lot of fluid on an average day when they're not having a migraine, but they do need to make sure they don't get dehydrated.

However, when they're having a migraine, part of that migraine can cause nausea and even vomiting. Even if they're not vomiting—which is a pathological way in which you can lose a lot of water and electrolytes—

the fact that they don't feel like eating or drinking—they have anorexia and nausea from the migraine—means that they can quickly become dehydrated.

In essence, it's a pathological situation in which the normal feedback loops of thirst and urination are short circuited by the nausea. Even in the course of half a day, a patient with a migraine can become severely dehydrated—enough that it actually worsens their headache and may make it last for two or three days. One of the most effective treatments for a migraine is to force fluids even if they don't really feel like eating or drinking in order to stave off the dehydration that would otherwise occur.

I'm going to talk about a couple of questions that frequently come up with respect to water. One is bottled water. Should we buy bottled water? Is there an advantage to it? Is it healthier? Does it taste better? Interestingly, bottled water costs about 1900 times as much as good, old fashioned tap water. It's more costly than gasoline. But, bottled water, if you look at it statistically, is no better than tap water. It's no more healthy and often, in taste tests, it doesn't taste any better. In fact, some cities have better tasting tap water than most brands of bottled water. Also, some bottled water is literally tap water. They're bottling tap water and selling it to you at almost 2000 times the cost. Bottled water, overall, is basically a scam. You're better off just buying containers that you can reuse and filling them from your own tap.

What about your water purifiers, things you install in the sink or your home in order to filter out organisms, impurities, or heavy metals from your water? Most modern industrialized countries, like the United States, have agencies like the Environmental Protection Agency, the EPA. They monitor and regulate water very closely. Currently, there are no major safety issues with tap water in the U.S. or other industrialized countries. However, this is largely regulated at a city and regional area. If you have any questions or concerns, you can look up—at the EPA or a similar organization—what the report says about the quality of the water in your local area to reassure yourself that the water you're drinking is safe.

Some people have well water. Well water is a different matter altogether because it's not on any kind of citywide system. Well water does need to be tested first to initially certify that the well water is safe. Also, if it's been many, many years and your home has well water, you may want to get it occasionally retested to make sure there's nothing leaching into the water. If there are any problems with your well water, you may want to have it filtered. There is no evidence, however, for most people—as long as you are on a city system—that water purifiers improve the safety of water. Most publicly available water is perfectly safe.

The primary or legitimate use for water purifiers is to increase the taste of water. There, you can just follow your own taste. If your tap water tastes fine to you, then don't worry about it. If it doesn't taste right, if it tastes a little chlorinated or a taste that you don't like, you may want to get a water purifier just to improve the taste of the water—even though it won't necessarily be more healthful. Even there, you can usually attach those purifiers to the sink that you drink out of—your kitchen sink for example—or you can have a water purifier on the water that you get out of the refrigerator door, the cooled water. The water that you're going to drink you're going to purify. But, you don't necessarily have to put a water purifier on the entire home for all of the water—the water that you use for doing your laundry, for example.

Also, the studies show that the inexpensive or modest purifiers perform just as well as the systems that cost many thousands of dollars. Don't believe the hype of the salesman who's telling you that you have to spend five or more thousand dollars on some expensive system wide or house wide water purifier system. There are organizations that review such products. You can go to them to see if the product you're thinking of buying—for not too much money, $50 or $100—how well it works.

What about ionized water? Some companies will try to sell you ionized water that has either health benefits or will make your blood more acidic or more alkaline. These are pure scams. Pure water cannot be ionized. There's H+ and OH- to a certain amount in all water, but they are constantly recombining with each other to make H_2O. It's in an equilibrium steady state. You can't ionize water and have it stay ionized for more than a very short period of time. The bottom line is there are no proven health benefits to it—or oxygenated water or any other kind of magical miracle water. Just don't believe it.

That was a quick trip through our precious bodily fluids, the elixir of life, water. Hopefully I corrected some common misconceptions that are out there. The bottom line I want you to come away with is that you should trust your thirst. Your body knows that it needs water; it carefully regulates water, and in most situations, if you just listen to your thirst, you'll do fine.

Vitamin and Nutrition Myths
Lecture 3

Even in ancient history, people understood that there was some connection between nutrition, the food that we eat, and health. For example, the ancient Egyptians wrote about the fact that liver could be used to cure night blindness. Although they didn't understand at the time that it's because liver contains vitamin A, they were treating a vitamin A deficiency.

One of the most common concerns patients have is about vitamins. Should they take a multivitamin every day, or can they get all the nutrition they need from the food they eat? Vitamins are those nutritional substances that are essential to health in tiny amounts but that an organism cannot manufacture in sufficient quantities itself. Therefore, you have to get vitamins from food.

Vitamins are only part of the nutritional content of food that we need to be concerned with, the micronutrients. Then there are the macronutrients, those parts of food from which we get calories or energy and also structural components, the stuff that we actually build our bodies out of. The three main types of macronutrients that we get in our diet are carbohydrates, lipids, and protein. Food also contains minerals, including calcium, phosphorus, magnesium, iron, zinc, copper, sodium, and potassium.

So how do we get optimal nutrition? There is general

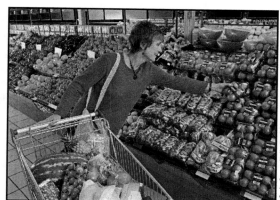

The best way to get good nutrition is through a well-balanced, varied diet.

© JupiterImages/Polka Dot/Thinkstock.

agreement in the scientific community that the best way to get good nutrition is through a well-balanced, varied diet. You should avoid highly restrictive or narrow diets that are dependent on just a few different kinds of food. The USDA food pyramid goes over the rough proportions of different types of foods that would be contained in a healthful diet. A healthful diet should contain and should emphasize the following:

- You should eat about 2 cups of fruit and 2.5 cups of vegetables per day. Try to pick from the different subgroups of vegetables, including dark green vegetables, orange vegetables, legumes, and starchy vegetables.

- You should get 3 or more ounce equivalents of whole grain products per day, with the rest of your carbohydrates coming from either enriched or whole grain products.

- You should have 3 cups per day of fat-free or low-fat milk or equivalent milk products.

- To round out your diet, you should get protein from lean meats as well as eggs, nuts, and legumes.

Do we need to take vitamins every day? The big vitamin myth is that taking a daily vitamin is important for everyone's health and well-being. In fact, there is no evidence for any health benefit of routine supplementation. This is a very difficult question to study, but there have been observational studies that found no correlation between routinely supplementing with vitamins and health outcomes. Further, studies that show health advantage or a good outcome based on nutrition are only able to link those advantages to eating healthy foods—not to taking supplements.

So far, we have been talking about supplementation for healthy people with no medical conditions. But what about subpopulations? Children have increased nutritional needs because they're growing. Should we routinely give children vitamin supplements? It's probably still the best recommendation, based upon the evidence, that what's most helpful for growing kids is a healthy diet. But I know how difficult it is to get kids to eat their vegetables. If your children have a restrictive diet despite your best efforts, it is reasonable to consider supplementation as nutritional insurance.

Pregnancy is another situation in which there are increased nutritional demands. It is routinely recommended for pregnancy—and for women who are planning on possibly becoming pregnant—to take a prenatal vitamin because you need to boost your nutritional reserves before you know that you are pregnant. There are also a number of medical conditions in which our nutritional needs may be greater than at baseline and where supplementation may be beneficial. And there are specific conditions or diseases in which there isn't a deficiency, but taking extra vitamins may actually improve symptoms or outcome.

The best way to get good nutrition is through a well-balanced, varied diet.

Vitamins are, by definition, essential to nutrition to prevent deficiencies and improve many medical outcomes. But I want to emphasize that we need to avoid the myth that if some vitamins are good, then more must be better. This has led some to recommend very high doses, sometimes called megadoses, of vitamins. There is no theoretical reason, nor is there any evidence, to support the safety or the health effectiveness of megadosing. It is not recommended. Aside from the possibility of overdosing toxicity, regularly supplementing with high doses of certain vitamins actually correlates with an increased risk of certain diseases.

The best advice is to keep it simple: Don't get overwhelmed with the complexity of the different types of nutritional advice that people are willing to give. A few simple rules are enough. Eat a variety of foods; eat plenty of fruits and vegetables. For most people in most situations, you will be in perfect health in terms of your nutrition. ■

Suggested Reading

Eades, *The Doctor's Complete Guide to Vitamins and Minerals.*

Shils et al., *Modern Nutrition in Health and Disease.*

Questions to Consider

1. Should everyone be taking vitamin supplements?

2. What is the best way to achieve healthful nutrition?

Vitamin and Nutrition Myths
Lecture 3—Transcript

One of the most common questions I get is about vitamins. Should I take a multivitamin every day? Should anyone be taking routine multivitamins? Are vitamins really risk free? Can't we just get all the nutrition we need from the food that we eat? That's what I'll be discussing in this lecture, all about vitamins and nutrition. In general, this lecture will cover a lot about what you should be eating. In an upcoming lecture, I'll talk more about what you should not be eating.

Even in ancient history, people understood that there was some connection between nutrition, the food that we eat, and health. For example, the ancient Egyptians wrote about the fact that liver could be used to cure night blindness. Although, they didn't understand at the time that it's because liver contains vitamin A. They were treating a vitamin A deficiency.

Nutrition really entered the scientific era in 1747 when ship's surgeon James Lind conducted what is considered to be the first modern medical experiment. He discovered that citrus fruit can cure scurvy and that scurvy is a deficiency of vitamin C—although vitamin C wasn't discovered until 1920. Lind did an actual controlled experiment where he fed citrus fruit to sailors suffering from early signs of scurvy. He compared that to vinegar and also to a weak acid. He thought maybe it was acid that was deficient in scurvy. It turns out that the sailors who received the citrus fruit did much better. They actually were cured of their symptoms of scurvy.

What is a vitamin actually? In the early 1900s, chemists were busy identifying various substances that would cure nutritional diseases. It was a Polish biochemist Kazimierz Funk who proposed the name vitamine, which was a combination of the words vital and amine. However, later it was learned that not all vitamins contained a chemical group called amine. Therefore, that final e was dropped and we're left with the word vitamin.

Specifically, vitamins are those nutritional substances that are essential to health in tiny amounts, but which an organism cannot manufacture in sufficient quantities for themselves. Therefore, you have to get vitamins from food by definition. Therefore, of course, which substances are vitamins depend on the species. Human beings, for example, need to get vitamin C from food but most other mammals can make vitamin C for themselves.

Vitamins are also defined by what they do. In fact, most vitamins are actually a group of compounds or chemicals that all have the same biological activity. Most vitamins are cofactors for enzymes, which means they help biochemical reactions occur. Some vitamins like vitamin D also have some hormone-like properties.

We also classify vitamins based upon their solubility. Water soluble vitamins—vitamins C and the B vitamins—are soluble in water and will be really quickly excreted in the urine. If you eat more than your body needs over a short period of time, you'll just get rid of the extra. However vitamins A, D, E, and K are all fat soluble vitamins. That means that they are stored long-term in the fat of your body. This also means that, in order to get a deficiency of this vitamin, you have to have a deficiency in your nutrition, usually over a long period of time.

Every vitamin is associated with a deficiency syndrome. In fact, that's how they were first discovered. But, many of them are also associated with known and sometimes very serious overdose syndromes as well. I'm going to quickly run through the different vitamins, their overdose and deficiency syndromes, and the common sources in food—starting, of course, with vitamin A, which are the retinols.

The RDA stands for the recommended daily allowance. Essentially, what the RDA is the minimum amount you need to get of a vitamin on a daily basis in order to prevent a deficiency syndrome. The RDA for vitamin A is 900 micrograms. Deficiency causes night blindness, as I mentioned previously. An overdose causes what we call hypervitaminosis A, which is actually a very serious medical condition that can ultimately be fatal. Common sources of vitamin A include fruits and vegetables like mango, broccoli, carrots, spinach, and beef liver.

Next we have the B vitamins. There are many B vitamins starting with B1 or thiamine. The RDA there is 1.2 milligrams. A deficiency of thiamine can cause a very serious neurological disorder called Wernicke-Korsakoff syndrome where, in the end stage, people actually completely lose their short-term memory. Overdoses will tend to cause drowsiness. Common sources of thiamine include spinach, green peas, tomatoes, watermelon, sunflower seeds, and other vegetables.

Next we have B2 or riboflavin. The RDA is 1.3 milligrams. The deficiency syndrome is ariboflavinosis, which causes changes to the skin and the oral mucosa—sores and bleeding, for example. Common sources include spinach, broccoli, mushrooms, eggs, milk, liver, and some seafood items like oysters and clams.

B3 or the niacin group has an RDA of 16 milligrams. A deficiency causes a syndrome that has been recognized for centuries called pellagra. We remember this by the three Ds—dementia, diarrhea, and dermatitis. Overdose can cause liver damage. Common sources include vegetables like spinach, also potatoes, tomato juice, lean ground beef, chicken breast, and tuna.

B5, or the pantothenic acid group, has an RDA of 5 milligrams. A deficiency causes paresthesia; that's a tingling sensation in the nerves. It's a mild form of nerve damage. Overdoses can cause nausea and diarrhea. B5 is common in many foods, so it's very difficult to get a deficiency of it.

Next we have B6 or pyridoxine. The RDA there is 1.3 milligrams. Deficiency of B6 causes anemia or low blood counts and also neuropathy or nerve damage. Ironically, overdoses of B6 also can cause nerve damage or neuropathy. Common sources include bananas, watermelon, tomato juice, broccoli, spinach, acorn squash, potatoes, rice, and chicken breast.

B7 or biotin has an RDA of 30 micrograms. Deficiency causes dermatitis and dementia. It is also a vitamin that is common in many foods.

Next we have B9 or folic acid. The RDA is 400 micrograms. Deficiencies of folic acid are most important in pregnant women where they can cause a serious neurological developmental disorder called neural tube defects, such as spina bifida. Pregnant women should definitely take folic acid. Deficiencies in other populations or in anyone can also cause anemia.

Sources include tomato juice, green beans, broccoli, spinach, asparagus, and black-eyed peas, and lentils.

B12 or cyanocobalamin has an RDA of 2.4 micrograms. A deficiency causes a megaloblastic anemia—again, a low blood count of a specific type that can be diagnosed simply by doing a blood test. Common sources include meats, poultry, fish, shellfish, milk, and eggs.

Now we're off the B vitamins; we're on to vitamin C or ascorbic acid. The RDA is 90 milligrams. Deficiencies cause scurvy, which I talked about previously. Sources are very common in fruits and vegetables such as spinach, broccoli, red bell peppers, snow peas, tomato juice, kiwi, mango, orange, and actually, there are very high levels in strawberries.

Vitamin D, or the cholecalciferols, have an RDA of 5 to 10 micrograms. A deficiency of vitamin D is called rickets, something that's be recognized for a long time—longer than we've known about vitamin D. That causes abnormalities in bone development. The most common source of vitamin D is simple sunlight. Most people can get all the vitamin D they need just from everyday exposure to the sun. However, vitamin D is also fortified in milk and can also be found in egg yolks, liver, and fatty fish.

Vitamin E, or the tocopherols, have an RDA of 15 milligrams per day. Deficiencies can cause neuropathy and ataxia, which is poor coordination or poor ability to walk. Common sources include nuts, oils, sunflower seeds, whole grains, wheat germ, and spinach.

Finally, we have vitamin K or the menaquinones and phylloquinones. They have an RDA of 120 micrograms. A deficiency of vitamin K causes bleeding because vitamin K is very important in the clotting cascade, the sequence of biochemical reactions that allows your blood to clot off and to stop bleeding from occurring. You can find vitamin K in the dark green, leafy vegetables including brussels sprouts, spinach, broccoli, kale, and liver.

Vitamins are only part of the nutritional content of food that we need to be concerned with. They are part of what we call the micronutrients. Let's turn now to the macronutrients. Macronutrients are those parts of food from which we get calories or energy and also structural components, the stuff that we actually build our bodies out of. There are some essential fatty acids and amino acids, but these are not technically vitamins because we need them in more than tiny amounts so they're still considered part of the macronutrients.

Let's discuss the three main types of macronutrients that we get in our diet. These include carbohydrates. Carbohydrates are sugars and also starches like bread or pasta. There's also lipids. Lipids are, essentially, fats and oils. There's also protein. Protein comes from meats as well as nuts and legumes.

Food also contains, in addition to vitamins and the macronutrients that I just discussed, many minerals or "trace minerals" as they're often called. These include calcium, phosphorus, magnesium, iron, zinc, copper, sodium, and potassium. These are also sometimes referred to as electrolytes. Electrolytes are simply minerals that exist in our bodies in their ionic form. For example, sodium with a positive charge is the electrolyte sodium. But, it is still considered a mineral that we get from our food.

Incidentally, you can overdose on minerals as you can on many of the vitamins. The most common mineral overdose is iron. In fact, this is the most common childhood overdose of all. This is because children will often get iron from vitamins which they may think of as candy, not necessarily medicine. Adult males do not need to supplement iron at all. In fact, we recycle almost all of our iron. Therefore, the only people who really need to supplement are those who are anemic or women who are menstruating because they need to replace the iron they lose each month.

Let's talk a bit about optimal nutrition. How do we get all the things that I spoke about in our food? There is general agreement in the scientific community that the best way to get good nutrition is through a well-balanced, varied diet. Variety is the key. You should definitely avoid highly restrictive or narrow diets that are dependent on just a few different kinds of food. The USDA food pyramid goes over the rough proportions of different kinds of foods that would be contained in a healthful diet.

Here's a basic overview. A healthful diet should contain and should emphasize these things: about 2 cups of fruit and 2-1/2 cups of vegetables per day. You don't have to measure these out precisely. This is really just a rule of thumb, a guideline to help you estimate that you're getting enough of the different kinds of food you should be eating. When you do eat vegetables, you should try to pick from the different subgroups of vegetables. These include dark green vegetables, orange vegetables, legumes, starchy vegetables, and other vegetables.

In addition, you should get three or more ounce equivalents of whole grain products per day with the rest of your carbohydrates coming from either enriched or whole grain products. You should also have three cups per day of fat free or low-fat milk or equivalent milk products. Of course, to round out your diet, you're also going to be getting protein from lean meats as well as eggs, nuts, and legumes.

Do we need to take vitamins every day? That question, of course, is related to the deeper question of do we get enough of our vitamins that we need from the food that we eat? There are only minor differences in nutritional quality of food depending on the production methods. Meanwhile, in modern times—and for the first time in human history due to globalization, for example—we have access to a variety of fresh fruits and vegetables year round. It's important to take advantage of that. Year round, you can get tomatoes, strawberries, and bananas—a variety of fruits and vegetables that will have a much greater impact on your overall nutrition than the mild differences between different food production methods.

One topic that comes up frequently among those who are concerned about the nutritional quality of our food is soil depletion. There are reports that perhaps due to modern agriculture, we are depleting our soil of the minerals that are necessary. Therefore, we're losing those trace minerals from our diet. Most people who make this point or who are concerned about this will refer to a 1936 Congressional statement. It turns out that, when you look at it closely, this was an article that was written in Cosmopolitan magazine, a literary magazine. This was inserted into the Congressional Record by Senator Duncan Fletcher from Florida. But, that becomes a primary reference for those who argue that our soil is depleted. They say, hey, if it was that depleted in 1936, imagine how bad it must be today.

Reports that our soils are depleted of minerals are often misinterpreted. It turns out that soil is actually frequently tested for its mineral content. Minerals are added in the farming process, in the fertilization process of the soil. The plants need the minerals to grow as well. Agricultural companies want to replete those minerals so that their yields will be maximal. That mineral content is in the food.

Which different types of food are most nutritious depending on how it's prepared and packaged? It is true that cooking decreases the nutrient content of food—not too much, but it is measurable. It does decrease the nutritious content. It is important to eat fresh fruits and vegetables to get maximal nutrition—or just lightly steam them. You should avoid thoroughly boiling food because that does leach out much of the vitamins and minerals.

What about frozen versus fresh and canned? Frozen food is definitely better than canned in terms of its nutritional content. In fact, frozen vegetables may be slightly better than fresh if they are picked at the peak of ripeness and frozen at that time—versus vegetables which are allowed to ripen in transport or in the stores, for example.

What about organic food? I'm going to be talking in a lot more detail about organic farming and food in a future lecture. But, suffice it to say that reviews of published evidence show that there are only negligible differences in the nutritional quality between organic and non-organically grown food.

This brings us to our first big vitamin myth—that routine vitamin supplementation or taking a daily vitamin is important for everyone's health and wellbeing. In fact, there is no evidence for any health benefit of routine supplementation. This is, admittedly, a very difficult question to answer if you want to know if there are long-term health advantages to vitamins over decades. Those studies are very difficult to do.

However, we have done observational studies. The biggest is a Swedish study that looked at hundreds of thousands of people that had enrolled in various different clinical trials. They found no correlation between those who routinely supplemented with vitamins and health outcomes. In fact, there was a slightly increased risk of death among those who supplemented. No one interprets this study as establishing cause and effect. It could possibly be—and, in fact, is probably true—that people who are taking vitamins are doing so because maybe they're not as healthy to begin with and that's why their outcomes weren't as good.

But, the bottom line is if we look at all the research that we have, experimental or observational, there is no evidence to back the claim that routine supplementation is important for health. For most people, eating a balanced diet is enough. Further, studies which show health advantage or a good outcome based upon nutrition are only able to link those advantages to eating healthy foods—not to taking supplements. Therefore, we come back to the conclusion, based upon the evidence, that the best thing to do is to have a healthy diet full of fruits and vegetables and variety.

There are many special situations to consider. When I refer to routine supplementation, I'm talking about in a healthy person with no medical conditions. What about sub-populations? Let's, for example, first go to children. Children certainly do have increased nutritional needs because they're growing. Should we routinely give children vitamin supplements? It's probably still the best recommendation, based upon the evidence, that what's most helpful for growing kids is that they have a healthy diet. In fact, you should get children in the habit of eating lots of fruits and vegetables and a generally varied and healthy diet, even from a young age.

However, I have kids. I know how difficult it is to get them to eat their vegetables, how difficult it is to get them to eat a variety of things. If your children do have a restrictive diet despite your best efforts, it is reasonable to consider supplementation as nutritional insurance.

Pregnancy is another situation in which there are increased nutritional demands. Pregnant women have incredibly high nutritional demands. It is routinely recommended for pregnancy—and for women who are planning on possibly becoming pregnant—to take a prenatal vitamin because you need to boost your nutritional reserves before you know that you are pregnant. Specifically, folic acid has been shown to be important, as I mentioned earlier. Supplementing with folic acid reduces neural tube defects like spina bifida.

What about some specific vitamins? For example, there is vitamin D. Vitamin D insufficiency and deficiency is being increasingly recognized in Western and developed countries. As many as two-thirds of the population in recent studies has been shown to be vitamin D insufficient—not fully deficient, not the kind of deficiency that would cause rickets, but maybe not getting as much vitamin D as they should.

Most of our vitamin D does come from exposure to sunlight. The vitamin D gets manufactured in reaction to exposure to the sun. For the average person, 15 minutes of sunlight exposure per day is sufficient to meet your vitamin D needs. However, that's an average person. This will obviously vary based upon your latitude, where you are in the world. People in Florida, for example, don't need as much sun exposure as those living in Alaska.

It also depends on your pigmentation, how dark-skinned you are. The darker your skin, the more sunlight you need. There is also the time of year—people do tend to become relatively insufficient in vitamin D during the winter months and have more vitamin D during the summer months. Therefore, for more people than we had previously thought, it may be necessary to supplement vitamin D if you're not getting enough from sunlight and fortified foods.

Calcium is another special situation. Adult women, especially those approaching menopause, may need to supplement calcium and vitamin D in order to optimize bone density and prevent osteoporosis. Osteoporosis is a relative decrease in the calcium content of bones. Once women go through menopause, they steadily lose bone content so it's important to build up as much bone density as possible prior to menopause. The ways to do that are with supplementing calcium, perhaps vitamin D, and of course, with weight bearing exercise. That's important as well.

Vitamin B12 is another one that deserves special consideration. As we age, we actually have a decreased capacity to absorb vitamin B12 just from our food. B12 can't be passively absorbed like most nutrients in food. It needs to be actively carried into our blood system from the food. That system can decrease as we age. A lot of people do become relatively or absolutely vitamin B12 deficient as they get older. That's the kind of thing that a primary care doctor will check routinely, just to make sure your vitamin B12 levels are sufficient.

If they are on the low side, oral supplementation is enough for most people to replenish your B12 supplies. However, if the ability to absorb the B12 has decreased too much, you may actually need monthly vitamin B12 injections in order to keep your levels up in the normal range.

Vegetarians also have special nutritional needs because they have chosen to narrow the range of foods that they will eat. You can get everything you need from a vegetarian or vegan diet. But, you have to know what you're doing and you have to be very careful. Vitamin B12 specifically can be a problem because a lot of the B12 that we get comes from animal sources. If you are choosing to have a vegetarian or vegan diet, be careful that you're eating foods that contain a lot of B12. You may have to have your B12 levels checked and supplement if necessary.

There are also a number of medical conditions in which our nutritional needs may be greater than at baseline and where supplementation may be beneficial. There are also specific conditions or diseases in which there isn't a deficiency, but taking extra vitamins may actually improve symptoms or outcome. For example, there is reasonable evidence to support that vitamin B2 reduces the frequency of migraine attacks. Therefore, in people with mild to moderate migraine headaches, supplementing B2 may improve the number of headaches that you have.

Also, there's evidence to support vitamin B6 for nerve healing. For those who have, say, carpal tunnel syndrome—a very common compression of the median nerve in the wrist—long-term healing and outcomes will be better if you take moderate supplements of vitamin B6. Again, I have to caution you that even slightly overdosing on B6 can actually cause nerve damage. Thus, be sure you're taking the proper dose.

It's been long recognized that vitamin C is important for wound healing. As I mentioned previously, vitamin C is important for making structural proteins, the kind of things that hold our cells and tissue together. Therefore, if you've just had surgery or if you're healing from an injury, taking extra vitamin C for a period of time will help you heal faster.

While vitamins are, by definition, essential to nutrition to prevent deficiencies and improve many medical outcomes, I do want to emphasize that we need to avoid the myth that if some vitamins are good, then more must be better. This has led some to recommend very high doses, sometimes what we call megadoses of vitamins. However, there is no theoretical reason, nor is there any evidence, to support the safety or the health effectiveness of megadosing. It is not recommended.

Many water soluble vitamins, such as vitamin C, will be simply excreted in your urine if you try to megadose. It is not as dangerous as the fat soluble vitamins, but it is a waste of time and money. High doses of vitamin E, for example, which is a fat soluble vitamin, have been shown to correlate with an increased risk of heart disease. Aside from the notion of overdosing toxicity, regularly supplementing with high doses of certain vitamins actually correlates with an increased risk of certain diseases.

What about superfoods? Are there some foods that are so nutritious that we can get really great nutrition just from eating a small amount of them? The bottom line is that there is no food in a pill and there is no food that you can take in tiny amounts that will have a significant impact on your overall nutrition. Examples of some kinds of foods that are marketed as so-called superfoods include spirulina. This is essentially pond algae. There's also wheat grass juice, which I've actually tried and I don't recommend it. It's not very tasty. The notion is that it contains special nutrients like chlorophyll and high doses of vitamins that can act as a superfood. In reality, it has no more vitamins or nutritional content then common fruits and vegetables that are much more tasty.

There's also the latest fad tropical superjuice, like açaí juice, for example. It's claimed to have all kinds of vitamins and nutrients. But, again, when you actually look at the data, it's just another kind of fruit juice. What about natural vitamins? If you do supplement for whatever reason, should you look for natural vitamins instead of synthetic vitamins based on the notion that they will be more effective or that they will have more of a healthful effect?

It turns out that ascorbic acid is ascorbic acid, for example. If you have synthetic vitamin C versus vitamin C that is derived from say a plant source, the chemical structure is identical. Therefore, the chemical properties are identical as well. The source doesn't matter to the chemical properties of that molecule.

The best advice, if we try to boil down everything that I discussed in this lecture, is to keep it simple. Don't get overwhelmed with the complexity of all the different types of nutritional advice that people are willing to give. A few simple rules are enough. Eat a variety of foods. Eat plenty of fruits and vegetables. For most people in most situations, you will be fine. You will be in perfect health in terms of your nutrition. As you will see in the next lecture, the problem for most Westerners is not that we get too little of any kind of food—in many instances, it's that we get too much.

Dieting—Separating Myths from Facts
Lecture 4

You don't want to get involved in some kind of elaborate scheme that you're not going to be able to really maintain long term, like counting every single calorie. It's better to use something that is simple and easy, that you can do every day for the rest of your life, and that will help you estimate and keep general track of how many calories you're eating. This includes just writing down what you eat. If you do that—just record what you eat—that helps people lose an additional 10% or 20% of weight.

D o you want to know the secret to weight loss? There are quite a number of self-help books, videos, and other products all trying to sell you that secret. How many times have you heard the claim "lose weight without diet and exercise?" This lecture examines diet—what we eat, what we should eat, what we perhaps shouldn't eat, and how much we eat.

How many calories does an average person need on an average day? That depends on a number of variables, specifically height, weight, age, and level of activity. An average man needs to eat about 2500 calories per day in order to balance his energy expenditures; an average woman, around 2000 calories. Of course, somebody with a very high degree of activity or someone above average in size may need to eat as many as 3000 calories in an average day.

Basal metabolic rate measures how many calories we burn going about our business. This is calculated based on our height, weight, and age. The basal metabolic rate increases with increasing height and weight and decreases with age. You also have to adjust the basal metabolic rate for activity level. Somebody who is sedentary isn't going to burn as many calories as somebody who is highly active. Putting all those factors together can allow you to roughly calculate how many calories you burn each day.

Weight management simply comes down to calories consumed versus calories expended. Overeating by as few as 50 calories per day can result in as much as 5 pounds gained per year. That's a lot of weight gain for a very tiny difference in our eating habits. So what if you want to lose some excess weight? A conservative approach to weight loss is underconsuming—consuming fewer calories than you burn by about 500 per day. If you underconsume by 500 calories per day, that's 3500 calories, or 1 pound, per week. One pound per week is a good, healthy rate of weight loss.

At the more aggressive end of the spectrum would be underconsuming by about 1000 calories per day. Most people cannot sustain that significant a decrease in their daily food intake for any period of time. Even still, underconsuming by 1000 calories per day only results in a weight loss of about 2 pounds per week. What this also means is that, if someone is claiming you can lose 5, 10, 15, or 20 pounds in 1 or 2 weeks, they're being less than

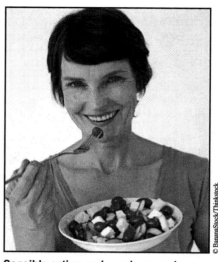

Sensible eating and regular exercise are the best ways to maintain a healthy weight.

honest. You can only burn about 1 to 2 pounds per week of fat, which is what you want to lose when you're trying to lose weight. Any weight loss above and beyond that is water weight or other things.

Lots of people claim to have tricks and tips for losing weight. Unfortunately, none of them are terribly helpful. One you may hear about is fasting, jump-starting a diet by fasting for a day or longer. There's really no evidence for any long-term or significant benefit from fasting, and it shouldn't be part of a weight control or weight management program. In fact, fasting may cause your body to try to conserve calories and lower its metabolic rate.

What about late-night eating? A lot of people give the advice that you shouldn't eat late at night if you're trying to lose weight because those calories turn directly into fat. This has been studied multiple ways in both animals and humans. It turns out that it really doesn't matter when you consume your calories; the net calories will still be stored if you have excess calories. It still comes down to calories in versus calories out.

What about restrictive diets? A lot of fad diets or weight loss diets are premised on the notion that if you eliminate certain things from your diet, the weight will magically melt away. This is not a helpful strategy or a helpful approach to weight loss. In the final analysis, it doesn't really matter what kinds of calories you're eating; the overwhelmingly important factor is how many calories you're eating. Also, by restricting the variety of food that you eat, you can compromise good nutrition.

Exercising definitely burns calories, but not as many as you may think.

In the last 20 years or so, there has been a huge fad of diets focused on either low fat or low carbs. The notion here is that if you adjust the proportion of macronutrients—fats, proteins, and carbohydrates—in your diet, you will get to some magical zone or magical balance in which you'll shift into a different kind of metabolism that will help you burn calories. After a lot of research, it turns out that there just isn't evidence to support these claims. It all still comes down to caloric intake.

I've spoken a lot about food and how much we eat. What about exercise? Isn't exercise important for weight loss? It turns out the answer is yes and no. Exercising definitely burns calories, but not as many as you may think. A reasonable exercise program is to do 30 minutes of cardiovascular exercise 3 days a week. That would burn about 450 calories. If you're trying to underconsume by 3500 calories per week in order to lose 1 pound per week, then burning off an extra 450 calories doesn't get you very far toward that goal. The bottom line is that you can't lose weight solely by exercising. You would have to exercise 90 minutes a day, 7 days a week, in order to burn off 1 pound per week. Thus you have to combine exercise with calorie control.

What about diet pills—is there any medicine or pill that will help in a weight loss program? There's no theoretical reason why there can't be a pharmaceutical, for example, that shifts us into more of a weight loss balance.

But nothing has been proven to be both safe and effective. That doesn't stop there from being many "weight loss pills" on the market that claim to melt away the fat without diet and exercise. I certainly wouldn't believe any of those claims.

The way I interpret that breadth of research is simple. Dieting doesn't work. Perhaps that's the biggest myth of all—that you can positively impact your weight maintenance by going on a diet. Rather, the focus should be on long-term, healthful strategies that you can maintain for the rest of your life. ■

Suggested Reading

Novella, "The Skeptic's Diet."

Rippe, *Weight Watchers Weight Loss That Lasts.*

Questions to Consider

1. Is there any way to achieve and maintain a healthy weight without diet and exercise?

2. What does the scientific evidence have to say about popular weight loss diets?

Dieting—Separating Myths from Facts
Lecture 4—Transcript

Do you want to know the secret to weight loss? There are quite a number of self-help books, videos, and other products all trying to sell you that secret. How many times have you heard the claim "lose weight without diet and exercise?" Even sensible weight loss advice sometimes is based upon questionable information. What's the truth about health maintenance and healthy eating?

I'm going to talk in this lecture about diet—what we eat, what we should eat, perhaps what we shouldn't eat, and how much we eat. There are many issues related to this. Specifically, it's weight loss, weight gain, weight maintenance, how to avoid and treat diabetes, heart health, overall health, and athletic performance. I'm going to start by talking about weight control.

I'm going to be referring to calories a lot in this lecture. I want to give just a quick background on what that word actually means. A calorie is a measure of energy. In fact, the term is used by physicists to refer to a specific and very small unit of energy. That's a calorie with a small c. When we talk about food calories, that's calories with a big C. That's actually a thousand small c calories or a kilocalorie. In the rest of this lecture, when I refer to the word calorie, I'm going to be referring to that food calorie.

There are 3500 calories in one pound of body weight. Sources of calories in our diet include carbohydrates like sugars and starches, which have 4 calories per gram; proteins, like meat and nuts, which also have 4 calories per gram; lipids, fats, and oils, which have 9 calories per gram; and alcohol, which has 7 calories per gram. That's it. Those are the only things in our diet that actually contain calories.

How many calories does an average person need on an average day? That depends on a number of variables, specifically height, weight, age, and level of activity. An average man, for example, needs to eat about 2500 calories per day in order to balance their energy expenditures. An average woman needs to eat around 2000 calories per day. Of course, an athletic person, somebody with a very high degree of activity, or someone above average in size may need to eat as many as 3000 calories in an average day.

We need to talk a little bit about basal metabolic rate. That is the calories out of the equation. That's how many calories we burn going about our business. This is calculated based upon our height, weight, and age. The basal metabolic rate increases with increasing height and weight and it decreases with age. You also have to adjust the basal metabolic rate for activity level. Somebody who is sedentary isn't going to burn as many calories as somebody who is highly active. You put all those factors together and you can roughly calculate how many calories are burned by a person each day.

Let's turn to weight management, an issue that many people are concerned with. Again, this comes down to calories consumed versus calories expended. That's really just basic physics, biology, and math. Overeating by as little as 50 calories per day can result in as much as five pounds gained per year. That's a lot of weight gain for a very tiny difference in our eating habits. It's very difficult to keep track of your caloric intake down to just a few crackers or a slice of bread. It's no wonder that people are able to maintain their weight over a long period of time.

Let's talk about weight loss. What if you want to lose some excess weight? A conservative approach to weight loss is under-consuming—this means consuming fewer calories than you burn by about 500 per day. Let's go back to our average adult male that burns about 2500 calories per day. If they under-consumed by 500 calories, eating about 2000 calories per day, they would lose 500 calories times seven days is 3500 calories or 1 pound per week. A pound per week is a good, steady, healthy rate of weight loss.

At the more aggressive end of the spectrum would be under-consuming by about 1000 calories per day. There, an average adult male would eat only about 1500 calories per day and an average adult woman even less than that, down to as few as 1000 calories per day. That's very challenging. Most people cannot sustain for any period of time that significant decrease in their daily food intake. Even still, that aggressive under-consuming by 1000 calories per day only results in a weight loss of about two pounds per week.

What this also means is that, if someone is claiming you can lose 5, 10, 15, or 20 pounds in a week or two, they're being less than honest. You can only burn about one to two pounds per week of excess body weight, of fat, which is what people really want to lose when they're trying to lose weight. Any weight loss above and beyond that is water weight or other things. It is not calorie burning; it is not fat burning.

These different amounts of calories per day are very tricky to estimate and it's very easy to accidentally overeat. For example, if you substitute cream cheese for butter on your bagel, swap mustard for mayonnaise on your sandwich, and have a baked potato instead of a vegetable, you can easily be overeating by as much as 500 calories.

Lots of people claim that there are tricks and special tips for losing weight and I'm going to go over a few of them. Unfortunately, none of them are terribly helpful. One you may hear about frequently is fasting, that people will jump start their diet or will help their diet by fasting for a day or for a longer period of time. There's really no evidence for any long-term or significant benefit from fasting. It really shouldn't be part of a weight control or weight management program. Slow and steady over the long haul is the approach that works. Fasting is not recommended. In fact, fasting may cause your body to try to conserve calories and lower its metabolic rate because it thinks it's starving—because it is.

What about late night eating? A lot of people give the advice that you shouldn't eat late at night if you're trying to lose weight because those calories turn directly into fat. This has been studied multiple ways in both animals and humans. It turns out that it really doesn't matter when you consume your calories. Whether you consume them right before you exercise or right before you go to bed, the net calories will still be stored if you have excess calories. You'll burn the calories that you need. It still comes down to calories in versus calories out. It just doesn't matter when you eat them.

What about restrictive diets? A lot of fad diets or weight loss diets are premised on the notion that if you eliminate certain things from your diet— you identify the bad food or the bad food group and you eliminate those things—the weight will magically melt away. This, again, is not a helpful strategy or a helpful approach to weight loss. In the final analysis, it doesn't really matter what kinds of calories you're eating. The overwhelmingly important or large factor is how many calories you're eating.

Also, by restricting the variety of food that you eat, you can compromise good nutrition. If you are trying to under-consume as part of a weight maintenance program, it's especially easy to get poor nutrition. Therefore, eating a variety of foods is especially important. Also, highly restrictive diets are just not sustainable. People find it extremely difficult to maintain a diet in general, especially one that has eliminated a lot of food choices.

In the last 20 years or so, there have been huge fad diets focused on either low fat or low carb. They seem to go back and forth in popularity. The notion here is that, if you adjust the proportion of macronutrients—fats, proteins, and carbohydrates—in your diet, you will get to some magical zone or magical balance in which you'll shift into a different kind of metabolism that will help you burn calories.

After a lot of research, it turns out that there just isn't evidence to support these claims. There is a lot of basic science that people draw upon. Sure, there are hormonal differences in how our bodies will handle proteins and fats versus carbohydrates—for example, how much insulin is secreted and how much insulin is necessary in order to deal with carbohydrates. That can have effects on our overall metabolism. However, these effects seem to be overwhelmed by the much greater factor of just how many calories are consumed. The bottom line here is there's no magic ratio of macronutrients. It still comes down to caloric intake.

The evidence for that is based largely on the clinical studies. Again, this has been studied in many different ways. What all these clinical studies show is that when diets do work, they work by reducing calories—regardless of the types of calories that are eaten. Some of these clinical studies do show that there are temporary effects on things such as hunger. For example, if you go on a very low carb diet, there is evidence to show that your hunger may be decreased over the first three to six months or so. That may lead you to consuming fewer calories. However, that effect appears to be temporary. After six months, it doesn't seem to make any difference. In fact, on all of these diets, most people will start to regain weight after six months. At the end of a year or so, the difference in weight loss is negligible or nonexistent. Usually, also, the overall weight loss is often not that much.

It turns out that going on a diet is not a great strategy. You shouldn't go on some special diet just to lose weight. You should, in fact, switch to a healthful diet that you can sustain for the rest of your life. It's always important to ask yourself, this diet that I'm going on for health reasons—whether it's weight maintenance or something else—is this something I can really live with? Is this something I could stay on long term? If it isn't, if it's just a short-term, quick fix, then it's not going to be a successful strategy. The clinical evidence pretty clearly shows that.

I've spoken a lot about food and how much we eat. But, what about the other end of this equation? What about exercise? Isn't exercise important for weight loss? It turns out the answer is yes and no. We have to put this in the proper context. Exercising definitely burns calories, but let's do a rough estimate of how many calories it does burn. A very reasonable exercise program, one that's recommended for overall health, is doing 30 minutes of cardiovascular exercise—like riding a stationary bike, for example—three days a week. That would burn about 150 calories; 30 minutes of exercise times three is 450 calories.

If you're trying to under-consume by 3500 calories per week in order to lose one pound per week—which is a conservative weight loss program—then burning off an extra 450 calories doesn't get you very far towards that goal. The bottom line is that you can't lose weight solely by exercising; you just can't burn off enough calories. You would have to exercise 90 minutes a day every day, seven days a week, in order to burn off a pound a week just through exercise. Thus, you have to combine that exercise with portion control and calorie control.

However, exercising is very important for cardiovascular health and overall health. It definitely correlates with improved health and longevity. It's important to maintain muscle tone especially in the older population. Therefore, it is recommended to get regular exercise. Also, it will help if you are trying to lose weight. Exercise does burn a little bit more calories for you so it does help in the bottom line equation of calories in versus calories out. But, it also prevents you from decreasing your caloric output in response to eating less.

I mentioned before that overeating or undereating by even a small amount can make a big difference in weight over the long term. How do people maintain their weight over long periods of time? When you eat less, your body compensates by burning less. When you burn more calories, your body compensates by making you hungrier so you'll consume more calories. We pretty much keep ourselves within a fairly narrow range. If you want to lose weight or shift to a different equilibrium at a lower rate, you need to simultaneously reduce the number of calories you eat and increase or maintain the number of calories that you're burning.

What about diet pills—is there any medicine or pill that will help in a weight loss program? Generally speaking, diet pills do not work. There's no theoretical reason why there can't be a pharmaceutical, for example, that shifts us into more of a weight loss balance. But, nothing has been proven to be both safe and effective. There's nothing currently available that's really a proven weight loss aid. That doesn't stop there from being many products on the market, herbal and otherwise, that are promoted as weight loss pills that will melt away the fat without diet and exercise. I certainly wouldn't believe any of those claims.

Some diet pills do have an effect. Their effect derives from the fact that they have stimulants in them, whether or not they're clear about that upfront or on the label. Sometimes you really have to hunt—look at the ingredients and see if there's any caffeine, which is a very common stimulant that's added to herbal or other diet pills or supplements. But, there are also other types of stimulants that you may not recognize—chemical names that are caffeine derivatives, metabolites, or other stimulants. Therefore, you really have to be careful and identify all of the chemicals that are any kind of herbal supplements.

I'd like to summarize what we've gone through on weight maintenance before I go on to other topics. There are many tricks that are promoted, but simply do not work. The bottom line is that there is no quick fix. What does work? There are lots of very common sense and healthy habits that you can engage in that will help you attain and maintain a healthful weight. For example, there are sustainable eating habits. Don't go on a diet; simply engage in more healthful eating habits with lots of vegetables, for example. Try to avoid very calorie dense food.

In addition, you need to do some type of method of estimating how many calories you eat. As I mentioned, overeating by a slice of bread a day can make you gain five pounds a year. You don't want to get involved in some kind of elaborate scheme that you're not going to be able to really maintain long term like counting every single calorie. It's better to use something that is simple and easy, that you can do every day for the rest of your life, and that will help you estimate and keep general track of how many calories you're eating. This includes just writing down what you eat. If you do that—just record what you eat—that helps people lose an additional 10 or 20 percent of weight when they're trying to lose weight.

In addition, it may be helpful to use some meal replacement products. For example, if you eat a breakfast bar that you know has exactly 160 calories, then you'll know exactly how many calories you're getting for breakfast. That will really help you estimate your total daily caloric intake. Continue routine daily exercise. It's good to walk when you can. Do some actual aerobic exercise at least three days a week.

If you do all of those simple things, it can help you maintain your weight long term. But, weight maintenance is not the only reason to have a healthful diet. There are other health reasons that you should be concerned about what and how much food you eat. For example, there is diabetes and glucose control.

Here we're interested in what we call the glycemic index of food, which is essentially a measure of how quickly a carbohydrate is broken down and turned into glucose in the blood. This relates to how much insulin you need to release in order to handle that glucose—to get it to go into cells, metabolize it, store it, and use it, for example. High glycemic index foods are rapidly metabolized into glucose while lower glycemic index foods are metabolized more slowly. High glycemic foods are therefore a higher risk of increasing your risk of developing diabetes. For people who are already diabetic—as they should know—they should avoid high glycemic index foods. This is because they don't have the insulin or they're resistant to insulin and they can't handle the rapid increase in blood glucose.

What are the high versus low glycemic index foods? High glycemic index foods are things like white bread, potatoes, white rice, and corn flakes—in fact, most breakfast cereals. These starches are rapidly broken down into glucose in the blood. Medium glycemic index foods would include foods like whole wheat, brown rice, whole wheat pasta, and sweet potatoes. Essentially, it's the darker, browner versions of the high glycemic index foods. That also includes plain table sugar. Table sugar, ironically, is not broken down as rapidly into glucose as are things like white bread. Low glycemic index foods would include things like cheese, nuts, legumes, seeds, or high grainy breads.

We talked about glycemic index and diabetes control. There's also heart health because we want to avoid atherosclerosis and heart disease. Diet is hugely important for heart health. Here the main concern is good fat versus bad fat and the overall amount of fat that we get in our diet. Good fats, the so-called good fats, are monounsaturated and polyunsaturated fats. The "saturated" refers to how many hydrogen atoms are on the carbon backbone of the fats. If they're saturated, that means there's a hydrogen atom everywhere there can be.

If it's mono or polyunsaturated, some of those hydrogen atoms have been replaced by double bonds. These are the good fats, mono and polyunsaturated fats. They're good because they increase what we call HDL, or high density lipoproteins, in the blood. HDLs are helpful because they actually transport cholesterol from blood vessels to the liver where it can be metabolized. So-called bad fats are saturated and these contribute to increases in low density lipoprotein or LDL. LDLs transport fats to the blood vessel walls. They actually deposit cholesterol on your arteries and they contribute to atherosclerosis.

Generally speaking, vegetable and fish sources of fat tend to be good. They tend to have a lot of HDL or increase your HDL while animal sources of fat tend to be bad and increase your LDL. More important than the absolute amount of either one of these is the ratio between the two. Generally, for heart health and to avoid atherosclerosis, you want to have a high ratio of HDL to LDL.

There's also another type of fat called trans-fats. This also refers to the structure of this carbon backbone that we talk about for fat molecules. Trans-fats are considered to be very bad. They should be absolutely minimized in the diet. They're bad because they both increase your LDL, the bad type of cholesterol, and they lower your HDL, the good type of cholesterol. They refer specifically to unsaturated fats where the carbon chains are on opposite sides of that double bond that I spoke about keeping the molecule straight. The opposite of trans is cis, which refers to chains that are on the same side of the double bond, which puts a little bit of a kink in the chain. Trans-fats are bad, cis fats are better.

What about cholesterol? Should you limit cholesterol in your diet? If you remember back in the 1980s, having a low cholesterol diet was all the rage. But, as we investigated this further, that turned into just another dieting myth. It turns out that the amount of cholesterol that you eat in your food doesn't contribute significantly to the amount of cholesterol in your blood. Again, it's the ratio of HDL to LDL that's important, not so much the cholesterol that you directly eat.

What about overall health? We talked about diabetes and heart health, but what about for overall health? There is actually some evidence linking certain kinds of foods to either an increased or a decreased risk of certain types of cancer, specifically colon cancer, for example. The evidence here is actually somewhat mixed and somewhat conflicting. Depending on which evidence you emphasize, you can decide that there isn't much of an overall effect here—or there might be a moderate effect in terms of what kinds of foods you should eat. But we can boil down this complexity to a couple of simple rules.

One is that it's clearly beneficial to regularly eat vegetables. This is the signal that consistently keeps peeking up out of the noise of all this complicated clinical research that we do on food and health. Remember to eat several servings of vegetables every day. You should also avoid certain kind of foods, specifically charred meats and highly processed or cured meats like bacon or cured ham. Again, a varied diet, all things considered, is the best.

How do we summarize everything that we discussed in this lecture today? For weight maintenance, the overriding philosophy is to keep it simple. Weight maintenance is by no means easy, but it can be simple and that means exercise portion control. Try to avoid high calorie or high calorie dense foods. Have some way of estimating how many calories you eat.

In addition, you can weigh yourself on a regular basis. The scale is the ultimate arbiter of your calorie balance. You shouldn't weigh yourself any more than once per week. This is because you're just going to see frequent fluctuations that really don't mean anything—fluctuations in things like water weight. Weigh yourself once a week under the same conditions and then average your weight over the last week or two. See what the trend is— are things stable which is where you want to keep them. If you're trying to lose about a pound or so a week, you want to see that basic trend on the scale. The scale will ultimately tell you if you are restricting your calories sufficiently or if you're exercising sufficiently to achieve your goals. If not, then you can make mild adjustments until you settle into where you need to be.

Also, for overall health, the one thing that consistently is shown by the evidence is that you should eat plenty of vegetables. There are also some things that you should avoid eating too much of. Avoid eating too many animal fats that are high in LDL. Avoid eating too many trans-fats. In fact, they should be minimized as much as possible. Make all of these simple adjustments to your lifestyle and don't focus on the short term. I think that is perhaps the single most counterproductive thing that people do. Unfortunately, most of the dieting advice out there—going on a fad diet or using some specific trick—it turns out to be a myth because they focus on short-term results. Focusing on short-term results is a recipe for long-term failure.

Most people who try to lose weight will long-term fail. About 95 percent of people who "go on a diet," over the short-term—no matter what kind of diet that they go on, just because they're paying attention to what they're eating—will lose weight. This shows that it doesn't really matter—fad diet A versus fad diet B. However, the same studies that show that there's some short-term weight loss by going on pretty much any diet—just because you're reducing your caloric intake—also show that there is no long-term weight maintenance. Ninety-five percent of those people who do lose weight on the short-term diets will gain it back.

The way I interpret that breadth of research is simple. Dieting doesn't work. Perhaps that's the biggest myth of all—that you can positively impact your weight maintenance by going on a diet. Rather, the focus should be on long-term, healthful strategies that you can maintain for the rest of your life.

The Fallacy That Natural Is Always Better
Lecture 5

> You could take a vitamin C molecule that is derived from rose hips and a vitamin C molecule that was synthesized in a laboratory. The chemicals are identical. There's no test you can do to distinguish one molecule from the other. Is one therefore natural and the other one not natural? If so, then what does that mean?

We all want the food that we eat to be wholesome and nutritious, the medication and supplements that we take to be safe and effective, and everything we come in contact with in our environment to be pure and safe. Often, the assurance that these things are true is covered by calling something natural. But what does it really mean to be natural?

Most people would assume that being natural means that it occurs in nature, which superficially is sound or reasonable. But what about a molecule that is manufactured or synthesized but is identical to a molecule that occurs in nature? Is the synthetic molecule natural because it's identical to a molecule that occurs in nature, or does its origin matter? Does the actual physical molecule itself, not just its chemical structure, have to derive from something natural like a plant or animal?

We can also consider degrees of processing. If you take something that derives from nature—a plant or an animal—and do stuff to it, is there any amount of processing that you can do that would make it pass over a fuzzy line into being no longer natural? What about, for example, just simple mechanical processing like chopping or grinding? And what about cooking, which changes the chemical structure of things to some degree? The point is there is no real clear demarcation line between something that is entirely natural and something that is completely artificial.

The deeper question here is what the implications are to human health of something being natural versus not. Being natural is no guarantee of being safe or healthful. There are many poisons in nature, including hemlock, cyanide, arsenic, and animal and insect venoms.

Many people use the notion of natural being better than synthetic as a justification for lifestyle choices even though the evidence may not support those choices. One group that takes the notion of being natural to a bit of an extreme is those who advocate eating raw food. They claim that raw food preserves the nutritious value and natural enzymes of food and that by cooking food, you are in essence killing the food. But scientific evidence does not support the claims behind this. For example, there are only minimal differences in the nutritional value of food that is raw versus lightly or even moderately cooked. Some advocates also claim that raw food is more digestible than cooked food. This claim also is not true. Some foods—like meats and starches—are easier to digest once they are cooked.

Another concern that comes under the banner of natural being better is the use of hormones in the production of meat, eggs, and milk. There are several kinds of hormones that are given to animals. Some are endogenous hormones—hormones that animals make for themselves ordinarily—and some are exogenous steroids. These hormones in meat have been banned in Canada and the European Union based on alleged health concerns. But

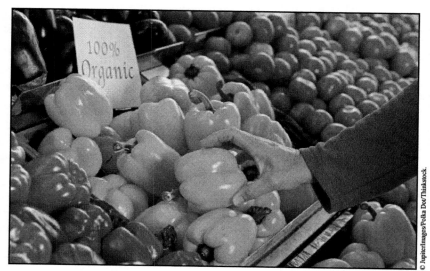

Organic produce has not been shown to be more nutritious than conventionally farmed produce.

this is largely based on theory and the popular notion that hormones are not safe—it's not based on any scientific evidence. In the United States and elsewhere, use of these hormones is carefully monitored and regulated.

There are only minimal differences in the nutritional value of food that is raw versus lightly or even moderately cooked.

Another issue is the use of antibiotics to minimize infection in animals in industrial settings. Do these antibiotics pose any risk or threat to human health? One concern is that extensive use might increase the risk of bacterial resistance to antibiotics. This is a very legitimate concern: There may be an indirect concern for human health there.

What about irradiating food? Again, some people oppose the notion of passing radiation through food because it's not natural and may alter the food from its natural state. However, the radiation passes through the food; there is no radioactive material in the food itself. Irradiating food is very effective in preserving food because it kills most of the bacteria. Irradiation may break down some nutrients, but the overall effect on the food is similar to that of cooking. The Centers for Disease Control estimates that if we irradiated 50% of the meat and poultry in the United States, we could prevent nearly 900,000 cases of infection, 8500 hospitalizations, and over 6000 catastrophic illnesses resulting in 350 deaths each year. The effectiveness of irradiating food is really not in question, but most of the opposition to it seems to be based on the notion that it's altering food from its natural state.

A very big issue with the notion of natural is organic food. Is being organic ultimately an appeal to this naturalistic notion, or are there legitimate concerns about organic versus conventional farming? One question that comes up is whether organic produce is more nutritious than conventionally farmed produce. A 2010 review, in the *American Journal of Clinical Nutrition*, of the last 50 years of research showed that there were no significant differences in nutritional value and no health benefits from eating organic food. There were only 12 studies that were most important in this review, but the evidence we have so far does not show any health or nutritional advantage. ■

Suggested Reading

Fallacy Files, "Appeal to Nature."

Gardner, *Fads and Fallacies in the Name of Science.*

Novella, "All Natural Arsenic."

Questions to Consider

1. What exactly does it mean to be "all natural"?

2. Are foods more healthful if they are organic, raw, or not genetically modified?

3. Why do you think the concept of "natural" has such widespread appeal?

The Fallacy That Natural Is Always Better
Lecture 5—Transcript

We all want the food that we eat to be wholesome and nutritious; the medication and supplements that we take to be safe and effective; and pretty much anything we come in contact with in our environment to be pure and safe. Often, the assurance that these things are true—that our food is safe, etcetera—is covered by calling something "natural," as if being all natural automatically comes will all of these virtues. But, is that really true and what does it really mean to be natural?

Partly, this appeal of being natural versus being artificial or synthetic comes from our exposure to this industrial society that we've build for ourselves. We're surrounded by chemicals and things that are artificial and synthetic. Therefore, being natural has an automatic appeal, although this appeal also goes back long in our history. There's something psychologically appealing about the notion of being all natural. It also partly stems from a fear of things being tainted. We have an emotion of disgust where we respond to things that feel as if they are contaminants or that they are artificial. The word "chemicals" is often used as a pejorative as if something that is a chemical is distinct from something that is natural.

Therefore, the word and the concept of "natural" is largely an emotional appeal. You may also be surprised that the word itself is very loosely regulated. There isn't much regulation or only very vague regulation about the use of the word "natural." It can therefore be applied to most things. There are no strict criteria for getting the label of natural. It doesn't mean as much as people think when it appears on packaging or marketing.

But, the deeper question here beyond what the word "natural" means or how it's regulated is how we would define it. Is there a specific definition that we can give that has real meaning to the word "natural?" Most people would assume that being natural means that it occurs in nature, which superficially sounds reasonable. But, when we dig a little deeper on that we realize that that's not a clear definition either. For example, all elements occur in nature— iron, oxygen, and carbon. Therefore, you might assume that anything made out of those elements is also natural. But, I don't think most people would accept that as a reasonable definition.

What if we take it up one level to molecules and chemicals? Therefore, any molecule which occurs in nature is natural. Those molecules that do not occur or are not found in things like plants and animals are therefore not natural. However, that leads to the question of what about a molecule that is manufactured or synthesized but is identical to a molecule that occurs in nature. Is the synthetic molecule natural because it's identical to a molecule that occurs in nature or does the origin also matter? Does the actual physical molecule itself, not just its chemical structure, have to derive from something natural like a plant or animal?

For example, this comes up with respect to vitamins. You could take a vitamin C molecule that is derived from rose hips and a vitamin C molecule that was synthesized in a laboratory. The chemicals are identical. There's no test you can do to distinguish one molecule from the other. Is one therefore natural and the other one not natural? If so, then what does that mean?

We can also consider degrees of processing. If you take something that derives from nature—a plant or an animal—and do stuff to it, is there any amount of processing that you can do that would make it pass over a fuzzy line into being no longer natural? What about, for example, just simple mechanical processing like chopping or grinding? What about mixing that with other substances or isolating a piece of it from its original source? If I take a plant, for example, and isolate one chemical or one molecule from the hundreds that occur within that plant, is that plant-derived molecule still natural or does the isolation process make it now something that's been manufactured?

We can also look at cooking. Cooking actually changes the chemical structure of things that are cooked, to some degree. Is cooking, therefore, making something natural into something unnatural? Is there any degree of cooking? What if we mix different ingredients together and cook them in a way that actually starts to combine chemicals into new structures that haven't existed before? The point of this is to make the point that there is no real clear demarcation line between something which is entirely natural and something which is completely artificial. There is actually quite a fuzzy line between these two depending on the degree of alteration or processing that occurs.

This process then could either be beneficial or harmful. For example, sometimes chemists will take a chemical structure that occurs in nature. They'll make a slight alteration to that chemical structure in order to make that chemical less toxic, absorbed better, or have better bioavailability. Therefore, making it less natural is not therefore a bad thing.

On the other hand, some changes that occur in this fashion, such as making hydrogenated fats, take fats and make them much less healthful. Hydrogenated fats will increase your risk of heart disease, for example. That's another case where processing makes something less healthful. It's not the processing itself or the degree to which something is natural that seems to matter, rather it's simply what the final chemical structure is and how it responds in our body.

But, the deeper question here—even deeper than what it means to be natural, what the definition of natural is—is what are the implications of being natural versus not being natural to the products that we use or to human health? There are many poisons in nature. Being natural is no guarantee of being safe or healthful. Hemlock, cyanide, arsenic, many venoms, both animal and insect, and other derivations from nature are terrible poisons. They evolve to be deadly poisons to humans and to other animals.

Many plants contain poisonous substances. I certainly wouldn't recommend that you go into your backyard and eat a random plant without knowing what it is. You're likely to get an upset stomach and if you choose poorly, you may even be seriously harmed by that. Only a small subset of plants encountered in nature are actually good for you and would make good food. Although, interestingly, a plant that many people think is highly toxic, poinsettias, turns out to be a myth. The toxicity of poinsettias is a myth. In fact, it's only very mildly toxic. It certainly isn't a food. I wouldn't recommend that you eat it deliberately, but there are numerous case reports of children and pets eating entire poinsettia plants without leading to any serious outcomes.

There are other poisons in nature still. Even the foods that we eat may have some hidden poisons. We eat mushrooms. But, if you're not careful about the mushrooms you eat, you may encounter the death cap mushroom, which is sometimes accidentally eaten. This contains a deadly poison that can lead to death in many cases. You may have heard that you shouldn't eat green potato chips, that they are poisonous. It turns out that, while one potato chip is not going to harm you, that's actually not a myth. Green potatoes contain a toxin called glycoalkaloids. There are case reports of people becoming very sick from eating green potatoes and even dying in some cases.

Raw cashews also contain a poison called urushiol. You may think you have bought raw cashews from the store. There are cashews marketed as "raw," but it turns out that raw cashews that you can buy are actually not entirely raw. They have been steamed and cooked to at least some degree. They're just not roasted, but they have to be at least steamed in order to eliminate or remove most of the urushiol from the cashews because that is a poison. It's the same poison that occurs in poison ivy and can result in a serious adverse allergic reaction.

Other foods like almonds, cherry pits, and apple seeds contain cyanide. Puffer fish or fugu, which is a delicacy in Japan and elsewhere, is a fish that contains a deadly toxin called tetrodotoxin. It can paralyze and kill you. The fish has to be prepared especially to make sure that none of the tissue which contains a significant amount of this tetrodotoxin is included in the final product. But, one error on the part of the chef can lead to accidental poisoning.

Tomato plants—the plants themselves, not the tomatoes—also contain a glycoalkaloid. Although some people use them as a spice in cooking, they must be careful to remove that plant from the final product so that nobody eats it.

In addition, there are some plants that are foods that are not poisons, but they have chemicals in them and these may actually have actions inside our bodies. For example, some plants, most notably soy, but also broccoli and wheat germ, contain what are called phytoestrogens. This actually has hormonal activity in humans. These are probably safe. There isn't much of a health concern about the estrogen-like effects of soy and other plants that contain phytoestrogens. However, there haven't really been definitive studies. For women, the evidence is sufficient to say there really is no health risk from phytoestrogens; however, the jury is still out a little bit for young children and also perhaps for male fertility. In those groups, more research is needed and there is some indication that there may be actual health effects. This could justify caution in using excessive amounts or large amounts of soy in prepubescent children, for example.

Now many people use the notion of natural being better than synthetic as a guarantee or a justification for certain lifestyle choices even though the evidence may not support those choices. One group that takes the notion of being natural to a bit of an extreme is those who advocate eating raw food. They claim that raw food preserves the nutritious value and natural enzymes of food and that, by cooking food, you are in essence killing the food. Eating "dead food" is not good for your health.

However, scientific evidence does not support the claims behind this. For example, there are only minimal differences in nutritional value of food that is raw versus lightly or even moderately cooked. In addition, the natural enzymes that occur in plant foods are plant enzymes and we don't need them. We can make our own digestive enzymes perfectly fine. Therefore, there's no health advantage or health benefit to the enzymes that you would find in your food.

What about digestibility? Some advocates of raw food claim that raw food is more digestible, that cooking it makes it harder for us to break it down and to absorb it. This claim also is not true. Some foods are easier to digest once they are cooked—meats, in particular, proteins, as well as starches. For example, a 1988 study done by Kataria et al showed that starches which are cooked are 2 to 12 times more digestible than raw starches.

What about the effect of cooking on brain size and population? We could take a historical view and I mean really far back in history to our ancestors. The invention of cooking food actually correlates, in the fossil record, with a great expansion of the human brain size and population size. With cooking, we had access to much better nutrition and greater calories mainly through increased digestibility, but also by expanding the number of foods that we can eat. There are some foods that are hard to eat at all if you don't cook them.

Therefore, the evidence shows that there are actually a lot of advantages to cooking. Though, some foods may be better digested if they are raw. In fact, it is recommended that you should try to include some raw fruits and vegetables in your diet or some lightly cooked or lightly steamed fruits and vegetables. It is true that extensive boiling can leach out vitamins and minerals from food. Therefore, you shouldn't heavily boil or cook all of your food.

Raw milk is a claim very similar to raw food. Milk that has not been pasteurized is called raw milk and again proponents claim that it is more healthful because it is natural. But, the nutritional value of pasteurized milk is actually the same as raw milk. There does not appear to be any advantages in clinical research to raw milk in terms of taste or health. Some people may prefer the way raw milk is produced because of better treatment of animals. But, those kind of claims are outside of the range of health and therefore I'm not going to be dealing with them.

A 2009 review showed that there are no health benefits to raw milk. However, it did link raw milk consumption to documented disease outbreak such as E. coli and listeria, being the most common. Sanitary conditions are important and are a partial fix to this risk of bacterial outbreaks from raw milk. But, pasteurization was introduced in order to minimize bacterial infections and outbreaks from milk. It works for that purpose.

Another concern that comes under the banner of natural being better is the use of hormones in meat production or other animal production such as eggs and milk. There are several kinds of hormones that are given to animals. This includes endogenous hormones, hormones that animals make for themselves ordinarily—such as estradiol and progesterone—and exogenous steroids, ones that animals do not make for themselves like zeranol.

These hormones in meat, for example, have been banned in Canada and the European Union based upon alleged health concerns. But, this is largely based upon theory and on just a popular notion that hormones are not safe—it's not based on any scientific evidence. In the United States and elsewhere, use of these hormones is carefully monitored and regulated. But, the scientific evidence has been enough to convince regulators that, at certain levels, it is safe for public consumption.

Antibiotics are another issue. The use of antibiotics in animals to minimize infection is an example. Whenever you crowd a bunch of animals together, they will spread infections around. Again, there are certain techniques you can use to minimize the need for antibiotics to minimize the risk of disease spread. But, for large industrial purposes, antibiotics are used to prevent infections in the animals. The question that comes up is, are these antibiotics posing any risk or direct threat to human health?

One concern is that extensive use might increase the risk of bacterial resistance to antibiotics. This is a very legitimate concern. While there does not appear to be any direct harm to humans, it is true that relying on antibiotics and using them heavily in animals does increase the number of bacterial species that are out there in the world that have resistance to antibiotics. Thus, there may be an indirect concern for human health there.

What about irradiating food? Again, some people oppose the notion of passing radiation through food because it's not natural and it may alter the food from its natural state. However, it's a myth that irradiated food is radioactive. It is not. The radiation passes through the food. There is no radioactive material in the food itself. But, that is not the extent of concerns that people have about irradiated food.

This is a quick review of what this technology entails. There are several different types of irradiation of food. There is gamma irradiation technology which uses very high energy gamma rays that are emitted from radioactive material like Cobalt 60 or Cesium 137. There's electron beam irradiation which uses beta rays. There's also x-ray irradiation which is deeper penetrating than electron beam radiation. It also doesn't require any radioactive material or source, therefore it is easier to use.

Irradiating food is very effective in preserving food because it kills most of the bacteria that's in the food. In fact, it's so effective that you can store irradiated milk in the cupboard. It doesn't even need to be refrigerated and it won't spoil for weeks. It is true that irradiation, because you are passing very high energy particles through food, may breakdown some nutrients like thiamine, for example. But, overall there is a minimal effect on the food itself. These effects are similar to cooking in terms of, for example, production of oxidants in the food. It's not much different than just cooking the food itself.

The CDC, the Centers for Disease Control, estimates that, if we irradiated 50 percent of the meat and poultry in the United States, this would prevent nearly 900,000 cases of infection, 8500 hospitalizations, and over 6000 catastrophic illnesses with 350 deaths each year. The effectiveness of irradiating food is really not in question. But, most of the opposition to it seems to be based upon the notion that it's doing something harmful to the food and altering it from its natural state.

Another concern that comes up very much within this notion of being natural tending to be better than being artificial or synthetic is the notion of genetically modifying food. Is GM, or genetically modified food, always a bad idea? Does it have real risks? How should we be concerned about this? It turns out that most of the food consumed by humans is not natural in the sense that it is not the form of that food that evolved in nature prior to human intervention, mainly through cultivation.

All of the plants and animals that you are familiar with and think of as food, just about, have been extensively cultivated over centuries or even thousands of years by human ingenuity. They never existed in nature before extensive human tampering. How much cultivation therefore is required, if at all, if you're going to make a distinction before a species is no longer considered natural? Is any amount okay?

Let's give the example of the carrot. This is a very interesting historical example because we still have wild carrots around today. You probably have seen them. They're a very common weed. In the United States, they're known as Queen Anne's Lace. It has a pretty white flower on top. If you've ever pulled one out of the ground—I remember doing this when I was even a young boy—and smell the root, it smells like a carrot. I recognize the familiar smell of a carrot on the root of this plant.

In the wild, these plants have a small, bitter, and nutritionally marginal root. You can eat it and gain some nutrition from it. But, parts of it are too fibrous to eat and the amount of nutrition you get out of it is minimal. However, this wild carrot has been cultivated over centuries to be larger, sweeter, and less fibrous until eventually, we end up with the carrot that we are familiar with today. Even then, by the 15th and 16th century, there were white, yellow, purple, and black carrots.

The orange carrot emerged at least by the 16th century, perhaps earlier; it's still not clear. At some point along the line, probably in a cultivar of yellow carrot, there was a mutation which dramatically increased the amount of beta carotene in this crop making the carrot orange. This became popular then because the orange cultivar is much more nutritious because of the beta carotene.

But, what about genetically modified food now? We can dramatically change plants by cultivating them. Is genetic modification any different? It is a lot quicker and more powerful. We can take genes even from distantly related species, like even bacteria. We can take a bacterial gene and put it in a crop plant. Therefore, there are definitely differences between genetically modifying food and just cultivating them. But, it is still just another technology or thing that humans do in order to alter, even significantly, food.

Some people object to the very notion of GM food. There are other issues and some political issues such as the ownership of that food. That's not what I'm talking about. I'm talking about just the health and safety of the food itself. The point is that, whether it's the result of natural evolution, cultivation, or genetic modification, the end product is what matters the most—not necessarily how we got to that end product.

A very big issue with the notion of natural is organic food. Is being organic ultimately an appeal to this naturalistic notion or are there legitimate concerns about organic versus conventional or chemical-based farming?

The regulations involve production, not the final product in order to get the label of organic in the U.S. and many countries. You need to go through a certain number of procedures. You need to use some methods and not use other methods and then you will get the label of organic. But the organic label does not say anything directly about the final product, only about the production method.

One question that comes up is whether organic produce is more nutritious than conventionally farmed produce. A 2010 review, in the American Journal of Clinical Nutrition, of the last 50 years of research showed that there were no significant differences in nutritional value and no health benefits from eating organic food. That's 50 years of evidence. Still, it wasn't a large number of studies. There were 12 studies that were most important in this review, but the evidence we have so far does not show any health or nutritional advantage.

What about organics and pesticides? I think this is a great example of the bigger issue of natural versus synthetic. The claim of organic farmers is that natural pesticides are safer and better to use than synthetic pesticides. Many people may be surprised to learn that pesticides can be used at all in organic farming. While there are different philosophies among organic farmers, the regulations allow for the use of pesticides from a list of what are considered to be naturally derived pesticides, but not a list of synthetic pesticides.

The distinction that's being made is one of natural versus unnatural, not necessarily safe and effective. In fact, there's no convincing evidence that current levels of the synthetic pesticides that are used in conventional farming pose any health risk. There are some residues of these pesticides on food and if you are interested in minimizing as much as possible this residue of pesticides, then organic farming does have fewer pesticide residues on it—according to the research. However, another option might be thoroughly washing vegetables which has been shown to also significantly reduce the amount of pesticides.

As I said, this alleged advantage to organic or natural pesticides is based upon its origin, but not necessarily evidence for actual superiority. One example of an organic pesticide is Bt, which derives from a bacteria, the bacillus thuringiensis bacteria. This releases a toxin that kills insects. Interestingly, there are some GM or genetically modified foods that put this gene from the Bt into the crop itself—so it makes its own natural pesticide. Here, we have a combination of an organic technology with a genetically modified technology.

But, let's get back to the question of are organic pesticides better? A 2010 Canadian study comparing several organic pesticides to several synthetic pesticides found that the organic pesticides were less effective. They were less effective at killing insects. Therefore, the farmers had to use higher doses and this actually had a broader environmental impact. In terms of the environment and amount of pesticides used, the organic pesticides fared worse than the synthetic pesticides.

Other organic pesticides that are used included one called Neem, which is a combination of chemicals AZA0 and liminoids. This disrupts the hormone cycle in insects. It is derived from seeds. Therefore, it's natural and okay for organic use, but it is a hormone disrupter and does kill insects. You can also get pyrethrins derived from chrysanthemums—again, a natural source. But, this is a very broad spectrum insect toxin. It's very toxic to honeybees, for example.

When you actually look at what makes up these organic pesticides, it turns out that the natural source is irrelevant to their chemical activity. The assumption that they are safe, better for the environment, or maybe even safer for human health, is based largely on this "natural" assumption. It seems to be more reasonable to base it simply on what the evidence shows about their chemical activity, how they're used, and the impact that they have on the environment and human health.

We could also take an evolutionary perspective from this notion of whether "natural" is necessarily better or safer. There is nothing special about those chemicals which happen to occur at the present time in nature that would lead us to believe, on a theoretical basis, that they are safe for human health or may have some specific advantage for human health. That's a bit of an egocentric view of evolution and of nature. Plants and animals evolve chemicals in order to serve their own survival needs, not our needs.

We can also take a view of evolution and apply that to medicine. There is in fact a branch called evolutionary medicine. This is based upon the notion that what is natural for people—especially what was natural for us millions of years ago, before we created our technological civilization—must therefore also be most healthy for us now. It is true that thinking about our evolutionary past does provide some insight into what lifestyles and what behaviors are likely to be more healthful for us.

For example, we evolved to eat certain kinds of foods in certain proportions and amounts. We are adapted to those food sources to certain levels of activity. In our modern society, we certainly have different access to foods and different amounts and kinds of food. We also largely experience different levels of activity. This certainly does have implications for human health. This one is a bit of a mixed bag in that there is reasonable theoretical reason to consider our evolutionary past, but that doesn't mean that we can automatically assume, without specific evidence, that anything our ancestors did must also be good for us.

As an interesting side question, we can ask are people still evolving or are we stuck in our evolutionary past? It's a common myth that people are not evolving, but it turns out that we actually are evolving. Studies that look at gene frequencies, the frequencies of genes in populations of humans, show that there is a continual steady rate of adaptation and changes in gene frequencies. It may become true that, at some point in the future, we will adapt further to the diet that is currently common among human populations.

This notion of adapting the diet to human health reaches its highest manifestation in what's called the Paleo diet. This is a diet specifically designed to mimic the diet of our Paleolithic ancestors, pre-agricultural. Therefore, it's no grains, dairy, salt, or refined sugar. It's comprised largely of meat, fruits, and vegetables. It's still a bit controversial and there's no convincing evidence of any health or other benefits to sticking to a Paleo diet. It is based on a small, short study of 20 young, healthy volunteers. It had a 30 percent dropout rate and complete data was only available for six people. Therefore, the claims made for the Paleo diet seem to be sourced on very, very few individuals in a small and somewhat flawed study.

To put all of this together, the term "natural" is often used as a substitute for concepts and virtues that we're really after—the notion that we want our food to be safe and nutritious, things to be effective, pure, and wholesome. But, replacing evidence and logic for those things—those virtues that we really want—with a shortcut, a label of being "natural," is actually counterproductive. It encourages us not to think carefully about the evidence behind the claims that we are hearing. It encourages us to accept uncritically things like the safety of organic pesticides as opposed to looking at the actual evidence. What does the evidence and science show about what is likely to be the case in terms of the safety and effectiveness of the things that we eat and the things that we use on our food?

Probiotics and Our Bacterial Friends
Lecture 6

People come to appreciate the bacteria that occupy their bodies and the role that they play when they're exposed to antibiotics. After a long course, or sometimes even not that long a course, of what we call broad spectrum antibiotics—antibiotics that kill a lot of different kinds of bacteria—this normal flora of bacteria can be decreased. When that happens, we become more susceptible to infection.

You've probably heard the phrase "no person is an island." That may be truer than you realize, for we are intimately close with billions of bacteria that coat every surface inside and out of our bodies. Soon after the discovery of bacteria in the early 20th century, the biologist Eli Metchnikoff suggested that some of these bacteria might actually be important to our health—and that maybe we could alter human health by altering these bacteria. He spawned the field known as probiotics, which is the topic of this lecture.

One of the core myths I'd like to address is the notion that all bacteria are bad. People tend to think of bacteria as germs—things that cause disease—when that is mostly not true. There are millions of different bacterial species in the world. The vast majority of those bacteria are completely neutral to human health. A very small minority are pathological; they will cause disease. Another small minority are actually useful; they aid in digestion, for example.

Every surface of our body that's exposed to the environment, inside and out, is occupied with layers of bacteria. Collectively, these bacteria are called the microflora, or the microbiota. There are 2 basic beneficial effects of the microbiota that we focus on. The first is that it's critical to the immune system. The carpet of bacteria actually crowds out harmless bacteria by taking up all the space and all the resources. Bacteria also aid in digestion. Bacteria break down foodstuffs like complex carbohydrates. They not only eat it for themselves, but they also break it down in a way that then we can further break it down and digest it ourselves.

Can we influence the ecosystem of bacteria in our body with what we eat? That's the basic concept of probiotics. However, that concept is a bit flawed. The primary conceptual problem here is that the ecosystem is easily altered. In fact, it's not easy to alter it at all. It's very difficult for a new bacterial species to work its way into that ecosystem.

Concepts aside, what does the evidence actually show? Do probiotic products work for any specific indication? There are some indications for which a mild benefit has been shown for some probiotic products. However, that is only the case when treatment is given very early and consists of probiotics with high colony counts that contain several species.

Let's talk about some specific uses. One use is preventing or treating diarrhea resulting from antibiotics. It turns out if you have an infection with *C. difficile*, the evidence shows that probiotics are of no benefit. What about irritable bowel syndrome, a very common disorder? There is weak evidence of a mild benefit, but the best that researchers could say at this time is that more research is needed. Probiotics have also been tested in allergies. A 2008 systematic review of the evidence for a specific type of allergy called atopic dermatitis found only mixed results. Do probiotics work for *H. pylori*? There's preliminary evidence for a mild benefit, not by itself, but as what we call adjunctive therapy. If you're taking the other treatments that have been shown to be effective for *H. pylori* and add probiotics, you may have a mild advantage.

People tend to think of bacteria as germs—things that cause disease—when that is mostly not true.

Most of the probiotic market is actually for routine use. Here I think the evidence is pretty clear: If you're a healthy individual with your normal bacterial ecosystem, then eating specific types of live bacteria simply doesn't have any benefit. It also should be noted that we are constantly exposed to bacteria from our environment. Adding a few extra bacteria in a specific yogurt doesn't really add much to our environmental exposure to bacteria. The bottom line is there is no evidence for routine use. While probiotics and prebiotics are more hype than help currently, there is evidence that there may be some potential symptomatic benefit for specific medical conditions. We may be able to affect human health with the probiotic approach, but we're not there yet. ∎

Suggested Reading

Crislip, "Probiotics."

Floch and Kim, *Probiotics.*

Questions to Consider

1. What is the role of friendly bacteria in human health?

2. Are there any proven uses for probiotics?

Probiotics and Our Bacterial Friends
Lecture 6—Transcript

You've probably heard the phrase "no person is an island." That may be more true than you realize for we are intimately close with billions of bacteria that coat every surface inside and out of our bodies. Soon after the discovery of bacteria in the early 20th century, a biologist by the name of Eli Metchnikoff suggested that some of these bacteria might be actually very important to our health—and maybe we could actually alter human health by altering these bacteria. He came up with many ideas that turned out to be wrong. However, he did spawn the field known as probiotics, which is what I'll be talking about mostly in this lecture.

Eli Metchnikoff won the Nobel Prize for medicine in 1908 for his work on the immune system, specifically phagocytosis. Later in life, he became a strong proponent of lots of claims surrounding probiotics. His career actually reminds me a lot of Linus Pauling, another biologist who won two Nobel Prizes in fact. But, later in life, he promoted ideas such as megadosing vitamin C for all kinds of health claims and orthomolecular medicine. Both of these gentlemen, in my opinion, represent two cautionary tales in science.

The first is that even though these were two giants of science and biology that we don't really invest authority in any individual person; any individual person, no matter how brilliant and famous, can be wrong. Rather, we are more likely to respect the authority of a consensus of opinion among many scientists. Don't get too fooled into thinking that an individual cannot be wrong no matter how famous or brilliant they have been.

The second is that both of these gentlemen later in life went outside of their field of expertise. They were basic scientists. They were brilliant in the lab. But, then they tried to make clinical medical claims that they were really not trained to deal with. Both, unfortunately, went horribly wrong in the conclusions that they were promoting.

Let's get back to the question of probiotics that Metchnikoff helped promote as a field. What are probiotics? It's the concept that not all bacteria are harmful, that there are many friendly bacteria. These live, friendly bacteria may actually be useful in human health. Therefore, products that contain these bacteria might actually enhance that bacteria living inside of us and promote health. Common sources of probiotic products, products with live bacteria in them, include yogurt, milk products, some juice products, and Miso, which is a Japanese spread made from fermented rice and other products.

The term probiotic is meant to contrast with antibiotic. Antibiotics are drugs and other things that are meant to either kill bacteria or keep them from reproducing whereas probiotics are promoting bacteria.

You may also encounter a term called prebiotics. That term was coined by Marcel Roberfroid in 1995. Prebiotics are essentially functional food. They do not contain live bacteria, but they contain food for bacteria. It's mainly non-digestible food components, mostly complex carbohydrates, like fiber or fermented products that are food for bacteria. These mostly include oligofructose and inulin. Those are the two most common prebiotic constituents. Inulin can also be found in things like bananas, flax, and barley.

These foods are not only meant to increase the bacteria in our stomachs, but also in our GI system. It also is meant to change the proportion of different bacteria to promote certain kinds of bacteria. Research into prebiotics is very preliminary. So far, there's no evidence to show any health benefits from taking prebiotics.

One of the core myths that I'd like to address in this talk, however, is the notion that all bacteria are bad. People tend to think of bacteria as germs—things that cause disease—when, in fact, that is mostly not true. There are many, many different bacterial species in the world, millions of species. By one estimate, there are 5×10^{30} individual bacteria in the world. That's a lot. That's by number or by mass more than any other type of living thing in the world.

The vast majority of those bacteria are completely neutral to human health. They really don't care about us one way or the other. They're neither helpful nor harmful. A very small minority is pathological; they will cause disease. Another small minority are actually useful. They aid in digestion, for example.

Every surface of our body that's exposed to the environment, inside and out, is occupied with a carpeting, layers of bacteria. Our skin, oral and nasal mucosa, conjunctiva of our eyes, lungs, and lining of our intestines are all coated with bacteria. Collectively, these bacteria are called the microflora or the microbiota. Every person is actually a superorganism, an ecosystem of this microflora.

How many bacteria are there in the average person? There are about 10 times as many bacteria in the average person as there are human cells. There are more bacterial cells in you than person cells. There are about 10^{14} bacteria whereas only about 10^{13} human cells. There are more bacterial genes in you than there are human genes in you. The large intestines contain the most bacteria. About 60 percent of feces is bacteria by dry weight. Every person, on average, contains about 2 to 9 pounds of bacteria in their bodies.

The bacterial ecosystem in your body contains about 1000 species. That's an estimate. About 40 to 50 different species make up about 99 percent of individual bacteria. There are about 50 species predominating, but as many as 1000 in total. These bacteria exist in a complex ecosystem in equilibrium with each other and also with the host, with the person. We share most of our bacteria with our family, meaning that the bacterial species that make up your microbiota are going to be most similar to other members of your family. That's rather stable throughout your lifetime.

In fact, we are coated with bacteria from soon after birth. The womb itself is completely sterile. There are no bacteria inside the womb. But, from the moment of birth, we are colonized with bacteria. Within 48 hours, you have an ecosystem of bacteria in you. Within that first 48 hours of your life, you have most of the bacteria that you're going to contain for the rest of your life. That bacteria makes up what we call a bacterial signature. Scientists have been able to distinguish one person from another by the list of individual species of bacteria that occupy them. These bacteria also differ by different places in your body. For example, you have one type of bacteria in your armpit and another different type of bacteria, or different species of bacteria, on your elbow, in your mouth, or on your back.

There are two basic beneficial effects of the microbiota that we focus on. The first is that it's critical to the immune system. The carpet of bacteria actually crowds out harmless bacteria by taking up all the space and all the resources. If an invasive bacteria tries to set up shop and cause an infection, this microbiota will crowd them out and prevent that from happening. If all of the bacteria on and in your body were suddenly killed, then you would be very susceptible to infection. You would get sick very quickly.

Bacteria also aid in digestion. Bacteria break down foodstuffs like complex carbohydrates. They not only eat it for themselves, but they break it down in a way that then we can further break it down and digest it ourselves. The bacteria in our intestines are also increasingly being recognized as playing some role—still to be further evaluated by research—in health and disease. For example, research has now correlated the risk of obesity with having certain species of bacteria in the intestines. We're not certain yet whether or not being obese causes you to have certain bacteria or—the more interesting possibility—that being colonized with certain species of bacteria actually contributes to or causes obesity. That, of course, would be a very interesting fact if it turned out to be true. It may be another way to treat obesity.

There are also certain inflammatory diseases possibly leading to other diseases, like metabolic disorders, that can correlate also with certain kinds of bacteria. Again, we may be able to decrease the risk of certain metabolic or inflammatory disorders by changing the bacteria that are occupying you. In the oral mucosa, bad breath or halitosis, tooth decay, and gum disease also correlate with certain specific bacterial species.

People come to appreciate the bacteria that occupy their bodies and the role that they play when they're exposed to antibiotics. After a long course, or sometimes even not that long a course, of what we call broad spectrum antibiotics—antibiotics that kill a lot of different kinds of bacteria—this normal flora of bacteria can be decreased. When that happens, we become more susceptible to infection.

The loss of the microbiota can be very critical. Fungal infections will tend to overgrow when you wipe out the normal bacteria coating the mouth and the tongue, for example. You can also get fungal infections like vaginal candida and opportunistic infections from other bacteria. Sometimes even bacteria that are part of the normal flora, that are kept in check, can become pathological and cause disease when too many of their comrades are taken out of the picture. Also, outside bacteria, bacteria that normally wouldn't gain access to your body, can gain access when the flora is gone.

One of the most common complications of broad spectrum or powerful antibiotics is diarrhea caused by a specific bacteria called clostridium difficile or C. diff as we call for short. It's a common pathogen that's normally present in our intestines, but it grows out of control after a course of antibiotics. It results in a very serious bacterial gastroenteritis. It's severe diarrhea and it can often complicate many hospital stays.

Now that we understand the bacteria in our systems and the role that they're playing for health—and a role that we're continuing to learn about—let's turn back to the products that are being marketed as probiotics. Can we actually influence the ecosystem of bacteria in our body just by what we eat? That's the basic concept of probiotics. However, that concept is a bit flawed. It's based upon the notion—the myth if you will—that we can significantly alter our microbiota, the bacteria in our intestines, just by what we eat.

Most of the products that are sold as probiotics contain a specific species or one of many species of bacteria called Lactobacillus. Another common type of bacteria in probiotics is bifidobacterium. The primary conceptual problem here is that the ecosystem is easily altered. But, in fact, it's not easy to alter it at all. I mentioned previously that, soon after birth, we start to form that ecosystem and that we have a basic assortment of bacteria in our bodies. We have 50 species predominating that make up our microbiota and it's stable throughout our lifetime. You share that assortment of bacteria with the people that you grew up with when you were younger; 40, 50 years later you still have the same bacteria that you got when you were a little child.

What that tells us is that the ecosystem is remarkably stable. It's remarkably resistant to change. It's very difficult for a new bacterial species to work its way into that ecosystem. With that concept as a background, imagine adding one, two, or three species of Lactobacillus or other bacteria to that ecosystem. The fact is they just do not take up shop. They do not work their way into the ecosystem and change the balance.

A colleague of mine named Mark Crislip, who is an ID specialist, made the perfect analogy in my opinion. He says that it's like planting corn in the rain forest. If you're trying to replace the bacteria that you lost from a course of antibiotics, it's like cutting down the rain forest and then planting rows of corn—thinking that that replaces the ecosystem. The evidence shows that it just doesn't.

But, concepts aside, we always like to see what the evidence actually shows. The biology is complicated, maybe we're not thinking about it in the perfect way, but let's just look at the evidence to say what does it actually do? What happens when people consume probiotic products? We can't just ask if probiotics work. We have to ask the more specific question—do probiotics work for any specific indication?

There are some indications for which a mild benefit has been shown for some probiotic products. However, it's only when treated very early, when using probiotics that have several species in them, and only ones with the highest colony counts. Products will actually say how many colony forming units or what the colony count is of that product. The only ones which have been shown to have any benefit have 10,000 or more. Again, what all of that says to me is, if there is a benefit, it's pretty mild. This is because we can only detect it when treated the most aggressively with the highest colony forming units as early as possible and with as many species as possible.

Let's talk about some specific uses. One use is preventing or treating diarrhea resulting from antibiotics. This is the one that makes some sense. You're losing the bacteria in your stomach, intestines, and GI system. Therefore, you're losing that carpet of resistance. Let's put something in its place. Even though it may not permanently take up residence, maybe it'll temporarily take the place of your normal bacteria while your own microflora is having a chance to recover. It turns out if you have an infection with C. difficile—remember I mentioned that was very common cause of diarrhea after antibiotics, the most serious complication—the evidence shows that probiotics are of no benefit to C. difficile infection. For that specific indication, the evidence appears to be pretty negative.

What about irritable bowel syndrome, a very common disorder? There is weak evidence of a mild benefit, but the best that researchers could say at this time is that more research is needed. What that means is we can't make any recommendations at the moment. If there is a benefit, it's very mild. If there was a big benefit, the research should have been able to show it by now. But, we can't rule out a smaller benefit without more research.

Preventing tooth decay—there is preliminary evidence only and no recommendations yet. Basically, more research needed. Traveler's diarrhea or Montezuma's Revenge as it's sometimes uncharitably called—there are mixed results with the literature. Again, there is no clear signal, no clear consensus among the research. Some products don't work at all. Some of the better products, the ones with the higher colony counts etcetera, may have some mild benefit.

Probiotics have been tested also in allergies. This is on the notion that the bacteria in your body is affecting your immune function. Maybe, if we can alter that, we can reduce the symptoms of allergies. There's been increasing interest in this. However, a 2008 systematic review of the evidence for a specific type of allergy called atopic dermatitis—essentially inflammation in the skin—found only mixed results. Again, there is no clear evidence for benefit. But, if you want to rule out a small benefit, you need to do more research. We cannot currently recommend probiotics based upon the evidence for any specific allergic indication.

What about helicobacter pylori? This is an interesting story in and of itself. Until about 20 years ago or so, the prevailing theory was that ulcers, peptic ulcers, were caused by stress and the overproduction of acid. It turns out that many people, not everyone, but many people with ulcers actually have a specific bacteria, which is part of the normal flora. This particular bacteria H. pylori, or helicobacter pylori, increases the risk of having peptic ulcers. If you take antibiotics to treat that bacteria, to kill it off or eradicate it, then the ulcer can be cured.

There's a little side myth here that is often repeated. That's the notion that the concept of H. pylori as a cause for ulcers was vigorously resisted within the medical community for years until it was finally accepted. But, actually reviews of the published evidence show that there was considerable interest in the H. pylori hypothesis from the beginning with vigorous research. But, scientists, because where we tend to be conservative, waited for sufficient evidence to come in. Once it did, it actually was rapidly accepted and treatment patterns changed.

Do probiotics work for H. pylori? There's preliminary evidence for a mild benefit, not by itself, but as what we call adjunctive therapy. If you're giving the other treatments that have been shown to be effective for H. pylori and you add probiotics with that, you may have a mild advantage.

However, most products that are sold as probiotics or prebiotics are for routine use. That means use in healthy people who are not treating some short-term or acute illness. They want to use it to simply promote health as an everyday product. Here I think the answer is the most clear. Up to this point, I've been saying that there's mixed results. There's preliminary evidence; there may be a mild benefit, but we need to do more research.

But, most of the probiotic market is actually for routine use. Here I think the evidence is pretty clear that there is no benefit to the routine use of probiotics. If you're a healthy individual with your normal bacterial ecosystem, then eating a specific type of live bacteria simply don't have any benefit. They don't affect that ecosystem. That's the bottom line. It also should be noted that we are constantly being exposed to bacteria from our environment. Adding a few extra bacteria in a specific yogurt or type of dairy product doesn't really add much to our environmental exposure to bacteria. The bottom line is there is no evidence for routine use. There is no real theoretical justification for routine use and I think that that one really should be put to bed.

There is a somewhat controversial treatment, although it's mainly controversial because it's unpleasant to consider. We've talked about ecosystems—bacteria exist in the ecosystem in your intestines. Your ecosystem is going to be most similar to your family member's because you both developed that ecosystem when you were all living together sharing bacteria, getting exposed to the same bacterial sources. If you have somebody who lived in the home with you when you were younger, like a sibling for example, or a parent, their ecosystem's almost identical to yours. If someone loses their ecosystem because they're very ill—they're in the hospital and getting frequent or broad spectrum powerful antibiotics—the idea is that maybe we can transplant or transfer something very close to their bacterial ecosystem to them.

How are we going to do that? The only thing that researchers could figure out is to do what they called a stool transfer. Stool is a polite medical term for feces, or waste. They don't make you eat it, of course; that would be completely unacceptable. They put a feeding tube through the nasal passageway and down into the intestine. They then pass stool donated from a family member through the feeding tube directly down into the intestines.

There actually has been a study looking at stool transfer showing some evidence of effectiveness. It actually is helpful; although, again, the evidence is still preliminary. There's not enough yet to say exactly how robust the benefits are. It's interesting to think whether or not this type of approach will take off as a treatment considering that it is somewhat of an emotionally upsetting type of treatment to consider. However, rather than leading to a very specific treatment—doing literal stool transfers to treat post-antibiotic gastroenteritis—it may just point in the direction of where we need to go in order to really help replace the ecosystem. You need to give an ecosystem in order to replace the ecosystem.

While probiotics and prebiotics are more hype than help currently, there is evidence that there may be some potential symptomatic benefit—not for routine use, but for specific medical conditions. It does point in the direction that maybe if we give more species, choose those species better, develop a little mini-ecosystem of microflora, and give them in high enough amounts to people at the right time in the right clinical setting, we actually may be on to something there. We may be able to affect human health with the whole probiotic approach, but we're not there yet. The treatments that we have now are just not at the point where they're having a significant impact on health.

But, the future looks very interesting. This mainly comes from genetically engineering bacteria, which we are making incredible progress with. One researcher, J. Craig Venter, has published a study in which he was able to take the instructions, the DNA, from a bacteria and remove them. He then completely manufactured a new set of instructions, a new DNA strand, that was mostly copied from an already existing bacterial species. He didn't invent it out of whole cloth. He took a bacterial species and made some interesting little tweaks and changes—some genetic engineering—to that bacteria, that DNA. He then put it into the bacteria whose DNA he had removed. That bacteria changed into the bacteria whose DNA they just gave it. That bacteria was able to reproduce. It was able to live, exist, digest, and reproduce to make more bacteria with a new set of instructions.

He only did this with mostly a preexisting bacterial genome. But, this is a very, very important proof of concept. This means that we can create completely synthetic bacteria. We may be able to design a bacterial genome from the ground up or we can make any number of changes—any change we want essentially—to the bacterial genome. Researchers have already been using more established methods of genetic engineering without completely manufacturing a genome. They've been able to insert very interesting genes into bacteria in your gut that will do things like alter the gasses that are produced by bacterial digestion. Some people may find that very interesting.

For research purposes, they've inserted genes that will label the bacteria and make them glow in the dark or phosphoresce. Therefore, we can better able follow where they go and which bacterial species are surviving. There are tremendous research applications. But, also, we are at the beginning of the point where we can imagine a future in which we can make designer bacteria. This designer bacteria will alter your breath, prevent tooth decay, increase digestion, help fight off obesity, and alter risk factors for autoimmune diseases and other metabolic disorders.

While we have the technology to glimpse this future, we are not there yet. The take-home message here is that the potential for probiotics—using this ecosystem, this other living organism that exists within us, in order to have maybe even dramatic effects on human health—is there and it's very exciting to think about. But, the products that are currently out there for routine use—

probiotics and prebiotics—and the ones that are being studied for specific medical indications either have no benefit or they have only very, very mild benefit. We have a long way to go in developing our research and our products before they would be of any use. For the time being, there doesn't really seem to be any reason to waste any resources on probiotics.

Sugar and Hyperactivity
Lecture 7

In fact—and this seems somewhat counterintuitive—because caffeine is a stimulant, it may improve attention and stimulate the frontal lobes to function a little bit better. It may, paradoxically, decrease hyperactivity or improve attention in children.

Every parent knows that kids have a ton of energy, and hyperactivity may just be a natural part of being young. But, in some children, it can actually be a disorder, a disability that hampers school performance and makes home life challenging. The search for a cause and a cure for excessive hyperactivity in kids has led down many blind alleys. It has led to an industry of self-help books leaving parents with a tremendous amount of information, including a lot of misinformation.

One of the biggest hypotheses—and perhaps the biggest myth dealing with childhood behavior—is the food hypothesis: Children behave the way they do because of the food that they eat. This notion that there's a link between food and hyperactivity goes back to the 1920s and has been controversial ever since. It was mostly popularized in the 1970s by Benjamin Feingold, who created the Feingold diet. This is a diet that removes many things, including food coloring, from children's diets to eliminate or reduce hyperactivity.

A comprehensive review of the evidence performed in the 1980s showed that there is no link between additives and food, and hyperactivity or behavioral changes. But a recent study showed a weak correlation between food coloring and parents noticing an increase in their child's activity. It is possible that there is a mild effect in a small subset, about 5%, of children.

There are also those who think that sugar is the culprit. Despite this common belief with its obvious source in casual observations that most parents would make, there is no link. There is no evidence to support a link between eating lots of sugar and any behavioral change.

What about allergies? I've had parents tell me that they think that their child has a food allergy, and that the allergic reaction is behavioral changes. Real allergies cause skin rashes, breathing problems, sleeping difficulty, and generally feeling under the weather. Allergies do not cause hyperactivity or other behavioral changes.

Attention deficit hyperactivity disorder, or ADHD, is diagnosed in children who are far enough to the hyperactive end of the spectrum that it begins to impair their ability to function at home, at school, and in other situations. ADHD is best understood as a relative deficiency of executive function in the brain. Executive function comes from our frontal lobes, which give us the ability to look at the big picture, to think about the consequences of our actions.

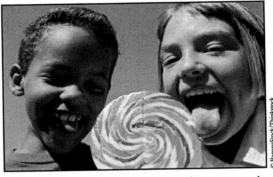

No link has been shown between eating sugar and behavioral change.

How do we diagnose ADHD? There's no blood test. There's no MRI scan. There's no definitive objective biological test to say who has ADHD and who doesn't. With spectrums, there's no absolute objective place to draw the line. To meet the criteria for that diagnosis, children or adults need to have at least 6 specific symptoms. The symptoms need to be of at least 6 month's duration and present in 2 or more settings.

How common is ADHD? By the strict diagnostic criteria, about 3% to 8% of children can be diagnosed with ADHD. About 50% of them will continue to meet those criteria into adulthood. It is a bit of a myth that all children with ADHD will outgrow their symptoms; only 50% do. A claim that comes up frequently is that ADHD is overdiagnosed. I think it is important that we do due diligence to make sure that we're using our diagnostic criteria appropriately. This has been specifically studied. If ADHD were overdiagnosed, you would expect that the false positive rate would exceed the false negative rate. But in specific studies, they find that there's no difference. ADHD is actually not overdiagnosed, despite the very popular belief that it is.

Is ADHD overtreated? There is an increase in the use of medication over recent years, but studies have shown that this increase is mainly because previously underserved populations are now being treated. A higher percentage of people with ADHD are being treated.

While ADHD is a genuine disorder, it is also part of a spectrum of typical childhood behavior and is highly treatable. We have very effective methods of improving behavior and outcomes in children. There's also a lot that we've learned about what to do for your typical child who has the typical range of hyperactivity—the kind of thing that all parents deal with.

There are a great number of myths out there about what triggers hyperactivity. A lot of it revolves around food—sugar, caffeine, and food additives. These serve as a distraction from the truth, and this is one of the big downsides of myths. Misinformation is often more harmful than just ignorance. Parents focus their efforts on highly restrictive diets that are very difficult and that may cause more problems for their child. They are better off focusing on basic parenting skills, forming a working relationship with their children, and focusing on the behavioral modification techniques that have been effective for decades. ∎

Suggested Reading

Hallowell and Ratey, *Driven to Distraction.*

MedlinePlus, "Hyperactivity and Sugar."

1. What is the evidence regarding the claim that eating sugar, or any food, makes children hyperactive?

2. What is the evidence to support the notion that ADHD is a real disorder?

Lecture 7: Sugar and Hyperactivity

Sugar and Hyperactivity
Lecture 7—Transcript

Every parent knows that kids have a ton of energy. I have two daughters myself and I love them to death, but sometimes it seems like they have more energy than they know what to do with. What parent hasn't seen their kids figuratively "bouncing off the walls" and wondered what could possibly be causing this behavior. More to the point, where's the off switch?

Hyperactivity may be a natural part of just being young. But, in some children, it can actually be a disorder, a disability that's hampers school performance and makes home life even more challenging. The search for a cause and possibly a cure for excessive hyperactivity in kids has led down many blind alleys. It has led to an industry of self-help books leaving parents with a tremendous amount of information, including a lot of misinformation.

One of the biggest hypotheses—and perhaps the biggest myth dealing with childhood behavior—is the food hypothesis: children behave the way they do because of the food that they eat. This link, this notion that there's a link between food and hyperactivity, goes back to the 1920s. It has been controversial ever since that time. It was first mostly popularized in the 1970s by Benjamin Feingold, who created the Feingold diet. This is a diet that removes many things from what children eat. It claims that it actually eliminates or reduces hyperactivity and many other problems as well. Many foods are erroneously linked to behavior. Going beyond just the Feingold diet, there are those who think that sugar is the culprit. Others think that it's food additives, caffeine, or some specific constituent of food like casein or gluten.

First, I'm going to give you a word on what we call confirmation bias. I think this largely explains why there's a big disconnect between what the scientific community thinks about food and hyperactivity and what many parents think about food and hyperactivity. Parents may, for example, observe that their child has a ton of energy and their activity level has vastly increased. They may think, well, what has caused this? Why are they suddenly bouncing off the walls? They'll think back to what they maybe ate most recently and note that they ate something sugary or sweet. Therefore, they make an association between the two things, and may then assume a cause and effect, that the sweets caused the behavior.

We call that confirmation bias because people tend to make observations which confirm things that they already suspect or believe. If a child's not acting hyperactive, you may not bother to notice or ask the question, what did they eat in the last 30 or 60 minutes? Therefore, you won't notice that kids eat a lot of sugar at times when they're not acting particularly hyperactive. Also, when there is a correlation, it may not be so simple to assume what the cause and effect is. For example, children may be more likely to eat sweets, cake, and sugary stuff at birthday parties or other events that themselves are likely to contribute to increased energy and hyperactivity.

Despite this common belief with its obvious source in casual observations that most parents would make, there is no link. There is no evidence to support a link between eating lots of sugar, the kind of things that children eat quite a bit of, and any behavioral change. There have been many specific studies and they've shown that there isn't even a correlation. The parents were absolutely convinced that their child will have a significant behavior change after eating sugar or sugary food. However, under controlled and blinded observation, when the children were fed one sugary food and another seemingly identical food that doesn't have nearly as much sugar, there was no correlation. The correlation turned out to be an entire illusion.

Other than the sugar, there's also food additives. Again, this gets back to the Feingold diet that I mentioned, which was more about food additives. A comprehensive review of the evidence performed in the 1980s showed that there is no link between additives and food and hyperactivity or behavioral changes.

There are many studies, but I want to focus a little bit on a recent one that did show a weak correlation between food coloring and the parents noticing an increase in activity. However, interestingly, the correlation was not noted by the clinicians or by any objective clinical assessment. It was only noted by the parents. We're left with, when we look at all the scientific evidence, two possible conclusions. Either there is no real causal link between additives and behavior or we see what we call "noise" in the data. If you do enough studies, you're going to get occasional weak positive studies only in certain circumstances. Unless it's a consistent signal in the research, we usually don't make too much of it. It's possible that there is a mild effect in a small subset of children, 5 percent or so. That would explain the effect that was seen in that one small study.

But, of course, proponents of the notion that food additives will cause hyperactivity will focus on those few studies that seem to support their notions. You have to really look at all of the data and put it into context. There, there's either a very small signal or no signal at all. However, once the belief was out there in the public, it took on a life of its own. Here we are again, decades later, and there's still this strong belief despite the fact that decades of research has failed to find it.

What about allergies? I get this one a lot. I've had parents tell me that they think that their child has a food allergy and that the allergic reaction is behavioral changes; they become hyperactive. Real allergies cause skin rashes, breathing problems, sleeping difficulty, and generally feeling under the weather. But, allergies do not cause hyperactivity or other behavioral changes. About 5 percent of children and 3 to 4 percent of adults have actual food allergies. Food allergies are real and they can actually be very, very serious. Many people, for example, have allergies to peanuts or other nuts. If they get exposed to it even a little bit—even being exposed to somebody else who was exposed to peanut butter, for example—they can have a severe allergic reaction.

The most severe type of allergic reaction that people get is called anaphylaxis where their airways can close up and they can stop breathing. That can be actually fatal. In fact, the most common cause of animal death in the world is anaphylactic shock from bee stings. Bees kill many more people than sharks or any of the other things that we worry about.

What causes real allergies? It's a hyper-reaction in the immune system. The immune system is doing its job, reacting to things in the environment. But, in some people, they have a hyperactive reaction. That causes all of the consequences and symptoms that we talked about. But, it doesn't affect the brain or behavior.

Another common food behavior myth is dairy products. Similar to sugar, parents may observe behavioral changes. If they're thinking that dairy is the link, if that's their bias, that is the observation that they'll make. That will confirm their bias. They'll think, did my child have any cheese recently? They'll find that, indeed, they did. That will confirm their belief of a link between dairy consumption and either behavior problems generally or sometimes specifically, autism or autistic behavior.

Autism is a real neurological condition in which children do have behavioral changes. They have problems with social interaction specifically. They may or may not also have some mental retardation to go along with that or there may just be the decrease in social interactions. But, they do engage in sometimes repetitive behaviors and some other problematic behaviors. Parents of autistic children often believe that those behaviors are triggered by certain kinds of food. Dairy is one of the ones that is currently a belief that is out there and is very common.

Once again, this has been examined scientifically. A 2010 study done at the University of Rochester reviewed all of the existing evidence. It showed that there was no correlation between eating dairy and behavioral outcomes in autism. In fact, it showed that there was no benefit to a diet that excludes dairy.

Gluten is another compound that gets focus of attention for autism, hyperactivity, or behavioral problems in general. Gluten is a type of protein that is found in rye, wheat, and barley. In fact, there is a real and often serious medical condition that includes a sensitivity to gluten. It's called celiac disease. People with celiac disease need to be on a gluten-free diet. But, this is completely a separate syndrome from autism, ADHD, or behavioral disorders.

Celiac disease causes inflammation and damage to the intestines. It may lead to malabsorption syndromes, which can in turn lead to nerve damage and other neurological symptoms. But, celiac disease can be diagnosed with specific medical tests. We can fairly definitively diagnose it. If you don't have abnormal testing for celiac disease, then you don't have a gluten sensitivity and you don't have to worry about it. Further, despite whatever the theoretical connection might be between gluten and behavior, scientists have asked the question if we put children with autism or other behavioral problems on a gluten-free diet, does it help? That same 2010 University of Rochester review looked at all the studies that looked at gluten and the gluten-free diet. They found, again, the bottom line is there's no evidence of any benefit to a gluten-free diet and the behavioral issues of children with autism or other children.

Caffeine comes up frequently as well. Children have access to caffeine in soda, iced tea, and chocolate. Perhaps chocolate is their most common source of caffeine. People need to remember that that is a source of caffeine also. Again, it's very plausible that caffeine—which is a stimulant—may give kids more energy and make them more hyperactive. But, it turns out that that effect seems to be too minor to detect clinically when you study it. Thus, it doesn't cause hyperactivity itself.

In fact—and this seems somewhat counterintuitive—because caffeine is a stimulant, it may improve attention and stimulate the frontal lobes to function a little bit better. It may, paradoxically, decrease hyperactivity or improve attention in children. High doses, however, can cause jitteriness, nervousness, and sleep difficulty—especially in those who haven't been taking caffeine for a while. You do become tolerant to the effects of caffeine over a while. Even after a few weeks of regular caffeine, you don't respond as much to all of these effects. No one's recommending that caffeine in high doses be used in kids to treat any of their symptoms. But, if anything, caffeine may reduce inattention or hyperactivity—not make kids bounce off the walls.

This leads us to the disorder, as I spoke about, of hyperactivity and inattention or ADHD, attention deficit with hyperactivity disorder. Of course, there is a spectrum of behavior among kids. Some kids are more hyperactive than others. There is a typical spectrum of behavior that we see in children. But, between 3 and 7 percent of children will be far enough to the hyperactive end of that spectrum that it begins to impair their ability to function at home, school, and other situations. That's when it gets this label of ADHD and becomes the focus of treatment.

This is best understood—in terms of what ADHD is—as a relative deficiency of what neuroscientists call executive function. Executive function comes from our frontal lobes, the most recently evolved and therefore, we think, the most developed part of the human brain. The frontal lobes give us the ability to essentially control our lives—to look at the big picture, think about the consequences of our actions, and inhibit our more primitive emotions and instincts in order to strategically plan the kinds of activities that we do in our lives.

Primarily, you could think about it as a filter by which we inhibit behaviors which may be self-destructive or inappropriate. That actually is a very energetic, demanding function that uses up a lot of our brain resources. People—children and adults—with ADHD, when we look at their brain function—with either an electroencephalogram to look at the electrical activity or function MRI scan to look at how active different parts of their brain are—have a relative decrease in the activity in those parts of their frontal lobes that are responsible for this executive function. Therefore, all the pieces do fit together fairly nicely, that ADHD is an executive function disorder.

How is it diagnosed? This is the tricky part. There's no blood test. There's no MRI scan. There's no definitive objective biological test to say who has ADHD and who doesn't have ADHD. Further, as I said, it's a spectrum. With continuums and spectrums, you do have that problem where there's no absolutely objective place to draw the line. But, that doesn't mean that there aren't some people who are far enough to one end of that spectrum that we can't identify them as having a disorder worthy of attention.

ADHD is what we call a clinical diagnosis. Clinical diagnoses, like migraines and many other things in medicine, are diagnosed by having a certain number of symptoms which are characteristic of that disorder. For ADHD, it's impulsivity, hyperactivity, and inattention. Children or adults who have ADHD, in order to meet the criteria for that diagnosis, need to have at least six specific symptoms. The symptoms need to be at least six month's duration and present in two or more different settings. If they're only observed at school, but nowhere else, you do not meet the criteria for the diagnosis of ADHD. If you have just four of those symptoms, you don't meet the criteria. You need to have a certain threshold.

Yes, it's a little arbitrary, but again, you have to draw the line somewhere. What researchers and scientists do is say, well, does this correlate with anything? If this is the criteria that we have, yes, it's fuzzy around the edges. But, if we use this criteria, does it predict outcome? Does it predict who's going to do well in school? Who's going to be successful in the workplace? Does it predict things like divorce rate and the risk of being imprisoned? It turns out that, when you strictly apply these clinical diagnostic criteria, it does predict those things.

Studies like the EEG and the MRI—and also now we're finding genetic links to susceptibility to ADHD—these are important for research to help us understand the disorder. However, none of them are specific enough yet to be useful in the clinical setting.

What do we mean by a disorder? I called ADHD a disorder. It's not a pathological disease; you can't look at cells under a microscope and see that they're pathologically abnormal. What a disorder means, in the psychological or psychiatric context, is that people with a disorder lack some function—in this case, executive function—that is typically possessed by most people. The relative decrease or lack of that functionality leads to demonstrable harm. That's the definition of a disorder and ADHD meets that definition.

For example, one-third of people with ADHD drop out of high school. Also, only about 5 percent complete a university degree compared to 40 percent of the population of their peers—their peers matched in other ways. That's a 35 percent absolute decrease—from 40 down to 5 percent— of getting a university degree. That's a pretty significant difference in educational outcome.

How common is ADHD? The name ADHD arose in 1980. However, if you look back in the medical literature, you will find clinical descriptions of ADHD going back to the 1800s. This is very common. We have modern names for medical entities, but if you just look at the actual details, you will see that physicians and scientists were describing these same syndromes even a hundred or more years ago.

By the strict diagnostic criteria—which would be found in what we call the DSM or the Diagnostic and Statistical Manual, now on the 4th edition going on to the 5th edition—about 3 to 8 percent of children will meet the criteria for the diagnosis of ADHD. About 50 percent of them will have symptoms and will continue to meet that criteria that persist into adulthood. It is a bit of a myth that all children with ADHD will outgrow their symptoms. Only 50 percent do, which means 50 percent will continue to have the full-fledged ADHD sufferers even into adulthood.

Is ADHD a uniquely American disorder? That is another myth I hear quite frequently. I think it's intended to say that it's not a real disorder because if it were real, then people would have it in every country. It must be cultural because we only see it in the United States. In fact, in January of 2002, an international consortium of scientists signed a consensus statement. Here again, we have a consensus of experts reviewing all the evidence up to that point. They said, and I'll read you the full quote of their statement, "We fear that inaccurate stories rendering ADHD as a myth, fraud, or benign condition may cause thousands of sufferers not to seek treatment for their disorder. It also leaves the public with a general sense that this disorder is not valid or real or consists of a rather trivial affliction." Their concern was that the myth that ADHD might not be real is causing demonstrable harm, meaning it's keeping people from treatment which may be helpful or may ameliorate the downside of having ADHD. They also recognized it as a truly international disorder. It is not uniquely American.

Another claim that comes up quite frequently—and it's a perfectly legitimate question to ask—is whether ADHD is overdiagnosed. I think we need to ask similar questions about anything that is diagnosed in 3 to 7 percent of the population. You might argue that's especially true for children. They are an especially vulnerable population. We need to do absolute due diligence to make sure that we're using our diagnostic criteria appropriately. Specifically with clinical criteria, where is this fuzziness around the edges, we want to really ask the question in every way possible—are we using this diagnosis properly? Are we diagnosing it when it should be and not overdiagnosing it, especially if overdiagnosing it could lead to inappropriate treatment.

This has been specifically studied. For example, you can compare the false positive rate to the false negative rate. False positive means that you give someone the diagnosis when they don't really have it. False negative means that you fail to diagnose somebody when they do in fact have the disorder. If ADHD were overdiagnosed, you would expect that the false positive rate would exceed the false negative rate. But, whenever this has been looked at in specific studies, they find that in essence there's no difference. ADHD is actually not overdiagnosed despite the very common popular belief that it is.

Of course, this is looking at physicians diagnosing ADHD by the published, established criteria. This doesn't mean the casual diagnosis of parents, teachers, or other people. That's a different story. Perhaps that's where we need to reign in the diagnosis. We can't just assume that because a child superficially seems hyperactive that they have ADHD. They really do need to have a medical assessment.

This is all especially important because ADHD is very treatable. One type of treatment involves CNS stimulants. If you remember when I was talking about caffeine, stimulants can paradoxically inhibit hyperactivity. That, again, seems like the exact opposite of what you would expect to happen. But, when you drill down a little deeper, we understand now that what's happening is that these stimulants are increasing the activity of the frontal lobes. This is a huge part of our brains and a very, very demanding energy-intense part of brain activity. It uses up a lot of our brain resources. Stimulants increase that amount of brain activity, enabling us to better inhibit our behavior. You increase inhibition; that results in decreased hyperactivity. We now have a vast literature to show that this approach—using short-term stimulants during parts of the day when people need to have increased attention and need to be able to inhibit their behavior, like at school or even at work—is a very successful strategy in coping with this disorder and in reducing the negative consequences.

There is also evidence that behavioral modification is very helpful as well. In fact, we may combine these approaches of using medication when necessary and behavior modification. What type of behavioral management is helpful? Whether or not your child is under the care of a physician who's treating a disorder, these are some useful rules of thumb that are helpful in getting children less hyperactive and better under control, if you will.

These are the recommended and proven methods that work. One is a daily routine. Kids respond well to specific and clearly delineated boundaries and consistency. If the rules are changing every day, that just makes them anxious. It makes them ignore the rules because they're not consistent. Positive reinforcement is also very important. When kids do behave well, they should be positively reinforced for that. However, on a side note, interestingly, many parents will reward children for doing a "good job" when in fact the evidence shows that telling a child "good job" can be counterproductive. It actually makes them anxious—that if they don't do a good job, then the next time, they won't get the praise or the positive reinforcement. It's far better to tell a child they've made a great effort, to reward their effort. Effort is one thing that children are 100 percent in control of. They're not always in control of the outcome, but they are in control of how much they try. Therefore, praise children for making a good effort, not necessarily for the net outcome.

Also, children need clear rules, instructions, and expectations. If there's any uncertainty, that really will short-circuit your attempts at controlling their behavior or giving them positive feedback. There needs to be consistent consequences to their unwanted behavior. Essentially, you can't let them get away with it. If you tell them, if you do this behavior, you have to make the consequences something you will follow through with. You can't make unrealistic consequences. You have to absolutely follow through with them every time and children will respond to that consistency.

You should communicate with the child's teachers. Children may spend a large part of their waking life in school under the observation of their teachers. As parents, if you have any issues about your child's behavior, make sure that you communicate with all of their teachers. Finally, it is recommended that you just set a good example for your children.

Is ADHD overtreated? This is a related question to whether it's overdiagnosed, but not necessarily the same thing. We have certain criteria for diagnosis, but that doesn't mean that everyone who meets that criteria needs to be treated. In a 2007 review published in the Journal of Attention Disorders, it showed that children were not generally overmedicated for ADHD and that the indications that are evidence-based are generally being followed.

There is an increase in the use of medication over recent years, but studies have also shown that this increase in use is mainly because previously underserved populations are now being treated. People who should have been treated but weren't because they weren't seeking medical care are now increasingly being treated. Therefore, the number of people being treated is going up, but that doesn't mean it's being overtreated. A higher percentage of people with ADHD are being treated, that's all.

There are individual cases of improper treatment. I'm not suggesting that there isn't anyone out there who is being overtreated or being inappropriately treated. Of course, if you have any concerns about this for yourself or a loved one, you should seek a second opinion and make sure that you're doing the right thing. But, there is no systematic overdiagnosing or overtreatment that we can detect in the research literature for ADHD.

While ADHD is a genuine disorder, it is also part of a spectrum of typical childhood behavior and it is highly treatable. We have very effective methods of improving behavior and outcome in children. There's also a lot that we've learned about what to do for your typical child who has the typical range of hyperactivity—the kind of thing that all parents deal with. But, it's important to note what does not cause hyperactivity or behavior changes in children.

There are a great number of myths out there about what triggers it and what causes it. A lot of it revolves around food—sugar, caffeine, and food additives. These serve as a distraction from the truth and that is one of the big downsides of myths. Misinformation is often more harmful, more pernicious, than just ignorance. Not knowing something is often not as bad as thinking you know something that turns out not to be true.

Parents focus their efforts on highly restrictive diets that are very difficult and that may cause more problems for their child. This is because now they're spending their time trying to get their children to be compliant with a very restrictive diet. The Feingold diet, for example, removes hundreds of things that children normally eat, that they're not allowed to eat under that diet. You're better off focusing on basic parenting skills, forming a working relationship with your children, and focusing on the basic behavioral modification that we've known for decades is very effective.

Antioxidants—Hype versus Reality
Lecture 8

Basic science tells us what kind of directions we should go in with clinical research but ... can't be used to make clinical claims. More often than not, we're going to be wrong when we guess what the outcome should be based upon just our basic understanding of basic biochemistry and biology.

The term "antioxidant" has become a marketing term synonymous with healthful. But does the hype really hold up to reality? Will that green tea or Acai juice make you live longer and be healthier? Let's examine the biochemisty a bit. We have something called oxygen free radicals inside our body, going around destroying our cells and DNA. This may sound scary, but actually, they exist in an equilibrium. They serve some beneficial effects inside our bodies. For example, they are used by some cells of the immune system to attack and destroy bacteria and viruses. Oxygen free radicals are also used as chemical signals that trigger important functions inside the cell. Therefore, you wouldn't want to completely get rid of them.

Because these oxygen free radicals are an unavoidable by-product of energy production in the mitochondria in all of our cells, it stands to

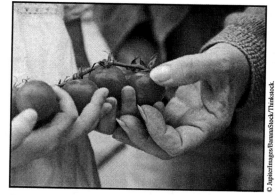

Eating several servings per day of fruits and vegetables is associated with a decrease in cancer risk.

reason we would have evolved mechanisms to sop up those oxidative free radicals and keep them from doing damage. Substances that do that are called antioxidants. There are a number of naturally occurring antioxidants in the body, including vitamins E and C and many specific enzymes. They exist in part to reduce these oxygen free radicals and keep the whole system in equilibrium.

What about eating antioxidants or taking supplements? Beginning in the 1990s, the possibility arose that cellular damage from oxidative stress was actually the underlying cause of not only normal aging, but also many neurodegenerative diseases like Alzheimer's disease, Parkinson's disease, and amyotrophic lateral sclerosis (ALS). This was cutting edge and very interesting science. Many of us were very excited by the prospect that antioxidants in some dose would become very effective in slowing down the progression of these diseases, maybe even halting it.

The public perception that antioxidants are healthful and a net good for health has persisted—despite the fact that the scientific evidence just did not turn out that way.

It turns out that as we get older, we lose some of our naturally occurring antioxidant capacity. It makes sense that replenishing antioxidants would be beneficial. Also, the brain is particularly susceptible to oxidative stress because the brain consumes a lot of oxygen. It therefore produces a correspondingly increased amount of oxygen free radicals. However, it's possible—and this was raised as a cautionary concern—that the oxidative stress leading to cell damage may have been a secondary effect. It may not have been the primary underlying cause of cell death in these neurodegenerative diseases. In other words, it's just one of the many things that happen when cells are dying, not the original or underlying cause of those cells dying.

So what did that research show? For Parkinson's disease, in human trials, antioxidants had no detectable beneficial effect in preventing the development of the disease or slowing its progression. The story is very similar for Alzheimer's disease. Human trials showed mixed results at best; there wasn't any compelling evidence for benefit even at high doses. For ALS, too, the results were disappointing. Studies of vitamins E and C, especially in high doses, did not affect the outcome of the disease. The

Lecture 8: Antioxidants—Hype versus Reality

114

scientific community was humbled by this experience. We had every reason to think that antioxidants were going to be a huge cure for many serious illnesses. Yet 15 or 20 years of clinical research completely disappointed us.

What about cancer prevention? We think that oxidative stress may damage DNA, in turn leading to cancer. In fact, there is evidence that eating several servings per day of fruits and vegetables is associated with up to a 30% decrease in overall cancer risk and greater longevity.

Fruits and vegetables contain antioxidants; eating them helps prevent cancer and improves longevity. However, we can't necessarily conclude that it's the antioxidants that are doing this. The exact mechanism of this clear benefit from fruits and vegetables has yet to be determined. High antioxidants may be playing a role, but there are other variables as well. Perhaps there are other things in fruits and vegetables that are healthful. Perhaps people who eat fruits and vegetables engage in other activities that are healthful. Perhaps if you eat lots of fruits and vegetables, you're not eating as much of other kinds of foods that may increase your risk of cancer.

There are simply too many variables to know whether it's the antioxidants or what exact role the antioxidants are playing in cancer prevention. But one clue we have comes from antioxidant supplements. The research shows that taking antioxidant supplements does not decrease cancer risk. That would argue against antioxidants being the definitive factor.

The public perception that antioxidants are healthful and a net good for health has persisted—despite the fact that the scientific evidence just did not turn out that way. What's the bottom line of all this? There's no evidence to support the routine use of antioxidant supplements or so-called superfoods—like Acai, Noni, blueberry, or pomegranate juice—that are loaded with antioxidants. There's simply no evidence that taking pills or eating superfoods has any health benefit. The evidence keeps leading us back to the common wisdom that most of us know to be true: You should eat your fruits and vegetables—especially your vegetables—every day. ∎

Suggested Reading

Denisov and Afanas'ev, *Oxidation and Antioxidants in Organic Chemistry and Biology.*

Novella, "Antioxidant Hype and Reality."

Questions to Consider

1. What role does oxidative stress play in health and disease?

2. Are there any proven risks or benefits to foods or supplements high in antioxidants?

Antioxidants—Hype versus Reality
Lecture 8—Transcript

Will that green tea or açaí juice make you live longer and be a lot healthier? The term "antioxidant" has become a marketing term synonymous with healthful. But, does the hype really hold up to reality? Before we discuss antioxidants, we need to go back and look at a little biochemistry to put this all into context.

First, I want to describe to you what a free radical is or we could just call it a radical. Radicals are molecules that are highly reactive. To review some really basic chemistry—I apologize if this is too basic, but just so we're all starting at the same point—atoms have positively charged protons along with uncharged neutrons. The number of protons in an atom determines what element it is. Those are both in the nucleus. Around them are electrons, negatively charged electrons. Generally speaking, there will be one electron for each proton in an atom. Ions are atoms that have fewer or more electrons than protons so they carry a net electrical charge.

Electrons aren't just whizzing around their nuclei in some chaotic or random fashion. They are very highly organized and structured. They fill what we call electron shells. First are the innermost shells. When the inner shell is full, then electrons will go to the next shell. When that gets filled, then they start filling up the shell after that—filling one after the other in a sequence. Atoms are in their most stable state, which means their lowest energy state, when their outermost shell is full of electrons.

In addition to liking to fill their outer shell, atoms also like to have all of their electrons paired. Again, this puts them into the lowest energy state. Specifically, by spinning in opposite directions, paired electrons balance each other out. A free radical is essentially any atom or molecule that has an unpaired electron in its outermost shell. Atoms with unpaired electrons like to form bonds with other atoms or molecules. The way atoms do this, the way they bind together is by sharing electrons; they form an electron bond. Two atoms that are each missing electrons from their outermost shell can share an electron and fill their outermost shells. That forms a lower energy or more stable state. In essence, that forms a bond between those two atoms. That's one of the bases of molecules, of basic chemistry.

How does that apply to the human body or any living organism? Animals have organelles in every living cell called mitochondria. These mitochondria are actually like little bacteria. They probably were—at one point in the distant evolutionary past of all animals—an actual separate organism that formed a symbiotic relationship with the eukaryotic cells that went on to form multicellular life. Now there are what we call organelles. There are many of them in every living cell and they are the energy factories. Mitochondria use oxygen to burn fuel and create energy in the form of ATP or adenosine triphosphate.

ATP are the little batteries of our cells; that third phosphate bond is very high energy. Then they contribute that energy to other reactions like contracting your muscles and doing all the things that cells do by breaking that phosphate bond and going back down to a DP or adenosine diphosphate. Again, that chemical bond is where the energy for our cells comes from.

In the process of making ATP from essentially the macronutrients in food, mitochondria generate a lot of oxygen—what we call oxygen free radicals, a byproduct of oxygen energy production. These free radicals are oxygen molecules that are also free radicals in that they have an unpaired electron in their outer shell. Some of these specific reactive oxygen species, as we also call them, include superoxide, hydrogen peroxide, and hydroxyl radical.

Some of you may have hydrogen peroxide in your drug cabinet. You may notice that, when you pour it onto a fresh cut, it fizzes. That's because, again, it's very, very highly reactive. It will kill bacteria and viruses because it is an oxygen free radical. These reactive oxygen species can cause damage. They can cause damage to the cell. They can cause damage to DNA. They are particularly reactive to lipids, which form the membranes of all living cells. They do this by reacting very aggressively with other molecules.

That may sound very scary, that we have oxygen free radicals inside of our body going around destroying our cells and DNA. But, actually, they exist in an equilibrium. They also serve some beneficial effects inside our bodies. For example, they are used by some cells of the immune system to attack and destroy bacteria and viruses. Oxygen free radicals are also used as chemical signals that trigger important functions inside the cell. Therefore, you wouldn't want to completely get rid of them. They actually do serve a function in the body.

Finally, this is where antioxidants come in. Because these oxygen free radicals are an unavoidable byproduct of energy production in the mitochondria in all of our cells, it stands to reason we would have evolved—animals in general—mechanisms to sop up those oxidative free radicals and to keep them from doing damage. Substances that do that are called antioxidants. Essentially, when you have a free radical, like an oxygen free radical, it causes a chain reaction. It steals an electron from another molecule to fill its outer shell turning that molecule into free radical. That molecule then steals an electron from a different molecule in order to fill its outer shell, but turning the next molecule into a free radical.

You have what is potentially an endless chain of stealing electrons from molecules. This can potentially be disruptive and can break down DNA, membranes, and other components of the cell. An antioxidant is any molecule that can donate a free electron to a free radical without itself becoming a free radical. Thus, it ends the chain. It ends this chain reaction of oxidative damage.

There are a number of naturally occurring antioxidants in the body. The two most common are vitamin E and vitamin C. They're the most abundant that we use. There are also many specific enzymes, specifically superoxide dismutase and others such as glutathione. They're there partly to reduce these oxygen free radicals, to end these chain reactions, and to keep the whole system in equilibrium.

We've described some of the basic science. Now we know what free radicals are, we know why we have oxygen free radicals in our body. We know what antioxidants are and why they are a critical biochemical component of the normal biochemistry of our bodies. But, what about taking antioxidants themselves? What about eating antioxidants or taking supplements?

Beginning in the 1990s, the possibility arose that cellular damage from oxidative stress was actually the underlying cause of not only normal aging, but many neurodegenerative diseases like Alzheimer's disease, Parkinson's disease, and amyotrophic lateral sclerosis or Lou Gehrig's disease—which proposes a serious scientific notion. This was cutting edge and very interesting science. It was perfectly legitimate. Many of us were very excited by the prospect that antioxidants in some dose would become very effective in slowing down the progression of these diseases, maybe even halting the progression of these diseases.

We all anticipated greatly the clinical trials that would show that antioxidants were effective. This turns out to be a very interesting and illuminating story of how science develops and how sometimes our initial, somewhat naïve, and simplistic notions don't pan out. The story of antioxidants didn't turn out the way any of us thought or hoped it would. What did that research show?

Like I discussed previously, there are different kinds of scientific research. Once we had sorted out the basic science about oxidative stress and antioxidants, we moved on to animal studies. The animal studies were encouraging. They showed that oxidative stress is playing a role in cell damage and death. When a cell dies, we call that apoptosis. Oxidative damage or free radical damage was playing a role in apoptosis or cell death.

It also turns out that as we get older, we lose some of our naturally occurring antioxidant capacity. It makes sense that replenishing them would be beneficial. Also, the brain—where many of those diseases that I talked about, those neurodegenerative diseases where the damage is taking place—is particularly susceptible to oxidative stress because the brain consumes a lot of oxygen. It therefore produces a correspondingly increased amount of oxygen free radicals. Lipids especially responsive to oxidative damage and there's a lot of lipids in the structure of the brain. A lot of pieces were fitting together and again, we were all very excited about the prospects here.

However, the stories are always more complicated than we at first assume. It's possible—and this was also raised as a cautionary concern—that the oxidative stress leading to cell damage, leading to apoptosis, may have been a secondary effect. It may not have been the primary underlying cause of cell death in these neurodegenerative diseases like Alzheimer's disease. In other words, it's just one of the many things that happens when cells are dying. But, it wasn't the original or underlying cause of those cells dying.

Let's go to some specific diseases that I mentioned. For example, there is Parkinson's disease. Parkinson's disease is a neurodegenerative disorder where people may have a tremor. They have difficulty walking and moving. They become very stiff. The part of the brain that enables us to move smoothly and fluidly is what's being damaged. Specifically, neurons in the substantia nigra that produce a neurotransmitter called dopamine start to slowly die off. As they die off, the disease gets more and more severe. In the end stage of the disease, the dopaminergic or dopamine producing neurons in the substantia nigra are completely gone. Patients have a very severe manifestation of the disease.

In animal models of Parkinson's disease, antioxidants showed that they were beneficial. It slowed down the progression of the disease. As a side note, I do have to mention that animal models of human diseases while sometimes very good are never perfect. We could never be sure that what's happening in a rat with Parkinson's disease is identical to what's happening in a human who develops sporadic Parkinson's disease. Oftentimes animal models are genetic. We find a mutation that mimics the disease. But, in humans it's not genetic. It's sporadic. It occurs without any specific genetic disorder. The animal models are not perfect. But, when animal models do work, it's an important proof of concept.

Once again, we were on track—antioxidants were looking very favorable. However, when we finally got to the definitive human trials—the only point at which we really know if something is going to work or not—antioxidants had no detectable beneficial effect in either preventing the development of Parkinson's disease or slowing its progression. Unfortunately, it just didn't work. It was actually quite a disappointment.

The story is very similar for Alzheimer's disease, a disease that causes progressive dementia or difficulty with memory, concentration, and cognition. Animal models, again, suggested that there might be benefit from vitamin C and vitamin E—the two most abundant antioxidants in the body.

However, human trials showed mixed results at best. Some were positive, some were negative. There wasn't any compelling evidence for benefit even at high doses. Again, we're left with maybe there's a tiny benefit that we can't really detect statistically. But, there certainly is no big effect from antioxidants with Alzheimer's disease.

A third example is ALS or Lou Gehrig's disease, a disease that I treat myself quite often as a neurologist. There are animal models of ALS. Again, this is a very interesting story, that we have developed an animal model for ALS. It's mice who have a mutation called a SOD1 mutation. It's a mutation in the gene for superoxide dismutase—which is one of the enzymes that's a naturally occurring antioxidant.

That was very promising. Now we have a mutation in a gene for a naturally occurring antioxidant being associated with causing a neurodegenerative disorder, ALS, in these SOD1 mice. That was huge support for the antioxidant or the oxidative stress hypothesis of ALS. But, again, biology always turns out to be more interesting and more complex than we initially think. It turns out that the mutated SOD1 protein, was not only not doing its job as an antioxidant, it was also directly toxic to motor neurons, the neurons that are dying in ALS.

Now we couldn't really separate out how much this mutation was killing off motor neurons because it's directly toxic and how much it was killing off neurons because it wasn't doing its job as an antioxidant. We were left with just studying antioxidants in people with ALS to see if they work. The results, again, were disappointing. Studies of vitamin E and vitamin C, especially in high doses, did not affect the outcome of the disease. It did not slow the progression of the disease. Vitamin E was studied to see if it prevented the disease from occurring in the first place and again, it was completely negative.

The scientific community was very humbled by this experience. We had every reason to think that antioxidants were going to be a huge cure for many serious illnesses with potential even going beyond that. Yet, 15, 20 years of clinical research completely disappointed us.

What about cancer prevention? That's another entity in which we think that oxidative stress may damage DNA and DNA mutations lead to cancer—a very plausible mechanism. In fact, there is evidence that eating several servings per day of fruits and vegetables is associated with up to a 30 percent decrease in overall cancer risk and greater longevity. Fruits and vegetables contain antioxidants. Eating them prevents against cancer and improves longevity.

However, we can't necessarily conclude that it's the antioxidants that are doing this. The exact mechanism of this clear benefit from fruits and vegetables has yet to be determined. High antioxidants may be playing a role, but there's other variables as well. Perhaps there are other things in fruits and vegetables that are healthful. Perhaps people who eat fruits and vegetables engage in other activities which are healthful or avoid activities which have a higher risk of cancer. Perhaps if you eat lots of fruits and vegetables, you're not eating as much of other kinds of foods that may not be healthful that may increase your risk of cancer.

There are simply too many variables to know if it's the antioxidants or what exact role the antioxidants are playing in cancer prevention. But, one clue we have is antioxidant supplements. If it is the antioxidants in the fruits and vegetables, then taking a pill with antioxidants in it should have the same benefit. However, the research shows, overall, that taking antioxidant supplements as opposed to eating fruits and vegetables with antioxidants does not decrease cancer risk. That would argue against antioxidants being the definitive factor.

Beta carotene, vitamin A, was associated with a higher risk of cancer in smokers—a paradoxical outcome. It probably still needs to be replicated in further studies, but the evidence we have so far shows that vitamin A may be counterproductive in smokers—specifically in those who have lung cancer. Selenium was associated with a reduced risk of cancer in men, but not women. That difference can't be explained on the basis of antioxidant effects alone.

What about hearth health? Here, the story is really interesting. Antioxidants do reduce cholesterol plaque buildup. Therefore, they may reduce atherosclerosis and the risk of heart attacks. Again, eating fruits and vegetables is definitely associated with a lower risk of cardiac disease.

There was a recent meta-analysis. A meta-analysis is when you take multiple studies, pool the data, and analyze all the data together. Essentially, it's an attempt at turning a few small to moderate size trials into one large trial. It's not a perfect technique, but it is helpful to try to get a sense of what is the consensus of data in a large number of studies. This meta-analysis of studies of vitamin E and heart disease showed no benefit at any dose. This was especially true for secondary prevention—preventing your second heart attack after you've already had the first one. Studies of beta-carotene actually showed an increase in cardiac disease and mortality. Here again, like with the vitamin A and smokers with lung cancer, we're seeing a paradoxical increased risk. Taking beta-carotene is therefore not recommended for those with heart disease or with significant risk factors for heart disease. Far from antioxidant vitamins being a panacea or even being very, very useful for health, they either don't work or, in some cases, they even increase risk.

What about longevity? Of course, we all want to live longer. We all want to live as long as we can. In addition to causing cellular damage, oxidative stress contributes to DNA damage, which is considered a very important part of aging. In addition to the evidence I've already mentioned, healthy centenarians—people who live over 100—tend to have higher levels of vitamin A and E than other people who are older, but not quite as old. That's some observational data that suggests that having higher amounts of antioxidants in your body is correlating with living longer. Great—who doesn't want to live past 100?

But, other kinds of observational studies are mixed. We're not seeing a clear example here. What we really need are good experimental studies. However, those are really hard to do. If you imagine, how long would a trial need to be to see if you can live 5, 10, or 20 years longer from taking antioxidants for the majority of your life. Those studies would have to be 30, 40 years long. They're incredibly impractical. You would have to monitor compliance with taking supplements or placebos for example throughout that whole period of time.

For purely practical reasons, we don't have really good, very long-term experimental studies. We have short-term experimental studies. We have some medium to long-term observational studies. There, the results are basically mixed and therefore, there's certainly no huge effect. We can't rule out that there may be a small beneficial effect, but certainly we would argue against taking high doses because of the potential increase heart risk.

What are the broad lessons from the antioxidant story? I think it's a really fascinating story and I actually lived through it in my career. I graduated medical school in 1991, right at the beginning of the antioxidant craze. Here we are, 19 years later. The story did not turn out the way I thought it was going to or the way the scientific community thought it was going to. Interestingly, the public perception that antioxidants are healthful and are a net good for health has persisted—despite the fact that the scientific evidence just did not turn out that way.

Let me pull back and explain what I think are some of the really broad lessons for understanding medical science and avoiding the trap of medical myths. One is that we cannot easily rely on animal studies. While animal studies are critical in the process of designing human trials, our animal models of the diseases that we're studying are not perfect. They do not always— in fact, they often don't—predict the outcome of later definitive human trials. Also, we cannot easily or simplistically extrapolate from the basic science research.

Always beware when someone's trying to sell you a product and justifying clinical claims based upon interesting things that happen in test tubes and Petri dishes. Basic science tells us what kind of directions we should go in with clinical research, but they can't be used to make clinical claims. More often than not we're going to be wrong when we guess what the outcome should be based upon just our basic understanding of basic biochemistry and biology.

Also, clinical data is often conflicting. There is very rarely a single definitive and be-all of all studies. There's different kinds of clinical data with different kinds of strengths and weaknesses. You need to put it all together and see what the consistent consensus of those studies is. If you focus on one study or one slice of information, you can tell pretty much whatever story you want to. It won't necessarily, however, be the correct story.

Also, another take-home message is that we shouldn't assume that vitamins are risk-free. Vitamins, like anything else, are an intervention. It's something we put into our bodies that will affect the biochemistry. Everything needs to be considered as risk versus benefit. We should not assume a zero risk for vitamins just because they're things that our body needs naturally. This is especially true when we get to "megadoses," where you're taking 10 to 100 times the dose that is the minimum necessary to avoid a deficiency or the kind of things you would find in most multivitamins.

I remember very distinctly in the late '90s and around the turn of the millennium when the initial clinical data was not really turning out positive for antioxidants. The proponents were telling me that it was because we're not studying it at a high enough dose. The reason why these results are negative is you need to push the dose up higher. But, of course, that was just an assumption used to explain away the negative evidence. It turns out that, when you push the dose higher, you start to get into toxicity. You actually started to get into an increased risk of heart disease and cancer in some situations.

Also, to some degree, we have to respect our own evolutionary history. Animals have had to deal with oxidative stress for literally hundreds of millions of years. That's powerful evolutionary selective pressure to work out as optimal a way as biochemically possible to deal with this. The story turned out to be much more complicated than we thought. Again, back in the early '90s, you might've thought that oxidative stress is bad; it causes damage. Antioxidants are good because they minimize damage—and that was pretty much the end of the story.

But, it turns out that oxygen free radicals and other free radicals in the body serve a useful purpose too. They also are signaling proteins. Essentially, the cell will detect the amount of free radicals that it has. That will trigger other downstream protective effects like producing what we call heat shock proteins which protect the cell from damage. If you take large amounts of antioxidants from the outside—what we call exogenously, basically pills

126

with antioxidants in them—that disrupts the balance that naturally evolved between oxidative stress, antioxidants, and all the other signaling and things that are happening in response to that.

When you disrupt that equilibrium, we shouldn't assume that we can easily predict what the effects are going to be. We need to be very cautious before we do things like taking megadoses to disrupt what the evolved equilibrium that has been there. We have been humbled. It turns out that taking large doses is not only not beneficial, it may, in fact, be harmful.

What's the bottom line of all this? There's no evidence to support the routine use of antioxidant supplements or so-called superfoods—like açaí, noni, blueberry, or pomegranate juice—that are loaded with antioxidants. There's simply no [evidence] that taking pills or taking these specific superfoods has any health benefit. The evidence keeps leading us back to a few common bits of wisdom that most of us know to be true. What your mother said was true. You should eat your fruits and vegetables—especially your vegetables—every day.

Also, another bottom line is do not take megadoses of vitamins. There is no evidence for benefit. There is increasing evidence and concern about possible toxicity and negative side effects to megadosing. However, it should be noted that foods that are rich in antioxidants, like fruits and vegetables, have proven health benefits. They're also a lot cheaper than most expensive tropical fruit juices or expensive supplements that somebody may be trying to get you to buy.

You probably cannot fix a poor diet with a pill. That's another take-home message. You can't sprinkle it on your steak. You have to eat a well-rounded diet with plenty of vegetables. To conclude this lecture, I would say, first of all, that there are things that we can do to extend our life. The news is not all bad and not all negative. Here are some things that have been proven over and over again and a recent review of the evidence shows that these things are all extremely important.

Eat your fruits and vegetables every day. Exercise regularly—20 to 30 minutes at least three days a week. Don't smoke and avoid excessive drinking—no more than two drinks per day for men and one per day for women. If you do these four things—things that, let's face it, we all know we should do—then you can prolong your life on average by 12 years. You will be 12 years younger biologically than somebody who doesn't exercise, smokes, drinks, and doesn't eat their fruits and vegetables.

We have the knowledge and the means to live a longer, healthier life by focusing on those things that we clearly know have a huge effect on health. We shouldn't get distracted by little things that may have a tiny effect, but the evidence really doesn't show anything definitive.

This lecture concludes the first series of lectures in this course. Starting with the next lecture, we're going to start discussing specific diseases and treatments.

The Common Cold
Lecture 9

The common cold has been with us, obviously, for a very long time. It was known to many of the ancient civilizations according to historical records. In fact, the Egyptians even had a hieroglyph for it.

The common cold is, well, common. We all get it, we want to prevent it, and we want to shorten its duration. Therefore, it's no surprise that myths about the common cold are just as common as the cold itself.

Probably the biggest myth is that cold weather causes the cold: You can't get a cold from being exposed to cold weather or being wet or being out in the rain. You need to get exposed to a cold virus in order to catch the cold. However, there's a separate question of whether being cold or wet makes you more susceptible to catching the virus if you are exposed to it. Largely speaking, the evidence for that is negative. But it's still slightly controversial.

It is generally recognized that the cold is more common in the winter. This is probably mostly due to the fact that in the winter months, kids are back at school. In essence, kids and their less than ideal hygiene make schools perfect breeding grounds for cold viruses. The viruses then spread to the rest of the population through multiple pathways.

What about vitamin C? You may have heard for years that taking vitamin C can either treat or prevent the common cold. But it's been researched for decades now and not shown much impact. Does it prevent you from catching the cold? The answer is very clearly no. What about decreasing the severity of the cold once you catch it? There, the answer is no as well. What about reducing the duration of the cold with vitamin C? Here the evidence is not as conclusively negative. It still is trending negative, but there is some weak evidence for a slight decrease in the duration of a cold by about a half a day—if you took vitamin C at the very beginning of the cold or were already taking it before you got the cold.

Herbal remedies have become popular for the common cold. A few years ago, Echinacea was the most common herbal remedy. But extensive clinical research in people with Echinacea clearly shows no benefit for either prevention or reduction of severity. What about other types of supplements—vitamins and minerals to help boost your immune system? One product in particular called Airborne is basically just a multivitamin. The notion of Airborne is that it will prevent you from catching a cold on an airplane. It turns out that there's really no theoretical basis for the notion that taking a short-term supplement will improve or increase your immune activity and make it more robust or better able to fight off a cold. There is no evidence to show that taking Airborne or any other multivitamin or supplements reduces either the risk of developing a cold or its severity or duration. It's also interesting to point out that Airborne has very high levels of vitamin A. If you take it as recommended, you actually will get what is considered to be an overdose of vitamin A.

You should also avoid exposure to people known to be sick, especially in the first 3 days of their illness when they have a fever.

Let's talk a bit about preventing the common cold. The most effective measure for preventing a cold is to avoid getting exposed to the virus in the first place. That means frequent hand washing with soap and water. That will clear the viruses or bacteria off your skin before you have a chance to infect yourself with them. You should also avoid exposure to people known to be sick, especially in the first 3 days of their illness when they have a fever. When you are sick or when you are around other people who are sick, avoid touching your eyes and nose. You also may avoid crowds when you are sick. That way, you'll do everyone a favor by not spreading the virus around. When you do have to sneeze or cough, do it into your elbow or a disposable tissue.

Dry air can also dry out the nasal mucosa making it more vulnerable to viruses. Using a humidifier—if the air in your environment or in your home is too dry—may actually reduce your risk of getting a cold in addition to making you more comfortable. Do not smoke: A history of smoking may increase the duration of a cold by an average of 3 days. Sleep deprivation generally runs down the body and makes you more susceptible to infections, including the cold. Finally, recent evidence suggests vitamin D may be helpful in preventing the cold.

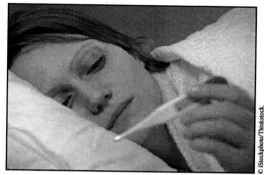

Contrary to myth, treating a fever with medicine will not interfere with your body's immune response.

What are the symptoms of the common cold? Most of the symptoms of the cold are actually not caused by the virus itself; they are caused by your immune system fighting off the infection. Should you treat the symptoms of a cold, or by doing so, are you suppressing your immune system's attempt to fight it off? If you reasonably treat your symptoms, your body can still fight off the infection without any problem.

Are there any over-the-counter medications you should keep on hand for when you get a cold? Certainly, you can have acetaminophen or nonsteroidal anti-inflammatory drugs, which means aspirin, ibuprofen, or naproxen. They will treat a fever, if you've got one. They are also analgesics, so they can reduce sinus pain, general discomfort, or the pain of a sore throat. What about cough suppressants? Interestingly, a lot of common products will mix together a cough suppressant and an expectorant. That makes no sense when you think about it. If you are having a somewhat productive cough and you want to get the phlegm up, then take an expectorant. But over-the-counter cough suppressants are really not very effective in suppressing a cough.

You can also adjust your behavior in order to reduce the symptoms of a cold. Drinking a lot of fluids will help prevent dehydration, including that of the mucous membranes. If you can eat, that will make you feel better as well. A good night's rest is also important in fighting off the infection, but there's no reason to stay bedridden. Finally, avoid smoking or exposure to smoke, as that can irritate and dry the membranes and extend the duration of symptoms in a cold. ■

Suggested Reading

Eccles and Weber, *Common Cold.*

Tyrrell and Fielder, *Cold Wars.*

Questions to Consider

1. Why is the common cold so common and yet so difficult to treat and prevent?

2. Is vitamin C, or any other food or supplement, effective in preventing the cold?

The Common Cold
Lecture 9—Transcript

The common cold is, well, common. We all get it, we want to prevent ourselves and others from getting it, we want to minimize spread, reduce our symptoms, and shorten the duration. Therefore, it's no surprise that myths about the common cold are just as common as the cold itself.

The common cold has been with us, obviously, for a very long time. It was known to many of the ancient civilizations according to historical records. In fact, the Egyptians even had a hieroglyph for it. But, of course, none of those ancient civilizations knew what caused the common cold. The term "common cold" itself dates back to the about the 16th century.

In the 18th century, Benjamin Franklin, after years of study, wrote, "People often catch cold from one another when shut up together in small close rooms, coaches, etc. and when sitting near and conversing so as to breathe in each other's transpiration." Ben got it just about right, but he wasn't the first one to recognize that colds and other diseases were spread by germs. In fact, the first notion of a contagion was first proposed in 1546 by Girolamo Fracastoro, who wrote that epidemics were probably caused by seed-like entities that spread from one person to another.

Then, in 1835, Agostino Bassi proposed the first clear germ hypothesis. He proposed that tiny living creatures caused the silkworm epidemic that was occurring at the time. This turned out to be true. The silkworm epidemic was caused by a fungus. The germ theory of disease didn't really gain acceptance, though, more widespread until about the second half of the 19th century.

Of course, it was thought that germs of one type or another must be causing the cold. The cold is an infection; it spreads from person to person as was known about for centuries. Although scientists first thought that the cold was caused by a bacteria—and there were efforts to develop vaccines against the common cold based upon this notion that it was a bacteria—that turned out not to be the case. In 1914, a biologist by the name of Walter Kruse, a professor in Leipzig, Germany, showed that viruses caused the common cold, not bacteria. However, his conclusions were not widely accepted until the mid-1920s, almost a decade later and not until they were replicated by other scientists.

What is the common cold, medically speaking? What is it specifically? We would refer to the common cold as a viral upper respiratory infection—an infection of the nasal passageways, oral passageways, and pharynx. We use other terms to refer to infections in other parts of the respiratory system. For example, pneumonia refers to an infection of the lungs themselves. Sinusitis is an infection of the sinuses. These are air-filled cavities in our skull, in the front, such as the maxillary sinuses in our cheeks. We also have some in the front of our skull above the eyes, for example. These are connected to the nasal passageways. You can get both acute, or short-term, and chronic, or long-term, sinus infections.

We also use the term "bronchitis" to refer to inflammation or infection of the airways that connect to the lungs, the bronchioles. Of course, these are not mutually exclusive. You can get an upper respiratory infection that then leads to a sinusitis or may lead to a bronchitis. If you ever had a really bad cough after a cold that seemed to be constricting your airways and making it difficult to breathe, you probably had a secondary bronchitis following a cold.

There are hundreds of separate viruses which cause the common cold. The most common type of virus is the rhinovirus. It's responsible for about 30 to 50 percent of colds. Coronaviruses are responsible for 10 to 15 percent and influenza viruses are responsible for 5 to 15 percent. The rest are caused by an assortment of other viruses including human parainfluenza, human respiratory syncytial virus, adenoviruses, enteroviruses, and metapneumoviruses.

The reason why you can get the cold multiple times—why you aren't immune for life once you've caught the cold once—is that, each time you get the cold, you're being infected with a new type of virus. It may be a different species, a different genus of a virus, or it may just be a different strain of a virus that you've encountered previously.

It is generally recognized that the cold is more common in the winter. Maybe that has something to do with the origins of the name of the common cold. This is partly due, if not mostly due, to the fact that in the winter months kids are back at school. People are also generally spending more time indoors, in close quarters, as Benjamin Franklin noted.

Parents will recognize the fact that, when their kids start coming back from either daycare or school, they often bring home viral infections. That tends to spread throughout the family who then may bring it to work. In essence, kids getting together with maybe less than ideal hygiene and spreading viruses around becomes a perfect breeding ground for these cold viruses. Then that spreads to the rest of the population through multiple pathways. That in and of itself is probably enough to explain why colds are so much more common in the winter months.

There is some evidence, however, that certain cold viruses may be actually adapted to the cold weather. They surround themselves in a protein coat that is more resistant to cold. They may actually have adapted to that. But, we can get colds in the summer. There are summer viruses that we're more likely to get in the warmer months. If you come down with a cold in July in the northern hemisphere, in the middle of the summer, that's more likely to be an enterovirus. If you get a cold in the winter, it's more likely to be a rhinovirus.

How does the cold spread? Colds spread largely through direct contact. Somebody who is infected and has the virus on their skin passes it on to someone else who then gets infected with it themselves. This often occurs from touching your mouth, nose, or even just your eyes. Rubbing the eyes is a very common source of infection. However, it is a myth that you can only get the cold through direct contact. In fact, you can get exposed to the virus and get infected through indirect contact. That means touching something that someone else who was infected touched. The technical term for that is a fomite. A fomite is anything on which a bacteria or virus can survive long enough to be spread indirectly from one person to the next.

You can also get exposed to the virus in water droplets in the air, which can be expelled by coughing or sneezing. You may catch a cold simply by being exposed to the virus from someone who sneezed maybe even across the room from where you are. That is, of course, why there is always the strong recommendation to sneeze or cough into a tissue, handkerchief, or into your elbow if nothing else is available to prevent that spread.

There are many myths, as I said, surrounding the cold. Probably the biggest one, however, is that cold weather causes the cold itself. How many times have you told someone not to go out—to be careful and bundle up before going out in the cold or in the rain—otherwise you may catch your cold. However, the weather itself does not cause a cold. You can't get a cold from being exposed to cold weather or being wet or being out in the rain. You need to get exposed to a cold virus in order to catch the cold.

However, there's a separate question of whether or not being cold, wet, or damp makes you more susceptible to catching the virus if you are exposed to it. Largely speaking, the evidence for that is negative. Being cold doesn't even increase your susceptibility. But, it's still, I would say, slightly controversial. That question has not been put fully to bed yet.

What about vitamin C? You may have heard for years—this has been a very common belief—that taking vitamin C can either treat or prevent the common cold. This was popularized by Linus Pauling and others. It has become so widespread in the culture that most people I speak to take it for granted that vitamin C can prevent or reduce the symptoms of a cold. But, it's been researched for decades now and we've broken it down into every sub-question that there is.

Does it prevent you from catching the cold itself? The answer there is very clearly no. The research shows that taking regular doses of vitamin C does not prevent you from catching the cold. Reviews of dozens of studies with thousands of individual patients show no benefit. What about decreasing the severity of the cold once you catch it—are the symptoms less severe because your body is better able to fight off the infection? There, the answer is no as well. There's no decrease in the severity of the symptoms of a cold.

What about reducing the duration of the cold, might you fight it off a little bit quicker if you take vitamin C? Here the evidence is not as conclusively negative. It still is trending negative. However, there is some weak evidence for a slight decrease in the duration of a cold by an order of magnitude of about a half a day, not much more than that—if you took vitamin C at the very beginning of the cold or were already taking it before you got the cold. There is a slight, if any, benefit and only a slight advantage to the duration of a cold. This is still controversial from vitamin C. But, there's no benefit to either the severity of the cold or the chances of catching it in the first place.

Herbal remedies have become popular for the common cold. A few years ago, echinacea was the most common herbal remedy. It was marketed for treatment of the common cold—to prevent infection, and reduce severity and duration. I'm going to talk about echinacea in more detail in my lecture on herbalism. At this point in time, I will say that after extensive research—clinical research in people with Echinacea—the evidence clearly shows no benefit for either prevention or reduction of severity from taking echinacea.

What about other types of supplements—not herbal remedies, but vitamins and minerals, nutrients to help boost your immune system and make you better able to fend off or fight off the cold or other viruses. One product in particular called Airborne, which is marketed as being developed by a school teacher, is really basically just a multivitamin. The notion of Airborne is that you take it when you're going to be on a plane. You're going to be in close quarters and exposed to a lot of people who are maybe spreading around viruses. It will prevent you from catching a cold if you're about to take that airplane trip.

It turns out that there's really no theoretical basis for the notion that taking a short-term supplement will improve or increase your immune activity and make it more robust or better able to fight off a cold. There is no evidence to show that taking Airborne or any other multivitamin or supplements reduces either the risk of developing a cold or its severity or duration. It's also interesting to point out that specifically, Airborne has very high levels of vitamin A. If you take it as recommended, you actually will get what is considered to be an overdose of vitamin A.

One interesting intervention that has become recently popular is called neti pots. This is essentially a little pot. It kind of looks like a teapot, but it has an elongated spout that you fill with warm water or salt water, and then irrigate out your sinuses. You pour the liquid into your nasal passageway. It then goes into the nasal sinuses and out the other side. It is meant to flush out the mucous and any bacteria or viruses.

Again, we need to break down to very specific claims. Does it prevent infections when used on a regular basis? Is it helpful when you get a cold or sinusitis? Regular use actually may increase your risk of sinus infections by cleaning out too much of the mucous, which is there for a purpose. It's there as part of the immune system. Also, you may be reducing the normal bacteria which inhabit the mucous membranes and are there to prevent infection from other bacteria or from viruses. Thus, routine irrigation of the sinuses is not a good idea. It's not helpful as many people claim and in fact, might increase the risk of sinus infections.

However, short-term use of a neti pot—or any method of nasal passageway irrigation, it doesn't have to specifically be a neti pot—sinus irrigation has been shown to decrease the duration of a sinus infection. There, the concept actually makes sense. If you have bacteria especially clogging up your sinuses, the most important thing to relieving that infection is just flushing it out, clearing out the bacteria that's getting stuck in there.

A healthy immune system should be able to fight off viruses and bacteria, but it can't do that if it's too clogged up and can't get access to the bacteria. Therefore, flushing it out does make sense. For an acute sinus infection, short-term use makes sense although there's nothing special about the neti pot. You can use a saline nasal spray, for example, and that will be just as effective. Routine preventive use is not helpful and may be a bad idea.

There's a homeopathic treatment for the common cold called oscillococcinum. I'm going to give a complete lecture on homeopathic remedies in detail, so I'm not going to go into background about homeopathy itself. But, I will say that oscillococcinum has been studied as a specific homeopathic treatment for the common cold and it has shown no benefit whatsoever. Regardless of the theory, the evidence is negative. Interestingly, oscillococcinum itself is made from duck liver. It has a fairly interesting if dubious theory behind it. It was based upon the mistaken microscopic studies that identified what was thought to be an oscillating bacteria—but it turns out that that was just an illusion. There was no oscillating bacteria there. It was an optical illusion of the microscope itself. Therefore, it doesn't really even exist, the oscillococcinum itself, that's supposed to be in the homeopathic remedies.

Let's talk a bit about preventing the common cold. Obviously, the best way to treat a cold is to just never to get it in the first place. That means frequent hand washing. You don't have to use any special antibiotic soap or anything; you just need to wash your hands with plain soap and water. That will clear the viruses or bacteria off your skin before you have a chance to infect yourself with it.

You should also avoid exposure to people known to be sick, especially in the first three days of their illness when they have a fever. That's the time when they will be shedding the most amount of virus. When you are sick or when you are around other people who are sick, avoid touching your eyes and nose. That is the most common route of infection. You also may decide to just avoid crowds when you yourself are sick. That way, you'll do everyone a favor by not spreading the virus around. Perhaps you shouldn't feel obligated to go into work when you're shedding virus with a cold. They might appreciate that.

When you do have to sneeze or cough, sneeze into your elbow or disposable tissue. Avoid personal contact. Especially wash your hands frequently when you yourself are sick. You will avoid spreading the virus around and onto other objects which then become fomites—something that will then transfer the virus onto other people. Clean counters and other surfaces that are frequented by people, especially if you have kids in the house or if there are sick people around. Kids' toys are often covered with viruses. Therefore, keep cleaning them. Keeping them sanitary will help when there are sick family members around.

Dry air can also dry out the nasal mucosa making it more vulnerable to viruses. Using a humidifier—if the air in your environment or in your home is too dry—may actually reduce your risk of getting a cold in addition to making you more comfortable. Incidentally, this may be yet another reason why getting the cold is more common in the winter. In the winter, when it's cold and you're using heat to heat the air in your home, that often will dry out the air in your home. This dries out your mucous membranes which reduces your resistance to infection. Use a humidifier if you have dry air in your home.

In addition to dry air and low humidity, other risk factors include smoking. A history of smoking may increase the duration of a cold by an average of three days. This is yet another reason why you shouldn't smoke—as if you need me to tell you that. Sleep deprivation generally runs down the body and makes you more susceptible to infections including the cold. Interestingly, recent evidence suggests vitamin D may be helpful in preventing the cold. This is a bit ironic in that there has been so much obsession with vitamin C. It turns out that vitamin C doesn't prevent the common cold, but perhaps another vitamin, vitamin D, may. At this point, we have just preliminary research and more research is needed. But, if your vitamin D levels are low, it certainly makes sense to supplement them.

What are the symptoms of the common cold? Most of the symptoms of the cold are actually not caused by the virus itself. It's caused by your immune system fighting off the infection. The immune system is what causes the inflammation. There are inflammatory compounds that are released by your immune system like histamine, prostaglandins, kinins, and interleukins. These cause the blood vessels to expand which is what causes the congestion. It causes the mucosa, the membranes to swell up, which also contributes to congestion. It also irritates the mucosa, activating the sneeze and cough reflexes. All of those things are caused by your immune system itself.

This actually brings up an interesting question then. Should we really go out of our way to treat those symptoms? Should we treat the symptoms of a cold or by doing so, are you just suppressing your immune system's attempt to fight it off? The immune system is probably overreacting a little bit when it's fighting off a cold and causing more symptoms than are strictly necessary in order to fight off the cold. If you reasonably treat your symptoms, your body can still fight off the infection without any problem at all. Don't worry about treating those symptoms. If you have a fever and it's making you uncomfortable, treat it. You don't have to be coughing and sneezing to get rid of the virus. You certainly don't need swollen membranes and congestion in order to fight off an infection. In fact, 25 percent of upper respiratory viral infections are asymptomatic. In other words, you can get a cold, an upper respiratory infection, and a quarter of the time, your immune system will fight it off without causing any symptoms whatsoever.

What about a fever? I mentioned fever as one of the symptom of a cold. There actually has been a little bit of a controversy over what the optimal way to treat a fever with a cold is. It is part of the body's immune response to the virus. But, do you need the fever to fight the cold? The answer to that is no. You can fight off the cold fine even you completely mask the fever with antipyretics, or medications which reduce fever.

Another little mini-myth here is that normal body temperature is 98.6 degrees. This is actually a very arbitrary figure. It was just what someone measured as the body temperature at one point in time. Subsequent evidence and research shows that there's actually quite a broad range of what is normal body temperature. Medical science, at this point in time, doesn't consider someone as having a fever unless their temperature goes greater than 100 degrees Fahrenheit.

Do fevers cause brain damage? Do we need to worry about fevers because they're going to heat up and damage the brain? Actually, the answer to that is mostly no. The kind of fevers that you are very likely to encounter, even what we would consider a high fever—up 104 and 105, the kind of fever that would make a parent somewhat nervous—is not going to cause brain damage. Only extremely high body temperatures like 107 to 108, which is not going to result from a common cold, can actually be at risk of causing brain damage.

What about the old adage of "feeding a cold and starving a fever?" That was sort of based on the notion that temperature comes from food, therefore if you take food, that's going to create more body heat and force the fever. It turns out that that simply isn't true. Your body is regulating its temperature neurologically and hormonally, aside from the food that you eat. Thus, short-term feeding a cold or starving a fever has no health benefit. That really is just an old wives' tale.

Also, what about taking an ice bath? Some people still feel that if someone has a high fever, you can make them feel comfortable by giving them an ice bath to quickly cool them down. But, that is not recommended. It's actually not healthy to chill the body to that degree. It's absolutely not necessary in treating a normal fever that would occur with a cold. Therefore, don't use ice baths.

Are there any over-the-counter medications you should keep on hand to treat you or your family members when you get a cold? Certainly, you can have acetaminophen or what are called non-steroidal anti-inflammatory drugs. We call them NSAIDs for short. That's aspirin, ibuprofen, or naproxen. Those are the generic names for common NSAIDs that you can get over-the-counter. One of the effects they have is an antipyretic effect. It will treat the fever. That will absolutely make people feel more comfortable. Again, you shouldn't worry about doing that. It also is an analgesic. That means it's a pain killer. If you're having sinus pain, are just generally feeling uncomfortable, or if your throat is sore and raw, the acetaminophen or NSAIDs will help reduce some of that pain. But, as I said, a lot of the pain, discomfort, and symptoms of a cold are caused by inflammation.

Acetaminophen is not an anti-inflammatory. Thus, if you have a lot of inflammatory symptoms, that's not going to be the optimal over-the-counter medication to take. You should take an NSAID. You should take an aspirin, ibuprofen, or naproxen. Although, I'll point out, do not give aspirin to young children. It has been linked with a rare but serious side effect called Rye's syndrome. For adults and children, you can take non-aspirin NSAIDs like ibuprofen. They're the best single thing to have on hand for treating most of the symptoms of a common cold and making you feel much more comfortable.

What about cough suppressants? Coughs can be a very annoying thing to have to suffer through with a bad cold, especially if you get a bronchitis. Interestingly, a lot of common products will mix together a cough suppressant and an expectorant. That makes no sense when you think about it. You shouldn't be trying to get up your phlegm with an expectorant, but then suppress the cough that's going to get rid of it at the same time. Generally, we don't recommend taking products that have a lot of different effects mixed together. If you are having a somewhat productive cough and you want to get the phlegm up, then take an expectorant. If your cough is dry and annoying, then you would want to take a pure cough suppressant. However, the over-the-counter cough suppressants are really not very effective in suppressing a cough. Recent studies in children essentially were unable to document any benefit to cough suppressant in children. They're of very limited utility.

You can also adjust your behaviors in order to reduce the symptoms of a cold. Drinking a lot of fluids is very helpful. It will help prevent dehydration. It will help prevent drying out the mucous membranes. But, you don't need to overdo it. You don't need to force fluids. Just don't let yourself get dehydrated. If you can eat, eat. That will make you feel better as well. You don't want to go hungry during an illness or cold.

Rest if necessary. But, again, you don't need to force rest. You just don't want to be sleep deprived. Another reason to treat the symptoms of a cold is so that you can feel more comfortable and get a good night's rest, which is important to fighting off the infection. But, undergo normal activity—perhaps nothing strenuous if you're really feeling under the weather. But, there's no reason to stay in bed or to be bedridden. Avoid smoking or exposure to smoke as that can irritate and dry the membranes—and extends the duration of symptoms in a cold.

What about chicken soup? Is it really beneficial to drink chicken soup during a cold? Any hot liquid will help moisten the mucous membranes, reduce a sore throat, help hydration—like any liquid—and may also loosen up the mucous in your sinuses and help expel it. But, there's nothing special about chicken soup itself. There is some evidence that there may be some anti-inflammatories in vegetables in hot soup. But, you could also get that—and at a much more optimal effect and dose—just by taking an aspirin-like drug.

I'd also like to distinguish between the cold and the flu. They have similar symptoms. The flu, however, is much more severe. It's of longer duration. It can last up to several weeks whereas a cold usually is less than a week in duration. Specifically, the flu is caused by influenza viruses, so you have to have an influenza virus in order to have the flu. Prevention and treatment is essentially the same for the common cold with the exception that the flu has vaccines that will prevent specifically influenza viruses.

There are seasonal flu vaccines. Occasionally, for flu epidemics, if we can get to them quick enough, we might be able to make a vaccine specific to a flu epidemic. But, for most people, getting a seasonal flu vaccine is a good idea to reduce your risk of developing the flu—which, as I said, is a really, really bad cold.

In conclusion, there are many myths surrounding the common cold. I think I've put most if not all of them to bed with this talk. Everyone, at some point, is likely to need this information either for you or for a loved one—or just to avoid getting a cold around the office or out in public. It is best to be armed with accurate information. There are a lot of things that you can do to reduce your risks and symptoms. It's also nice to know that, with correct information, you can avoid wasting your time and resources doing things that are not helpful—and maybe even avoiding a few things which might make the situation worse.

Vaccination Benefits—How Well Vaccines Work
Lecture 10

In 1796, British physician Edward Jenner coined the term "vaccination," derived from the Latin word *vacca* for cow. This is because he was using the cowpox vaccine in order to prevent smallpox.

Myths, misconceptions, and resistance to vaccines are as old as the modern vaccine program itself. In fact, myths and misinformation seem to be increasing today in our society. This is threatening the effectiveness of the vaccine program as a public health measure. It's also making it difficult for individuals to make informed decisions for themselves and their families about vaccines. We explore how vaccines work and how effective they are.

Vaccines work by provoking a targeted immune response. A primary immune response—a response to something that your immune system is encountering for the first time—peaks at about 5 to 10 days. That's a long time for a virus or bacteria to be reproducing and spreading throughout your body. With a subsequent exposure, your immune system's response will peak in only 1 to 3 days. That means your body can fight off that infection much earlier and much more robustly.

There are different kinds of vaccines; the technology has actually advanced quite a bit in the last 100 years or so. The most primitive type of vaccines, called inoculations, utilized living viruses or bacteria and were essentially just a controlled infection. There was always the risk that the inoculation could cause a serious infection.

The next step was the development of the attenuated virus or bacteria. An attenuated vaccine uses the exact species or strain of virus that you're trying to inoculate against, but the virus is attenuated. The process of attenuation essentially is to breed it in another species so that it will be less virulent in humans. Your body will have time to fight it off, but you will develop immunity. The disadvantage to the attenuated virus vaccine is that it may back mutate.

The next type of vaccine is the inactivated vaccine. Here you take a virus or bacteria and essentially kill it. You inactivate it so that it cannot reproduce, but it still has all the proteins on the outside. There is a small risk of infection with an inactivated vaccine—but only if the virus is improperly inactivated. With proper inactivation, there is zero risk of infection. Inactivated vaccines may not be quite as effective as a live vaccine. For this reason, they are more likely to require booster shots.

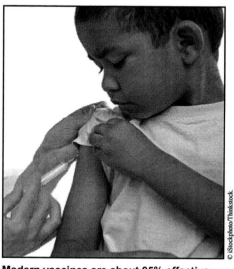

Then there are subunit vaccines. These contain not even an entire virus—just part of the protein shell, for example. Here, there is no risk of infection. Conjugate vaccines combine a toxin or an immunogenic protein to the coat, because certain coats

Modern vaccines are about 95% effective.

are not very immunogenic. But, if you couple it with something else—a toxin or something that's really good at stimulating the immune system—the immune system will be activated against it.

Toxoid vaccines are vaccines not against the organism of a virus or bacteria, but against a toxin that the virus produces. Toxoid vaccines do not prevent an infection, but the antibodies will bind and inactivate the toxin as it's being released. Therefore, it will prevent the negative health consequences of the infection while allowing the infection to run its normal course.

Do vaccines work? There are still today people who question whether vaccines work. But the evidence is extremely clear: Vaccines are about 95% effective. This means that 95% of people who are vaccinated with a vaccination schedule—which may involve boosters—will develop a functional immunity to the substance against which they're being vaccinated. Vaccines are less effective in elderly and immunocompromised people. That is a serious concern because those are often the very people that we need to protect the most.

This leads us to the concept of herd immunity. There are estimates that when about 90% or more of any population—people who are likely to be exposed to each other—are vaccinated against an infection, you achieve herd immunity. That infection cannot easily spread from person to person. Anyone who is harboring the virus or bacteria is very unlikely to encounter somebody else who isn't immune. Therefore, they'll be able to fight it off before they spread it around. This prevents outbreaks and also prevents infections from being endemic. ■

Suggested Reading

Allen, *Vaccine.*

Henderson, *Smallpox.*

Questions to Consider

1. How do vaccines work?

2. How much evidence is there for the safety and effectiveness of vaccines?

Vaccination Benefits—How Well Vaccines Work
Lecture 10—Transcript

Myths, misconceptions, and resistance to vaccines are as old as the modern vaccine program itself. In fact, myths and misinformation seem to be increasing, if anything, in our society. This is threatening the effectiveness of the vaccine program as a public health measure. It's also making it difficult for individuals to make informed decisions for themselves and their families about vaccines.

The history of vaccines goes back a long way. The notion that, once you're infected with a disease, you have a reduced chance of getting infected with it again—or you may never catch it again, you may be immune—goes back in the historical record for at least 1500 years or so in China and India. It was recognized that those individuals who came down with smallpox and survived would not get the smallpox infection again. In the late 1700s, several people were experimenting with this notion by using cowpox—a benign, but closely related infection—to inoculate people against smallpox.

In 1796, British physician Edward Jenner coined the term "vaccination," derived from the Latin word *vacca* for cow. This is because he was using the cowpox vaccine in order to prevent smallpox. Research into vaccines then was greatly enhanced by the work of Louis Pasteur, who pioneered the field of microbiology. In this lecture, I'm going to be talking mainly about the question of whether vaccines work and the misinformation or questions about whether or not they even work. In the next lecture on vaccines, I'm going to talk about mainly the safety concerns. Do vaccines cause harm?

First, here is a little background on how vaccines work. Vaccines work by essentially provoking a targeted immune response. The immune system will react to any foreign substance that it encounters. However, it takes time to build up the response. It doesn't have an immediate maximal response. In addition, the immune response is adaptive. It actually remembers what it's been exposed to in the past and it can mount a better response the next time around. The technical term for this is the anamnestic response. It means the immune system remembers and adapts to what it has been exposed to previously.

A primary immune response—that's what we call a response to something that your immune system is encountering for the first time—peaks at about five to ten days. That's a long time for a virus or bacteria to be reproducing and spreading throughout your body. A subsequent immune response—the second, third, or fourth time you are being exposed to a germ, virus, or bacteria—your immune system's response will peak in only one to three days. That's a lot faster. That means it can fight off that infection much, much earlier and much more robustly.

Also, the number of antibodies that your body produces is greater. They persist in your body for a longer period of time. Antibodies are one of the primary components of the immune system. They are proteins that will bind to foreign substances and target the other components of your immune system against those invaders. Antibodies are essential.

This anamnestic—or enhanced secondary or subsequent—response to infections is primarily caused by B-memory cells and T4-memory cells. The B cells are the cells in the immune system that make those antibodies. Once you have an infection, the B cells that make antibodies which react to the invading substance or organism will reproduce themselves. Those B cells that are more finely tuned to that invasion will reproduce further because the stimulation actually causes those B cells to reproduce. Eventually, you have that response, that optimal response, with B cells finely targeted against the invader producing lots of antibodies.

Once the infection goes away, most of those B cells go away, too—except for the B memory cells. They hang around. They stay in your body for months, years, or decades. They are able to produce antibodies that are finely targeted against an invading organism as soon as it's encountered. There are also the T cells. The T cells don't make antibodies. They respond to the antibodies binding to a foreign cell or a foreign substance. They will do things like attack it and eat it up. They are another important component of the immune system. They also can remember things that they've encountered previously.

The result of this anamnestic or secondary response to an infection is the ability to fight it off. Usually, if you have a robust memory for that organism, it can fight it off even before it can cause symptoms—and certainly before it can cause a sustained infection that gets out of control. Essentially, you will fight off the infection within a few days—without having to mount a huge inflammatory response—by making targeted antibodies and targeting the immune system very efficiently at that infection. Therefore, you will often have what's called a subclinical infection. Once you're immune to an infection, you'll still get exposed to it, but you'll fight it off so quickly, you won't even know it.

There are different kinds of vaccine that I'm going to be talking about. The technology has actually advanced quite a bit in the last hundred years or so. Let's talk about the most primitive or the earliest type of vaccines. These utilize living viruses or bacteria. They essentially are just a controlled infection. This is called inoculation. It's also called variolation or insufflation. The oldest disease that this was used against was smallpox.

In fact, smallpox was deliberately given to people in India. This is in the historical record as early as 1000 B.C.E. What they would do is they would try to give somebody a mild smallpox infection by giving them a small amount of exposure. That would give them an infection that they could survive. It would create immunity so that they would not get a severe smallpox infection later on. There are also records of this as early as the 17th century in Persia, Africa, and Europe. Thus, the idea spread to many, many cultures.

Three to five percent of people who were treated in this way actually went on to die from smallpox. Therefore, it wasn't a great technology, but it still accomplished the basic goal of preventing a much greater chance of dying from a full smallpox infection. This technology was then improved with the advent of the cowpox vaccine. What you're doing here is, instead of giving the actual virus or bacteria that causes the infection you're trying to prevent, you get a closely related virus or bacteria. This way, when your body is fighting off and develops an immunity to the cowpox, it'll be able to mount a more robust response to the closely related smallpox virus. It's not the same thing as full immunity, but if it gives your body any advantage of fighting off that virus more quickly, it reduces the risk of dying from the smallpox.

Protection, however, was poor. It was not that robust because the match wasn't identical. Your immune system had a leg-up, but it didn't have memory B cells that were already finely tuned to the very specific virus. It was better than nothing, but not great. There was always, of course, the risk that the inoculation itself can cause a serious infection. You were giving somebody an active infection and that could get more serious than was intended.

One advantage then, the next step, was the development of the attenuated virus or bacteria. An attenuated vaccine uses the exact species or strain of virus that you're trying to inoculate against, however it attenuates it. The process of attenuation essentially is to breed it in another species. If you breed the polio virus, for example, in a pig or chicken for a number of generations, the virus will actually adapt to that other species. Therefore, it will be less adapted to humans. It will be less virulent, less deadly in humans. That attenuated strain will cause a much less severe infection. Therefore, your body will have time to fight it off, preventing the consequences of the infection. At the same time, it's developing immunity because it is the same virus even though it's this attenuated strain.

One of the first attenuated virus vaccines was the Sabin polio vaccine. Other attenuated virus vaccines, some of which are still in use, are the measles, mumps, and rubella vaccine. Often those things are combined into what we call the MMR vaccine. Chicken pox and yellow fever are also other viral attenuated vaccines. Attenuated bacterial vaccines include typhoid and tuberculosis.

The disadvantage to the attenuated virus vaccine is that it may back mutate. You're culturing it in either a tissue culture or another animal. You're waiting for enough mutations to occur and be selected so that it will be adapted to something other than a human infection. But, when you then have the infection back in a human, it can adapt back to the human. You may just be unlucky and get a back mutation, as they're called. Suddenly, that attenuated polio virus may mutate into a virulent polio virus. That can cause a real serious infection.

In fact, that was the main drawback to the Sabin vaccine. About one in a million people who were vaccinated with that vaccine against polio actually got polio from the vaccine. That still is much less than the risk of getting it while there was endemic polio in the population. It was still a huge advantage, but again, not perfect. This is also the reason why we do not give attenuated vaccines to people who are immunocompromised. This is because it is a live virus. It may cause an infection and it may persist long enough to have a higher chance of back mutating.

The next type of vaccine I'm going to discuss is the inactivated vaccine. Here you take a virus or bacteria and essentially kill it. You inactivate so that it cannot reproduce. It still has all of the proteins on the outside. It's those proteins that your immune system is reacting to. One example of this is the Salk polio vaccine, which is different than the Sabin polio vaccine. This is inactivated and this is the reason why the Salk vaccine largely replaced the Sabin vaccine. Most flu vaccines are also inactivated though there are also attenuated flu vaccines. Examples of inactivated bacterial vaccines include typhoid, cholera, plague, and pertussis.

There is a small risk of infection with an inactivated vaccine—but only if the virus or bacteria is improperly inactivated. Essentially, the manufacturing process was suboptimal. But, with proper inactivation, there is zero risk of infection. There's another disadvantage in that the inactivated vaccines may not be quite as effective as a live vaccine. The reason for that is that an active infection causes a longer duration of exposure of the virus or bacteria to the immune system. Therefore, it causes a greater production of B cells and therefore, more memory B cells. For this reason—because the duration of exposure is shorter with inactivated vaccines—they are more likely to require booster shots. You may need a second or third vaccine in order to get up to full immunity whereas the live virus or bacteria vaccines usually don't require a booster.

Next there are subunit vaccines. This is like the hepatitis B vaccine and the human papilloma virus vaccine. These contain not even an entire virus— just part of the protein shell, for example. Here, there is no risk of infection. This is not an intact virus that's being killed or reactivated. It's just a piece of it. Often, these are made using recombinant genetic technology. We, for example, may put a gene from a virus into a yeast. We then purify that viral protein from the yeast. A full living virus is actually not part of the process at any point.

Conjugate vaccines combine a toxin or an immunogenic protein to the coat, like the polysaccharide coat of a bacteria. An example of this is the haemophilus influenza type B vaccine, often abbreviated as the HiB vaccine. The reason why we need to do this with certain types of bacteria is that the polysaccharide outer coat of the human influenza type B bacteria is not very immunogenic. This means that it does not stimulate the immune system very much. Therefore, it won't have much of an immune response. But, if you couple it with something else—a toxin or something that's really good at stimulating the immune system—the immune system will be activated against that immunogenic protein. It will also be activated against the polysaccharide coat, so that will develop the immunity against the bacteria.

Toxoid vaccines, such as tetanus and diphtheria, are vaccines against, not the organism of a virus or bacteria, but a toxin that the bacteria produces. This, therefore, would not prevent an infection. However, the antibodies will bind and inactivate the toxin as it's being released. Therefore, it will prevent the negative health consequences or the effects of the infection while allowing the infection itself to run its normal course.

I want to say a word about the herpes zoster vaccine. It's actually a little bit of an interesting story. Herpes zoster is an attenuated virus vaccine. It's recommended for those who are 60 years and older. The reason for this is to prevent herpes zoster, also known as shingles. This is the same virus, varicella zoster, that causes chicken pox. When you get the chicken pox, it causes an acute infection. When the infection runs its course, your immune system has fought off the virus, and the symptoms go away, the virus is not completely eradicated from your body. It goes dormant and it will live in, usually, the parts of your nervous system. It will go into what we call the dorsal root ganglia, the cells that give rise to your sensory neurons. It will live there but in a dormant state that's not activating the immune system. It's hiding from your immune system.

If you've had chicken pox and you have dormant varicella zoster in your cells, at any point subsequently in your life, those viruses can become reactivated. It's more likely to occur when your immune system is compromised for some reason. This could be because you're taking medications, you're having a chronic illness, or your body is generally just run-down and your resistances are low. But, it can also just happen in a completely healthy person without any problems.

When the virus becomes reactivated, it comes out into the nerves causing nerve pain. It can be extremely painful. Also, the virus can work its way all the way to the skin where it causes a rash—what we call a vesicular rash with little pimple-like lesions on the skin. That's often how people first know that they have herpes zoster.

Previously, older adults who survived chicken pox when they were children would have their immunity boosted by exposure to children who had the chicken pox. When you were 40 or 50, you may have had a child with chicken pox. You had partial immunity, so you may have had a subclinical infection to the chicken pox. This would boost your immune system to the chicken pox. Therefore, your immunity would be able to keep the zoster at bay and reduce your chance of getting the shingles.

However, today we inoculate children routinely against chicken pox, so children are not getting as much chicken pox anymore. Therefore, adults are not getting their immunity boosted by being exposed to children with chicken pox. Therefore, their immunity is slowly waning over time so that, by the time they get to 60 or older, their immunity has been reduced. Therefore, they need a booster shot of the attenuated virus vaccine in order to prevent or reduce their risk of getting shingles.

There is more in vaccines than just the viruses, bacteria, or the components of that. Those are what we call the antigens. The antigens are the things that activate your immune system. It's what your immune system is binding to. But, you have to put other things in vaccines in order to make them work as well. One type of thing that is put into vaccine is called an adjuvant. An adjuvant is anything designed to enhance the immune system's response to the antigen. They either stimulate the immune system, making it more active, or they might increase or prolong the exposure of the antigen to your immune system.

The advantage of using adjuvants is that it allows for a lower dose of antigen itself. You can give less virus, bacteria, or components. This may make the live vaccines a bit safer, but also, it enables manufacturers to have antigen go a lot farther. This is critical for certain types of vaccines like a seasonal flu vaccine where companies only have a few months to make the vaccine. This is because they're constantly trying to keep up with the strains that are out there. Therefore, having antigens go a lot farther will enable them to make more vaccines. Some example of adjuvants include aluminum salts, squalene, oils, and virosomes.

Another constituent of vaccines is preservatives. We have to both preserve the components of the vaccine itself and prevent contamination. Antibiotics are often used to prevent bacteria from growing in the vaccines themselves. There's also agents that are bacteriostatic. They prevent bacteria from growing.

One component is thimerosal, which is a mercury-based preservative that's been used for decades—although it was removed from most vaccines in recent years. Formaldehyde is also used to kill viruses and bacteria. But, they can only be used in toxoid or inactivated vaccines. Therefore, you can't use either thimerosal or formaldehyde in a live attenuated virus vaccines or bacterial vaccine because it would kill the virus or bacteria, rendering it inert.

There are also stabilizers. They prevent the degradation of the proteins in the vaccine and extend the shelf life of vaccines. Common stabilizers include monosodium glutamate or MSG, and glycine, which is a protein stabilizer. Some people may have concerns about MSG if you have an MSG sensitivity or allergy. But, the doses of MSG in the vaccines are completely safe and do not cause any demonstrated reaction.

Other constituents include things that the virus or the bacteria needed to be grown in. Many viruses are cultured in egg proteins. Some of those chicken egg proteins may get into the vaccine, such as some flu vaccines. If you have an allergy to egg proteins, you may get an allergic reaction to live virus vaccines that have been cultured in chicken egg. You do have to tell your doctor about that.

There is an interesting myth spreading around that some vaccines contain cells or tissue from aborted fetuses. But, this is not true. There is a kernel of truth to it, which is often then misinterpreted. The truth is that some live virus or bacteria vaccines are cultured in human cells that are what we call an immortal cell line. Forty or more years ago, these cell lines were originally started. They were originally derived from aborted fetuses, but those cells have been growing essentially in Petri dishes for the last 40 years. None of those cells get into the vaccine itself. It's just that the virus was cultured in those cells.

Let's get to the core question now. Do vaccines work? There's still to this day—all this time, after vaccines have been developed and with the advances in technology that have been made—those that question whether or not vaccines even work. But, the evidence is extremely clear. Vaccines are about 95 percent effective. This means that 95 percent of people who are vaccinated with a vaccination schedule—which, again, may involve boosters that have been shown to be effective—will develop a functional immunity to the substance against which they're being vaccinated. Ninety-five percent effectiveness—that's pretty good.

They're less effective in the elderly and they are less effective in the immunocompromised. That is a serious concern because those are often the very people that we need to protect the most. That, of course, leads us to the concept of herd immunity. Vaccines are safe and effective for the individuals who receive them. Each individual, averaged out, has about a 95 percent chance of being immune to the substance against which they are being vaccinated. In addition, being vaccinated protects those people around us.

There are estimates that, when about 90 percent or more of any population—people who are likely to be exposed to each other—are vaccinated against an infection, you achieve what's called herd immunity. That infection cannot easily spread from person to person. Anyone who is harboring the virus or bacteria is very unlikely to encounter somebody else who isn't resistant, who isn't immune. Therefore, they'll be able to fight it off before they spread it around. This prevents outbreaks and also prevents infections from being endemic, from just constantly being passed around a population.

This exact number, 90 percent, will depend somewhat on what we call the virulence or the infectivity of the virus or the bacteria, but that is an average figure. That also means that for those people who are immunocompromised, they depend upon herd immunity because they themselves are not going to develop a robust response.

We can go beyond herd immunity to what we call eradication. We can completely eliminate an infection by a very thorough vaccine program. This is only possible for those infections, those viruses and bacteria, that exist only in humans—meaning there's no animal reservoir. If viruses can also spread from humans to other animals—like chickens or pigs, animals that are in our world that we may be exposed to—it becomes much more difficult to eradicate it because even if there's no personal life with a virus, it can still come back to us from those animal reservoirs.

For those viruses without that, we can actually achieve eradication. So far, the one infection that we have eradicated from the world is smallpox. At its peak, smallpox killed 400,000 people a year in Europe. As late as 1921, there were 100,000 cases a year in the United States. Some have called smallpox a 12,000 year scourge on humanity and it was completely eradicated by vaccines against smallpox.

We almost achieved eradication for polio. Polio was down to just a couple of countries and we were on the brink of eradicating it. However, the program to eradicate polio was delayed by years because of rumors and misinformation being spread specifically in the African country of Nigeria. There were rumors about a conspiracy that the polio vaccine contained the immunodeficiency virus and was being used to spread AIDS or alternately, was being used to cause sterility in people. This caused enough people to be too afraid to get the polio vaccine that polio returned and became endemic again in Nigeria. Now, through education programs, we are back on track, but we're again years away from completely eradicating polio. However, it is in our sights if there are no other hitches along the way.

Vaccines can also prevent epidemics from happening or prevent epidemics from becoming pandemics. It reduces the spread of a disease around. Diseases do return and spread to unvaccinated populations. For example, the measles virus is no longer endemic in the United States. It used to be endemic, meaning it was spreading around. Now measles cases only come from other countries. You can still catch measles in the United States, but it has to come from somewhere else. It's no longer endemic.

What we are seeing is in local populations where because of concerns about vaccines or concerns that vaccines aren't effective, the vaccination rate is reduced below herd immunity levels—below 90. In some cases, it may be as low as 60 or 50 percent in these isolated populations or localized populations. In those populations, diseases that were once endemic but are no longer endemic are returning to those populations. We are seeing essentially outbreaks of vaccine preventable diseases in populations with low vaccination rates.

Some people still argue that there's no published scientific good experimental evidence that vaccines actually reduce the burden of disease in the population. That's simply not true. I want to quote from a 2007 study in the *Journal of the American Medical Association*. This article concluded that a greater than 92 percent decline in cases and a 99 percent or greater decline in deaths due to diseases prevented by vaccines recommended prior to 1980 were shown for diphtheria, mumps, pertussis, and tetanus. Endemic transmission of polio, measles, and rubella viruses has been eliminated in the United States. Smallpox has been eradicated worldwide and declined to 80 percent or greater for cases and deaths of most vaccine preventable diseases targeted since 1980. That sounds pretty effective to me.

I'm going to focus mainly on safety concerns of vaccines in the next vaccine lecture, but I'll quickly summarize how we test and monitor vaccines for safety. Vaccines, like any other drug that goes on the market, are extensively studied before they're marketed for safety. This testing often takes as long as 10 years with the usual three phases of human testing. First, it's done in healthy individuals, then in small to medium sized trials in people who are either at risk or in cases of treating diseases, people who have the condition.

Finally, it's done in large numbers of people, in hundreds or thousands, to make sure that statistically we have good safety evidence.

The safety record of vaccines is actually quite remarkable. There are, of course, adverse events. No one claims that vaccines are 100 percent safe or that there are no risks of side effects. There are adverse events reported in about 1 per 10,000 doses given of vaccines and a serious adverse event in about 1 per 100,000 doses. It may seem like you might not want to take that risk of being that 1 person in 100,000, but you have to keep a couple of things in mind.

First of all, these figures come from all reports. This is mainly due to the vaccine adverse event reporting system in the United States and other similar systems in other countries. These are not proven cause and effect so this is almost certainly an overestimate. In addition, we have to consider the risk versus benefit. If you consider only the risk of any medical intervention, it could seem scary and you might think why would I bother taking that risk? But, if you consider risk versus benefit, then it puts it into the proper perspective. The benefits of vaccine for the individual vastly outweigh the small risk of a real and serious adverse event, not even counting the advantages to the society at large with herd immunity.

In conclusion, vaccines are arguably the single most effective and safest medical intervention that our technology has come up with. It doesn't stop vaccines from being a victim, however, to myths and misinformation. In the next lecture on vaccines, we're going to explore some of the real vaccine myths that are out there and the threats that they pose to human health by spreading misinformation.

Vaccination Risks—Real and Imagined
Lecture 11

> Rumors began to spread that squalene in the vaccines given to Gulf War veterans was linked to Gulf War Syndrome. The gaping hole in this hypothesis, however, is that squalene was never even in the vaccines that those soldiers were given.

Continuing our discussion of vaccines, I'm going to turn now to talking about some myths about fears and about the safety of vaccines. We begin with a well-known myth about autism. A UK physician named Andrew Wakefield published a 1998 paper in *The Lancet* that claimed that he found a correlation between autism, which is a neurodevelopmental disorder; gastrointestinal disorders; and infection with the measles virus. The paper did not directly implicate vaccines. However, in the subsequent press conferences and media contacts that Wakefield had, he specifically spread concerns about the MMR (mumps, measles, and rubella) vaccine being linked to this gastrointestinal-autism disorder connection. MMR fears spread from that point for the following decade and beyond.

In the UK, vaccination rates with the MMR vaccine dropped from about 92% in 1996 down to as low as 84% in 2002. In some parts of London, compliance rates were as low as 61% in 2003. That's a dramatic decrease in the number of people willing to take the MMR vaccine or give it to their children. These rates are low enough that they're below herd immunity. That's that magic number of people who are vaccinated—around 90%—that prevents the endemic spread of an infection. This subsequently led to outbreaks of diseases that had been previously removed as endemic in the UK, such as measles. A similar thing happened shortly after that in the United States: The rates dropped, particularly in certain populations, and those populations became susceptible to previously eliminated diseases.

Wakefield was later found to have undisclosed conflicts of interest. He was actually applying for a patent for a replacement measles vaccine. He was also being funded by lawyers who were engaged in lawsuits on behalf of parents who were claiming that their children's autism was caused by the MMR vaccine. Even later, there were allegations made that the data in his original *Lancet* paper, or some of that data, may have been faked. This is because it didn't square with hospital records that were then re-reviewed. In 2010, based on these undisclosed conflicts of interest and these allegations, *The Lancet* actually withdrew his paper from the published record. Wakefield was found guilty of professional misconduct in the UK and no longer has a license to practice medicine there. However, the damage had already been done. Fears about a correlation between the MMR vaccine and autism were already spreading.

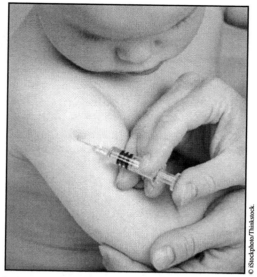

Independent studies in several countries found no connection between the MMR vaccine and autism.

A 2010 survey found that as many as 25% of U.S. parents think there is a link between vaccines and autism. In that same survey, 9 in 10 parents think that vaccines are important to the health of their children. This indicates that there's a certain amount of confusion in the general population about the safety of vaccines.

Ultimately the question of the safety of vaccines is not about the ethics or the research of one scientist; it's about the scientific evidence. There have been a number of studies on whether there really is a connection between the MMR vaccine and autism or other neurodevelopmental disorders. Data from Poland, the UK, Denmark, Finland, and Japan all independently found that there is no connection whatsoever between MMR and autism.

In the years following Wakefield, when research was progressively clearing MMR vaccine as a correlation with autism, those who were having fears about the MMR vaccine shifted to fears about thimerosal. Thimerosal is in some vaccines, but was never in the MMR vaccine. It is a mercury-based preservative added mainly to multidose vials or some inactivated vaccines to prevent bacterial contamination. It has been used for decades in many health and beauty products, not just vaccines.

I think of all the myths that I cover in this course, myths surrounding vaccines have the potential to do the most harm.

The question is whether the ethylmercury in thimerosal is toxic to people—and specifically to children—in the doses that you get from the vaccines. Mercury certainly is a neurotoxin; nobody denies that. The toxicology of mercury is pretty clear. However, autism does not resemble mercury toxicity. They're both neurological disorders, but the details of the signs and symptoms are different enough that we can say they're distinct disorders.

Over the last decade, there have been multiple studies in multiple countries looking at any correlation between exposure to thimerosal and the risk of developing either autism specifically or neurodevelopmental disorders in general. These studies have shown no correlation. Most significantly, in the United States the government decided to remove thimerosal almost completely from the routine childhood vaccine schedule. This removal was completed certainly by the beginning of 2002. The result of this was that the cumulative dose that children were exposed to from the entire vaccine schedule has been dramatically decreased. Those who were most vociferous about a connection between thimerosal and autism predicted that autism rates would plummet after the removal of thimerosal from the vaccine program. This did not happen. In fact, the autism rates continue to increase at exactly the same rate.

There are other vaccine myths that have cropped up as well. One myth is that we don't need to vaccinate against diseases that are no longer endemic. But the only time we can really safely stop using a vaccine is when a disease is

Lecture 11: Vaccination Risks—Real and Imagined

162

worldwide eradicated. So far, that's only happened with smallpox. Others have raised fears that vaccines weaken the immune system, that natural immunity is better. However, that's actually not the case. Vaccines strengthen the immune system by providing a challenge to the immune system against a very particular antigen or group of antigens.

These myths are not benign. I think of all the myths that I cover in this course, myths surrounding vaccines have the potential to do the most harm. People want and need to be able to make informed decisions about their own health care and the health care of their family. When armed with the correct, science-based information, people can make very effective health decisions for themselves and their loved ones. ■

Suggested Reading

Novella, "Vaccines and Autism."

Offit, *Autism's False Prophets.*

Questions to Consider

1. Why do fears and misinformation persist about vaccines?

2. What are the real risks of vaccines?

Vaccination Risks—Real and Imagined
Lecture 11—Transcript

Continuing our discussion of vaccines, I'm going to turn now to talking about some myths about fears and about the safety of vaccines. I'm starting with a story in the United Kingdom, the UK. In the UK, vaccination rates with the MMR vaccine—the mumps, measles, and rubella vaccine—dropped from about 92 percent in 1996 down to as low as 80 percent in 2004. In some parts of London, compliance rates were as low as 61 percent in 2003. That's a dramatic decrease in the number of people willing to take the MMR vaccine or give it to their children.

These rates are low enough that they're below herd immunity. That's that magic number of people who are vaccinated—around 90 percent—that prevents the endemic spread of an infection. This subsequently led to outbreaks of diseases that had been previously removed as endemic in the UK such as measles. A similar thing happened shortly after that in the United States with vaccination rates for the MMR. The rates dropped, particularly in certain populations, and again, those populations became susceptible to previously eliminated diseases. What is happening here is the spread—almost viral, if you will—of fears surrounding the MMR vaccine in particular, but also, of vaccines in general.

Fears began mostly with one physician, a UK physician by the name of Andrew Wakefield. He began with a 1998 paper published in *The Lancet*—which is a very prominent medical journal in the UK—in which he claimed that he found a correlation between autism, which is a neurodevelopmental disorder; gastrointestinal disorders; and infection with the measles virus. The paper did not directly implicate vaccines. However, in the subsequent press conferences and media contacts that Wakefield had, he specifically spread concerns about the MMR vaccine being linked to this gastrointestinal/autism disorder connection that he found.

MMR fears spread from that point for the following decade and beyond. This is what resulted directly in the spread of fears about MMR and the decreased compliance rates. Wakefield was later found to have what we call undisclosed conflicts of interest. He was actually applying for a patent for a replacement measles vaccine. He was also being funded—given money—by lawyers who were engaged in lawsuits on behalf of parents who were claiming that their children's autism was caused by the MMR vaccine. He did not disclose these financial ties.

Even later, there were allegations made that the data in his original *Lancet* paper, or some of that data, may have been faked. This is because it didn't square with hospital records that were then re-reviewed. In 2010, based upon these undisclosed conflicts of interest and these allegations, *The Lancet* actually withdrew his paper from the published record. Two other Wakefield papers were subsequently withdrawn from the record as well. Wakefield was found guilty of professional misconduct in the UK by regulators. He was subsequently struck off, which means he no longer has a license to practice medicine in the UK. However, despite the fall from grace—if you will—of Andrew Wakefield, the damage had already been done. Fears about a correlation between the MMR vaccine and autism were already spreading.

Following Wakefield's study, MMR uptake in the UK dropped to, at its lowest point, 79 percent in 2003, leading to outbreaks of measles. This was followed by lesser drops, to a lesser degree, in the United States. Herd immunity is about 90 percent, as I said. Vaccination rates in the United States overall never dropped below 90 percent. But, there were outbreaks in populations where the rate dropped below 90 percent. A 2010 survey found that as many as 1 in 4—or 25 percent—of U.S. parents think there is a link between vaccines and autism. Though, in that same survey, 9 in 10 parents think that vaccines are important to the health of their children. This indicates that there's a certain amount of confusion in the general population about the safety of vaccines.

While the story of Andrew Wakefield is very interesting and telling, ultimately the question about the safety of vaccines is not about the ethics or the research of one scientist. It's about the scientific evidence. In the decade following Wakefield's *Lancet* paper, there have been a number of studies—epidemiological, observational, and other types of studies. They have addressed specifically the question of whether there really is a connection between the MMR vaccine and autism or other neurodevelopmental disorders.

Data from Poland, the UK, Denmark, Finland, and Japan all independently found that there is no connection whatsoever between MMR and autism. The Japanese study was particularly interesting. This is because the MMR vaccine was withdrawn from use in Japan and it was not followed by what you would predict would be a decrease in the rate of autism if MMR were correlated with autism in any way. These studies show a remarkable concordance of evidence—what scientists really like to see. All the evidence points in the same direction—that there is a lack of association between MMR and autism.

It's also important to note that timing is very important in medical science. Obviously, causes need to come before their effects. If we're going to hypothesize that the MMR vaccine causes autism, then children should get exposed to that vaccine prior to the onset of their autism. It's also understandable that many parents whose children aren't diagnosed with autism until they're two or three, for example—after most of the vaccine will already have been given—may make the correlation in their mind that the vaccines are correlating with the autism. However, on careful examination, it turns out that autism actually has its onset long before the diagnosis is ultimately made.

A 2010 study published in *Child and Adolescent Psychiatry* showed that signs of autism mostly appear between 6 and 12 months of age. However, the first MMR vaccine in the series is not given before 12 months of age. It's usually given either right at, or shortly after, 12 months. Therefore, despite the timing of the diagnosis, autism has its real onset even before the MMR vaccine is given in those cases.

I'm talking a lot about autism. I mentioned that it's a neurodevelopmental disorder, but let me describe it in some more detail because it's so central to this one myth. Autism, as I said, is a neurodevelopmental disorder. This means that the nervous system does not completely develop normally. In some cases, it may be even regressive which means that, after developing to a certain point, children may regress or lose some of their development.

It primarily involves three areas of symptoms: social skills, language, and behavior. For a strict diagnosis, you don't need to have all of these symptoms; you only need to have a certain number of symptoms to meet the criteria. But, these are the things to look for in terms of an autism diagnosis.

Under the category of social skills, children with autism have what's called a "marked impairment in nonverbal behaviors." They don't make eye contact as well. They don't express themselves with facial expressions or gestures as well. They also may fail to develop age appropriate peer-to-peer relationships. They don't form friendships the same way that other children would, for example. They also lack a spontaneous seeking to share enjoyments, interests, or achievements with other people. They don't have that social connection where they will spontaneously ask someone else about something they're doing or that they're interested in. Also, they lack what's called social or emotional reciprocity. They don't respond to the emotions of other people.

In the arena of language, there is a delay. In some severe cases, there is perhaps even a total lack of the development of spoken language—although most children with autism can speak, there's just a delay in their language development. There may also be a marked impairment in the ability to initiate or sustain a conversation. Even in children who can speak fairly normally, they don't engage in conversation spontaneously. They'll tend to keep to themselves. They may engage in stereotyped or repetitive use of language. They may use words in their own peculiar way, not in a way that would be common to other people. They lack varied or spontaneous make-believe play or social interactive play.

In terms of behavior, there's another list of symptoms that clinicians will look for when they're considering the diagnosis. One is a preoccupation with one or more stereotyped or restricted patterns of interest. Children with autism may be fascinated with one particular thing, one particular stuffed animal, for example, or one type of toy. They will tend to focus on that. They will be very inflexible; there is adherence to what are called nonfunctional routines or rituals. They have to do certain things the same way over and over again even though there's no particular function to that routine; they're just stuck in it.

They may engage in stereotyped or repetitive motions or mannerisms. One common thing is called hand flapping, for example. They may flap their hands when they get excited as sort of a stereotyped or repetitive behavior. They may become preoccupied with the parts of objects. They may, for example, play with the button on their shirt over and over again.

The causes of autism are not fully understood. We do, however, have a lot of information about autism. Not knowing everything about the disease is not the same thing as knowing nothing. One thing that is most clear is that autism is strongly a genetic disorder; there is a large genetic component. In fact, researchers have discovered that children with autism are more likely to have certain variations of certain genes than children without autism. Many of those genes have to do with brain development, specifically how the brain communicates with itself—how certain parts of the brain communicate with other parts of the brain. It makes sense that those would be the genes that would be different or abnormal, if you will, in children with a disorder like autism.

There remains legitimate scientific controversy over the degree if any to which environmental factors trigger or exacerbate autism. I would say, at this point, that there is no clear environmental trigger or factor, but we haven't definitively ruled it out either. With the issue of what causes autism and whether it correlates with certain potential triggers is the question of how many children have autism. What is the diagnosis rate?

Let me first explain a couple of technical terms. One is incidence. When we use the term incidence, we specifically mean the number of new cases per year. You might express an incidence of a disease, for example, as 100 people being diagnosed per year. Prevalence is the total number of cases at any one point in time. There are a million people with disease X today. That's a prevalence. Now, let's talk about the prevalence, the number of children at any given time with autism.

Prior to 1990, prevalence estimates were about 3 children per 10,000. Three out of every 10,000 children had the diagnosis of autism. However, more recent estimates put the number closer to 100 per 10,000 or about 1 percent of the population. That's a very significant increase, a 33-fold increase in the prevalence of autism. This increase is partly what has led to fears about there being an environmental trigger of autism.

However, I need to point out that correlation alone is not enough to conclude causation. That's a common misconception. For example, A may correlate with B. That doesn't mean that A causes B. It could, but not necessarily. It's also possible that B causes A or that some other factor C causes both A and B. Scientists need to sort out exactly what the cause and effect is among all those possibilities. But, first we have to confirm that the correlation is real and not just a statistical fluke, fluctuation in the data, or some artifact of how we're looking at the data—which crops up quite a bit. In the case of autism, when you look at autism, the MMR vaccine, and vaccines in general, there is no correlation. The correlation itself is not real.

Is there an autism epidemic? There are some people who are raising the alarm bells, saying we're in the midst of an autism epidemic, and therefore, there must be an environmental factor. You can't have a genetic epidemic, right? Let's address that question.

Scientists have been trying to answer that question very specifically for years. What they found is that there are a number of important factors which are artifactually increasing the apparent prevalence of autism. An example is the expansion of the diagnosis, the loosening of the diagnostic criteria. This has, in fact, happened. There is the inclusion of a broader range of diagnoses under the autism umbrella. There is also the inclusion of milder forms of autism such as Asperger's Syndrome which is a mild form of autism—they are now included under the autism umbrella.

There's also something called "diagnostic substitution" where one diagnosis is being substituted for another over time. Research has shown that, 20 years ago, children may have been diagnosed with something like development delay or a primary language disorder. Those same children with the same constellation of symptoms today are being diagnosed as having autism spectrum disorder. There is diagnostic substitution going on. Further, we're getting better at making the diagnosis. It's being made at an earlier age. If you include younger children in the total number of people with the diagnosis, that will increase the prevalence.

Further, there is an influx of families with children with autism into high service areas where a lot of the counting of the autism prevalence is happening. Further, there is expanded surveillance and increased awareness. More doctors are aware of the diagnosis and how to make it. More parents are aware of it and are bringing their children to a doctor to make the diagnosis. In fact, recent research shows that, if you live near somebody who has a child with an autism diagnosis, you're statistically more likely to have a child with the diagnosis too. Those patterns follow only social connections, not any other environmental connection. Therefore, there definitely seems to be a long list of these artifactual observational factors that are creating the illusion, if you will, that there's an autism epidemic. But, it's just how we're counting up the numbers.

It is also possible that there is a small but real increase in the incidence or the prevalence of autism. That hasn't been ruled out. But, what we can say, based upon the data we have now, is that it has to be pretty small. There's always a limit to epidemiology. You can't count every single person. There are 300 million people in the United States alone for example, let alone other countries like the UK. We can't count everybody so there are always some choices you have to make when you do epidemiological studies. They are always limited in power.

When you read scientific studies, they'll always say something that's very conservative about the fact that they can't rule out a real increase in the numbers. But, what we can do is set limits on how much that can be. This all leads to the question of another component of vaccines called thimerosal.

In the years following Wakefield, when research was progressively clearing MMR vaccine as a correlation with autism, those who were having fears about the MMR vaccine shifted to fears about thimerosal. Thimerosal is in some vaccines, although interestingly, was never in the MMR vaccine. It is a mercury based preservative added to mainly multi-dose vials or some inactivated vaccines to prevent bacterial contamination. It has been used for decades in many health and beauty products, not just vaccines.

The question is whether the ethylmercury in thimerosal is toxic to people—and specifically to children—and in the doses that you get from the vaccines.

Mercury certainly is a neurotoxin; nobody denies that. The toxicology of mercury is pretty clear. However, autism does not resemble mercury toxicity. They're both neurological disorders, but the details of the signs and symptoms are different enough that we can say they're distinct disorders. It should also be noted that the form of mercury matters as well.

Thimerosal contains ethylmercury. Ethylmercury is far less toxic than methylmercury, which is the kind of mercury that is found in seafood like tuna. It is also the kind that's released into the air from coal-burning plants. Often, safety limits that are set for methylmercury are much lower than they would have to be for ethylmercury, but we still use them to be on the safe side. Toxicity is all about dose. If you look at the effects of even ethylmercury on cells in a Petri dish, the toxicology certainly does raise some red flags; it is concerning.

But, we need to know how our bodies handle mercury, specifically ethylmercury. Also, in a biological system, does a high enough dose get to any cell population enough to cause any measureable damage? When you look at the clinical data, we can say pretty clearly that regardless of the toxicity of ethylmercury in the toxicological studies, in clinical studies we can't find any evidence that it's actually caused any harm to anyone.

Over the last decade, there have been multiple studies in multiple countries looking at any correlation between exposure to thimerosal and the risk of developing either autism specifically or neurodevelopmental disorders in general. These studies have shown again—just like with the MMR data—a remarkable consistency in showing that there is no correlation with exposure to thimerosal with the timing of the dose, the total dose, or the removal of exposure from the population.

Most significantly, in the United States, based upon two things—the precautionary principle of trying to limit the overall human exposure to mercury and to deal with the increasing fears about thimerosal—the CDC and the FDA decided to removed thimerosal just about completely from the routine childhood vaccine schedule. This removal was completed certainly by the beginning of 2002. There does remain some thimerosal only in some optional vaccines and some flu vaccines, but not in most flu vaccines.

The result of this was that the cumulative dose, the dose that children were being exposed to from the entire vaccine schedule, has been dramatically decreased. At its peak, the cumulative exposure was 187.5 micrograms of ethylmercury. Now the cumulative exposure from all the vaccines in the child's routine are less than 3 micrograms. There is still a little bit of thimerosal used in the manufacturing process and trace amounts may be left behind in the vaccines. However, it is no longer added to the final product as a preservative.

Those who were most vociferous about a connection between thimerosal and autism predicted that autism rates would plummet after the removal of thimerosal from the vaccine program. This did not happen. In fact, the autism rates continue to increase at exactly the same rate—even ten years after the removal of thimerosal and the marked reduction in exposure of thimerosal to children. That was, as we say, the final nail in the coffin of the thimerosal autism hypothesis.

Fears then turned to other toxins in vaccines after the MMR vaccine and thimerosal were essentially cleared by multiple studies. Those who were anxious about vaccines turned to other toxins. As I discussed in the first vaccine lecture, there are other things in vaccines. One such thing is squalene. Squalene is used as a naturally occurring stabilizer in vaccines. It occurs naturally in our bodies at certain levels and has been used for years in many products. The evidence shows that it's completely safe and the doses that occur in vaccines are well below safety limits.

However, rumors began to spread that squalene in the vaccines given to Gulf War veterans was linked to Gulf War Syndrome. The gaping hole in this hypothesis, however, is that squalene was never even in the vaccines that those soldiers were given. There is no evidence of course linking squalene to anything like Gulf War Syndrome.

Other alleged toxins that have been pointed to include formaldehyde. Formaldehyde certainly is a scary sounding chemical, but it needs to be noted that formaldehyde is also a natural byproduct of our own biochemistry. We all have a certain amount of formaldehyde inside of us just from our cells going about their business. We have much more formaldehyde, in fact, than the tiny amounts that occur in vaccines. Remember the overarching concept here is that toxicity is always about dose. We need to know if the dose that people are getting is actually toxic.

Aluminum is another one. There's been a tremendous amount of research looking at the safety of aluminum. Again, there's no evidence for toxicity from the doses that children are getting in vaccines. Another type of fear has been raised—maybe if the adverse effects are not being caused by the chemicals that are in vaccines, maybe it's the vaccines themselves. Maybe children are getting too many vaccines, too soon and it's overwhelming their young immune systems.

Some people advocate what they call an alternative vaccine schedule, spreading out the vaccines and giving fewer vaccines in order to avoid any concerns about this overwhelming of the immune system. However, there is no evidence that there is any advantage to spreading out or reducing the vaccines. In fact, a 2010 study published in *Pediatrics*, which is a medical journal, showed no health advantage at all to delayed or reduced vaccine schedule.

We also need to point out that the working components of vaccines are the antigens. Antigens are the things that stimulate the immune system. Some have raised fears that artificially stimulating the immune system may have its own dangers and that, as we increase the number of vaccines, that's when problems started to occur. However, while the number of vaccines was being increased, vaccine technology was also improving.

A hundred years ago, a single vaccine, the smallpox vaccine—which is no longer given—contained 200 proteins. Now, the 11 different vaccines in the childhood schedule combined contain only 130 proteins. It's much less than what children were getting in the past. Also, 130 different antigens over the years of the vaccine program is a tiny amount compared to the antigens that children are being exposed to just going about their day-to-day lives.

There are other vaccine myths that have cropped up as well. One myth is that we don't need to vaccinate against diseases that are no longer endemic. In industrialized nations that have benefitted from vaccines, we are a bit the victim of our own success. The public, families, and parents no longer know what it's like to have to fear a polio epidemic—or a real epidemic of measles, mumps, or other diseases that have been reduced or eliminated by vaccines. They think they don't need the vaccines. However, the moment vaccine rates begin to drop, diseases that have been previously eliminated that do come back from other countries. The only time we can really safely stop using a vaccine is when a disease is worldwide eradicated. So far, that's only happened with smallpox.

Others have raised fears that vaccines weaken the immune system, that natural immunity is better. However, that's actually not the case. Vaccines strengthen the immune system by providing a challenge to the immune system against a very particular antigen or group of antigens. They increase the immune system's ability to fight off those invading organisms. That represents an actual increase in immune function.

However, there's a little kernel of truth here in that when the immune system is challenged, it does have limited resources. It can't fight off multiple infections all at once. That's why we don't give vaccines to people who are already sick and fighting off an infection. We are very cautious about giving vaccines to people who have immune dysfunctions, who are immunocompromised.

There is still another myth about vaccines. There are many that claim that the duration of immunity from vaccine is shorter than from a natural infection. Therefore, the risk of vaccines is that you will have a false sense of security because the immunity won't last. It's far better, some argue, to get the actual infection; the immunity will last much longer. Again, there is a kernel of truth here in that if you sustain a long infection, your immune system will get exposed to the antigens in that infection for a much longer period of time. You will develop more immunity that will last for longer.

However, that's taken into consideration when we design the vaccine schedule. For those vaccines that don't have long-lasting immunity, the requirement is to give booster shots. This is either over a short period of time or sometimes every interval of time. For example, every ten years or so, you need to get your tetanus booster in order to prolong immunity. But, many of the common vaccines have perfectly fine duration. Again, this is a question that scientists address. We don't just make assumptions.

Half-life is the time it would take for half of the immune cells that are providing the immunity to go away for certain infections. For varicella zoster, the half-life is 50 years. For measles, it's 200 years. For smallpox, it's 75 years. For tetanus, as I mentioned, it's shorter—it's only 11 years. To me, 200 years for measles sounds like a pretty adequate duration of immunity.

These myths are not benign. I think of all the myths that I cover in this course, myths surrounding vaccines have the potential to do the most harm. One myth is that the people who are vaccinated have nothing to risk from the unvaccinated. If people choose not to vaccinate themselves or their children, they're not putting others at risk, only themselves. However, that's not true. This is because, while vaccines are 95 percent effective, there's still 5 percent of the population who don't develop immunity from the vaccine.

There are also people who can't be vaccinated, as I said. If you're immunocompromised, if you are sick, you may not be able to get a vaccine. The most vulnerable people who really need to be protected the most are the most at risk from those who are not vaccinated. Plus, there are also children who are just too young to be vaccinated, but they need to be protected as well.

There's also the myth that vaccines help the community, but they don't help the individual. It's as if you're taking a hit for the team. You are putting yourself at personal risk in order to do what's best for society. But, actually, if you look at the statistics, the benefits of vaccines are greater for the individual than the risks of vaccines for the individual. Even from just an individual point of view, it does make sense to vaccinate.

The cost of these fears is actually quite immense. The myth that vaccines are linked to autism or other neurodevelopmental disorders has caused unwarranted fear and a lot of confusion among parents. I still get people—friends, patients, and acquaintances—who come to me. They're new parents and they want to know if they should vaccinate their children. They've heard all these rumors about a possible connection and it really causes a great deal of distress. This has led to—and there's the potential that it can lead in the future to—loss of herd immunity in some communities and the return of serious infections like mumps, measles, and whooping cough.

The vaccine myths really are pernicious. They perhaps are the worst in terms of the harm that they cause of all the myths that I cover in this course. They also spread a great deal of misinformation. People want and need to be able to make informed decisions about their own healthcare and the healthcare of their family. Spreading the misinformation and rumors directly attacks that right to make informed consent. Fortunately, when armed with the correct information and real science-based information, people can make very effective health decisions for themselves and their loved ones.

Antibiotics, Germs, and Hygiene
Lecture 12

This is a war, if you will, that we are currently engaged in, the medical community. We are trying to preserve the effectiveness of our antibiotic armamentarium. Meanwhile, using antibiotics relentlessly is resulting in the development of more and more bacterial resistance—to the point that some fear we may enter what's called a post-antibiotic era.

We are awash in germs. Bacteria, viruses, fungi, and protozoa are all organisms that want to invade our bodies and cause infection. But we have evolved a defense against this—our immune system. We also have the advantage of technology, including antibiotics, that we can use to help our immune system in this fight.

There are several antibiotic and germ myths. The big one is that antibiotics work against many different types of infections, including the cold. This is not the case: Antibiotics work only against bacteria. Another myth is that all antibiotics kill bacteria. In fact, most antibiotics are bacteriostatic: They only keep bacteria from reproducing, giving our immune systems time to do the killing themselves. Some antibiotics, however, are bacteriocidal, which means they directly kill bacteria.

I often hear it said that people can become resistant to antibiotics. In fact, people themselves do not become resistant to antibiotics; it's the bacterial populations inside of our bodies that become resistant. The caution is not that you will become resistant, but that you can become a breeding ground for resistant species of bacteria. Another myth is that antibiotics weaken the immune system. This is not true. They do not have any effect on the immune system. The immune system, in most cases, still has to fight off the infection. Antibiotics just give the immune system a chance to do so.

Some people believe that if an antibiotic has not worked in a specific individual previously, that antibiotic won't work in the future. That is not necessarily true. The effectiveness of any particular antibiotic is specific to the infection—the strain and the species of bacteria—not the person.

One thing about antibiotics that is not a myth is that they should not be overused: Overuse of antibiotics increases resistance. Therefore, it is important to find alternatives to antibiotics. In other words, it's important to find ways to minimize infections rather than relying on an antibiotic whenever you need to. Some alternatives are true and effective. But there are a lot that are myths.

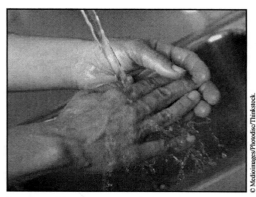

One common myth that is offered as an alternative to treating a bacterial infection with antibiotics is supplements or products that boost the immune system. If you are healthy, well-nourished, and not sick, your immune system will be functioning optimally. There is no way to boost it or increase its activity beyond its already optimal functioning. Only if there is something inhibiting or interfering with the activity of the immune system can you take steps to restore the immune system to its normal functional state.

Hand washing is the most effective way to prevent getting an infection.

One product that has been around for years as an alternative to antibiotics is called colloidal silver. This is actually the element silver, in a suspension that you are meant to drink. The claim is that silver has antibacterial activity. Silver is used externally to sterilize, for example, medical equipment—but it is not meant to be taken internally.

One alternative, however, is genuine: honey. Honey, while not an antibiotic when taken internally, does have antiseptic properties when used externally. Studies show that using honey as an antiseptic in a wound works quite well—almost as well as pharmaceutical creams that are designed specifically for that purpose.

Hand washing is the single most effective behavior to prevent getting an infection, such as the cold, flu, or more serious bacterial infections. This is especially true if you are exposed to people who you know to be sick. Health-care workers, for example, especially need to wash their hands. What about antibacterial soaps? These are very common on the market these days. What makes a soap antibacterial is that it contains a chemical, the most common one being triclosan, that has an antibacterial effect. But in 2007, a systematic review concluded that antibacterial soaps containing triclosan are not more effective than regular soap. However, there are some studies that show that it may be more effective if it is combined with other antibacterial agents. The jury is still out on whether we can develop an antibacterial soap that has advantages. ■

We do need to take reasonable measures to stay hygienic and free from infection. Knowing when to use an antibiotic is also very helpful, as is knowing when not to use an antibiotic. While basic hygiene is good, scientists are actually considering the possibility that our modern society may in fact be too hygienic for our own good. A little exposure to germs may not be a bad thing. ■

Suggested Reading

Brown, *Penicillin Man.*

Scientific American Readers, *Infectious Disease.*

Questions to Consider

1. How often, in what circumstances, and with what kind of products should you wash your hands?

2. Is it possible to have too much hygiene? Why or why not?

3. When is it appropriate to use antibiotics?

Antibiotics, Germs, and Hygiene
Lecture 12—Transcript

We are awash in germs. Bacteria, viruses, fungi, and protozoa are organisms that want to invade our bodies and cause infection. We have evolved a defense against this—an immune system—to fend off all of these invading armies of microscopic organisms. But, infection remains a serious concern both for humans and for most species. Fortunately, we have the advantage of having technology that we can use to help our immune systems in this fight.

Previously I spoke about vaccines which are one technology in helping our immune systems fight off infections. In this talk, I'm going to focus largely on other approaches including antibiotics. In a previous lecture on probiotics, I talked about the fact that, while most bacteria are neutral to human health, some are actually friendly. In this talk, I'm going to focus on the bad bacteria, the pathological ones that want to cause disease.

I'm going to talk about several antibiotic and germ myths. For example, there is the big one—many people think that antibiotics will work against many different types of infections. They think antibiotics work against the cold for example, but antibiotics work only against bacteria, not other kinds of germs.

To go over some terminology, the word "antimicrobial" refers to any drug or substance which will kill any kind of germ while antibiotics refer specifically to bacteria. Antiseptics are things that can kill bacteria or germs, but outside the body. They're not generally safe to take internally.

Let's also go over a few basic concepts, words that I'm going to be throwing out throughout the lecture. Another myth is that all antibiotics kill bacteria. In fact, most antibiotics are bacteriostatic. They only keep bacteria from reproducing, giving our immune systems time to do the killing themselves. Some antibiotics are bacteriocidal; they do kill bacteria directly.

The way that antibiotics work is by exploiting some aspect of bacterial biology that's different than human biology. Bacteria are prokaryotes. They are cells that do not have a nucleus, whereas humans, other vertebrates, and animals in general are eukaryotes. They are different kinds of cells. We're related but only very, very distantly. This creates the opportunity to discover something that's different about the biology. Therefore, we can create an intervention like a drug that will adversely affect the bacteria, but in a way that will not affect eukaryotes hopefully at all.

Different antibiotics are thought of clinically in terms of how they are used. For example, antibiotics are classified in terms of their clinical utility based upon which bacteria they have activity against. In addition, we think of them as being broad spectrum or narrow spectrum. Broad spectrum antibiotics are good against a large number of different bacterial species whereas a narrow spectrum antibiotic is active against only a few.

We also have to consider what parts of the body the antibiotic has access to. For example, if you have a bacterial infection in your cerebrospinal fluid, your CSF, you will need an antibiotic that penetrates into the CSF. It won't do any good if it can't get to where the bacteria are.

Quickly, I'm going to go through the different chemical classes of antibiotics and how they work. The first class is called the beta-lactams. These inhibit the biosynthesis of the bacterial cell wall. Therefore, the bacteria can't produce their wall and that encapsulates the bacteria. It interferes with the cross peptide linking of a protein called peptidoglycan. These are like the glue that sticks the different pieces of the wall together. It interferes with that so the wall doesn't hold together. When the bacteria try to divide, the bacterial cell wall will tend to collapse. Examples of beta-lactams include penicillins and cephalosporins.

Aminoglycosides are another important class of antibiotics. These inhibit protein synthesis so the bacteria cannot manufacture proteins, which are obviously a major constituent of all living cells. They do this by binding to part of the ribosome. For quick review, a ribosome is a small piece inside a cell. It's called an organelle. It's a little machine inside every cell. RNA is like DNA. DNA is where the genes are, where the codes for the proteins are. The RNA is a copy of the DNA and specifically, the transfer RNA is a copy of a gene in the DNA that then will transfer that information to the ribosome. It binds to the ribosome. Then the ribosome will read it off as a set of instructions and connect together the amino acids building the protein chain.

Aminoglycosides bind to what is called the 30s subunit of the bacterial ribosome. There are two pieces to the ribosome or subunit, the 30s and the 50s. The letter "s" stands for a Svedberg unit, which is just a measure of how big it is. By binding to the 30s subunit of the bacterial ribosome, it blocks the ribosome from turning that tRNA, the instructions for a protein, into a protein. The bacteria can't make proteins and eventually it dies. Thus, aminoglycosides are bactericidal. Examples of that include kanamycin, streptomycin, and gentamycin.

Tetracyclines also prevent protein synthesis, but they don't bind to the ribosome. They bind to the tRNA itself keeping it from binding to the 30s subunit. Tetracyclines are bacteriostatic so they prevent the bacteria from reproducing; they don't kill them outright. Examples of tetracyclines include, in addition to tetracycline itself, doxycycline and trimocycline. They're conveniently named with cycline at the end so you know that that drug belongs to that class.

The quinolones inhibit the bacterial DNA synthesis. When the bacteria try to reproduce, it needs to make another copy of its DNA. It can't do that so it therefore prevents any reproduction of the cell. However, the quinolones also tend to be bactericidal so this actually can kill the bacteria. They actually need to reproduce their DNA to live, not just to reproduce. The quinolones also tend to be very broad spectrum. They have activity over many different species of bacteria. Examples of the quinolones include nalidixic acid, norfloxacin, and ciprofloxacin.

The sulfonamides are one of the oldest types of antibiotics. They bind to a bacterial enzyme that is necessary for the production of folic acid. The bacteria can't produce folic acid, which is a necessary chemical for bacteria to survive. They tend to be very broad spectrum and therefore very useful. However, the one downside to sulfonamides as a class is that allergies are very common. In fact, 3 percent of the population will develop a rash in response to taking sulfonamides.

Interestingly, the sulfonamides were the first antibiotic available. They were available and being mass produced in 1932. Most people think that penicillin was the first antibiotic. Penicillin was discovered in 1928. It was the first antibiotic that was discovered, but we didn't figure out how to mass produce it until 1944. The sulfonamides beat penicillin to the market. An example of a sulfonamide is what is called sulfa drugs.

Now that we've done the quick overview of the different types of antibiotics that we have in our armamentarium, let's talk about some concepts about how to use these antibiotics. Bacteria rapidly reproduce. A generation time may be as short as 15 minutes. If you do the math, you double the number of bacteria every 15 minutes. It doesn't take long before there are millions or even billions of bacteria in an active infection. During an infection, those bacteria are mutating. The bacterial genes are mutating just like any other living organism. But because the generation time is so short, there are many mutations. That gives a bacterial population an opportunity to experiment, if you will, with different biochemical variations.

Occasionally, bacteria will hit upon a mutation that changes something about its biology that will make it resistant to an antibiotic. That is how antibiotic resistance both develops and evolves. The antibiotics are actually providing selective pressure. They're selecting those bacteria that happen to hit upon mutations, which make them resistant to some degree to the effects of that antibiotic. When fighting an infection, bacteria that are more resistant will tend to reproduce and thrive. Over the course of an infection, antibiotic resistance may emerge.

The story of bacterial resistance is actually worse than that. Not only do bacteria have the ability to evolve rapidly, they also contain their genes in a little circle, a circlet called a plasmid. These plasmids, these rings of bacterial genes, can be exchanged between different bacteria—even bacteria of different species. Bacteria can also share parts of their plasmids. It doesn't have to be an all or nothing exchange. This allows for genes that confer antibiotic resistance to be shared among bacteria and even to spread to other bacterial species.

There are some factors that worsen the chance of developing bacterial resistance. This is a war, if you will, that we are currently engaged in, the medical community. We are trying to preserve the effectiveness of our antibiotic armamentarium. Meanwhile, using antibiotics relentlessly is resulting in the development of more and more bacterial resistance—to the point that some fear we may enter what's called a post-antibiotic era where we are surrounded by bacteria that have evolved resistance to most or all of our antibiotics.

One factor that increases the risk of resistance is overuse. The more we use antibiotics, the greater that consistent selective pressure, the greater the emergence of resistance. Also, broad spectrum antibiotics—because they have effectiveness activity against more different kinds of bacteria—are more likely to cause resistance than narrow spectrum antibiotics. Therefore, it's important for physicians who are prescribing to select an antibiotic that has just the activity needed to fight a specific infection. We only use broad spectrum antibiotics when we don't yet know which kind of bacteria we're fighting.

Also, and this is what's most important for the average person who's just taking antibiotics, it's very important to complete a course of antibiotics. Don't stop just because you start to feel better. It really is true that you do need to complete the full course. Imagine, if you will, that while you're taking the antibiotic, the bacterial populations are being steadily reduced. Some of those bacteria may have partial resistance against the antibiotic, but if you complete your course you'll wipe them out. However, if you stop when the bacterial numbers are reduced to just a few, those few relatively resistant bacteria are allowed to then reproduce and spread again. That is a perfect set-up for creating or giving the opportunity to evolve even better resistance.

How do bacteria become resistant to antibiotics? There are a number of mechanisms that have been identified. This is a very interesting and significant scientific question. If we can figure out how bacteria are resisting our drugs, maybe we will be able to design better drugs that get around their resistance. One way that they evolve resistance is to change the binding target. Antibiotics have to bind somewhere on or in a bacteria in order to have effectiveness. If that target changes—for example, if the ribosome where an antibiotic is binding changed its structure so that the antibiotic is no longer able to bind there—it can't have activity.

Also, bacteria could evolve the ability to prevent drug from entering inside the bacteria where they have their activity or they can evolve a mechanism to pump out the drug faster than it can enter. They may allow the drug to enter the bacteria, but they will sequester it away. They'll block it off somewhere inside the cell, away from the target where it has its activity. They may evolve enzymes, proteins that have chemical activity, that inactivate the drug.

Let's go over a few interesting antibiotic myths in addition to the ones that I've already mentioned. I often hear people say that people can become resistant to antibiotics. In fact, people themselves or animals do not become resistant to the antibiotics like you can become resistant to other types of medications. It's the bacterial populations inside of you that become resistant. The caution is not that you will become resistant, but we don't want you to be a breeding ground for resistant species of bacteria. Even your friendly bacteria may develop resistance. Again, because they can transfer that resistance to pathological bacteria through their plasmids, that also can be a bad thing.

Another myth is that antibiotics weaken the immune system. This is not true. They do not have any effect on the immune system. The immune system, in most cases, still has to fight off the infection. It's just giving the immune system a chance to do so and not letting the body get overwhelmed by the infection before the immune system has a chance to do its job.

It also is a myth that antibiotics should be taken whenever you have a fever, illness, cold, or earache, for example. In fact, most infections are viral. Most of the infectious symptoms that the average person comes down with are going to be due to a virus. This means that you do not have to take an antibiotic for most colds or earaches or sinus infections. You only take an antibiotic when a bacterial infection specifically has been documented.

Sometimes it is believed that, if an antibiotic has not worked in a specific individual previously, that antibiotic won't work in the future. That is also not necessarily true. The effectiveness of any particular antibiotic is specific to a very specific infection, what strain of what species of bacteria you are infected with—not the person themselves.

Antibiotics should not be overused. That is absolutely true because overuse of antibiotics increases resistance. Therefore, it is important to find alternative to antibiotics. In other words, it's important to find ways to minimize infections rather than just relying on taking an antibiotic whenever you need to. Some alternatives—which I will talk about in a moment—are true and effective. But, there are a lot of alternatives that are not effective and that themselves are myths. One common myth that is offered as an alternative to treating a bacterial infection with antibiotics is supplements or products that boost the immune system.

Whenever you see that claim made for a product—that it boosts the immune system—you have to realize first that that claim is often not regulated. Companies do not have to provide evidence to support that claim. It's something they're allowed to do without evidence. But also, the term boosting the immune system is not a technical or medical term that scientists or doctors use because it doesn't really mean anything specific.

If you are healthy, well-nourished, and not sick, your immune system will be functioning optimally. There is no way to boost it or increase its activity beyond its already optimal functioning. Only if there is something inhibiting or interfering with the activity of the immune system can you take steps to restore the immune system to its normal functional state.

One product that has been around for years as an alternative to antibiotics is called colloidal silver. This is actually silver, the element silver, in a suspension that you are meant to drink, to take internally. The claim is that silver has antibacterial activity. It's actually bactericidal. Silver is used externally to sterilize, for example, medical equipment. But, it is not meant to take internally. There is no evidence that it's effective, that it actually gets to the bacteria, and has use in the doses that you can safely take. Also, colloidal silver has very serious risks. It can cause what's known as argyria. It actually turns your skin gray or silver. It's not safe and it doesn't work so don't believe claims for colloidal silver.

But, here's one that is true: honey. Honey, while not an antibiotic when taken internally, does have antiseptic properties when used externally. In fact, prior to modern technology, some cultures learned that if you spread honey in a wound, it would not get infected or it would heal better. Modern science has actually verified that. There are studies which show that using honey as an antiseptic in a wound works quite well, almost as well as pharmaceutical creams that are designed specifically to do that.

But, as I said, there are more types of germs than just bacteria. We should talk about the other types of invading organisms and the medications and other things that we have developed to fight against them. There are, for example, antivirals. However, anti-virals are limited to only certain families or types of viruses, not all viruses in general. Anti-virals generally inhibit the reproduction of viruses. They don't kill or inactivate them. Viruses are hard to kill.

One class of drugs called highly active antiretroviral therapy, which is often shortened as HAART, is active against the human immunodeficiency virus. They are so active that patients with HIV are now living almost normal life expectancies. Herpes viruses also are targeted by a medication called acyclovir and related anti-virals. There are anti-virals for hepatitis B, hepatitis C, and for influenza, like Tamiflu.

Some mechanisms for anti-virals are as follows. They can prevent the virus from entering into the cell. They can prevent the virus from uncoating itself and releasing its package of RNA or DNA, which is what causes the infection. They can inhibit enzymes that are used in replicating—the virus replicating itself—or in protein assembly.

Let's turn to funguses now. I mentioned that fungi can also be germs that invade our body. There are anti-fungal medications to combat them. Some common fungal infections include athlete's foot, ringworm, and candidiasis—like thrush in your mouth, for example. Cryptococcal meningitis is a very serious fungal infection.

Fungi are eukaryotes, like people, so it's a little bit harder to find a drug that is active against them that doesn't have as many side effects. For that reason, anti-fungal medications do tend to have more side effects than antibiotics or anti-virals. But, the one thing that is different about fungi is that they have a different kind of component of their cell walls. They have ergosterol where we tend to use cholesterol. One type of antifungal medication will bind to ergosterol and will break down the fungus cell walls without affecting the cell walls in people or vertebrates.

There are also anti-protozoans. Protozoans are eukaryotic single-celled animals like amoeba. There are drugs that are effective against them. There are also many parasites, like malaria. There are drugs like metronidazole, which are effective against that as well. In addition to drugs—to antibiotics, anti-virals, and anti-fungals—there are behaviors that you can use in order to minimize your chance of getting infected in the first place.

As I mentioned in the previous lecture, hand washing is the single most effective behavior to prevent getting an infection, such as the cold, flu, or more serious infections like bacterial infections. This is especially true if you are going to be exposed to people who you know to be sick. Healthcare workers like doctors and nurses, for example, especially need to wash their hands. But, this wasn't learned until the 19th century.

In fact, there was a physician, Ignaz Philipp Semmelweis, who was born in 1818 and lived until 1865. During his career, he proved that you could reduce the transmission of hospital infections from one patient to another patient if the healthcare worker, the doctor, simply washed their hands between each patient visit. He provided clear-cut evidence of a dramatic reduction in hospital acquired infections simply by doing this. However, there was tremendous resistance to his recommendations at the time which were thought of as draconian, having to constantly wash and rewash your hands.

Eventually, the scientific evidence won out. Today we recognize that aggressive hand washing and universal hand washing between patient visits is a critical part of minimizing hospital-acquired infections. For most cases, soapy water is adequate hand washing. However, alcohol based hand washing or sanitizers can also be effective.

What about antibacterial soaps? These are very common on the market these days. Everything seems to be antibacterial. What makes a soap antibacterial is that it contains one or another chemical, the most common one being triclosan. This has antibacterial effect. In 2007, if we want to look at the actual evidence, a systematic review concluded that antibacterial soaps containing triclosan are not more effective than regular soap. However, there are still some studies which show that maybe it's more effective if you combine it with other antibacterial agents. The jury is still out on whether or not we can come up with some kind of antibacterial soap that has advantages. But, most of the stuff that's on the market right now is no better than just regular soap.

Scrubbing seems to be the key component. You can't just put the soap on your hands and rinse it off. It's the scrubbing that actually does most of the work. There is evidence on the development of antibiotic resistance in response to antibacterial soaps. Again, we're not quite sure what the bottom line is there. It may be contributing to antibacterial resistance, but we're just not sure.

There are other ways to avoid infection as well. You can avoid intimate contact with those known to be infected. Blood transfusions are another way of getting infections. Certain viruses, for example, can be transmitted in the blood. However, this is exceedingly rare as the blood supply now is very carefully screened. However, healthcare workers are still at risk from blood exposure by doing procedures and drawing blood, for example. They could be accidentally exposed to the people with viral infections, for example, where the viruses generally replicate and live in the blood. For that reason, what we call universal precautions—meaning that you have to assume that any patient that you're dealing with is infected—is the standard of care at this time.

What about face masks for the flu or the cold? You might see, during flu season, a lot of people in public wearing a face mask. There's actually not much research, so not a lot of evidence to go on. However, there is some evidence that wearing a face mask while you're sick will reduce the risk of you spreading the disease to someone else. However, wearing a face mask will not protect you from getting infected from someone else.

Food is another important vector or mechanism by which infections can get into our bodies. Eating raw or undercooked food is the main culprit, the main risk. Eggs and meats, for example, can contain a variety of bacteria—salmonella or E. coli, for example. They can even contain parasites or protozoal infections. Raw food can also cross-contaminate. Perhaps you cook the food adequately, but before you do that, you prepared the meat on your counter. The bacteria then went from the counter to vegetables which you then ate either lightly cooked or raw. You have to be careful about everything the meat and eggs touch, not just the food itself.

Interestingly, I looked into the question of cutting boards. Are plastic cutting boards better than wooden cutting boards in terms of being a place where bacteria can form and can pass from one food item to another? It turns out that the research is remarkably mixed. It's not clear. Wood is more porous. It absorbs the water—and therefore bacteria—like a sponge, more than plastic. However, it also seems to absorb it so deep that it sequesters it away from the surface. Therefore, it may not get back out and on to food. However, plastic cutting boards are less porous. They don't absorb the bacteria in the first place. But, when you cut into a plastic board and you make a nice little cut, that becomes a recess where bacteria can collect. It is still superficial and able to be passed on to another food item. It seems that maybe the best type of cutting board in terms of reducing the chance of cross-contamination are glass or ceramic cutting boards, but they're not widely used.

Animals are also an important vector. Insects and ticks are the most common. Mosquitoes, for example, can pass malaria and other infections along. There, the use of mosquito netting in endemic areas is one of the most, if not the most, effective measures. Essentially, avoid exposed skin when out of doors during tick season or during mosquito season.

Good hygiene, of course, is important. Louis Pasteur, who was a brilliant biologist and greatly advanced microbiology, became a little obsessed with hygiene, however. In fact, after investigating the effects of germs causing disease, he became so obsessed that he refused to shake anyone's hand for fear of catching a germ. While basic hygiene is good, that level of obsessive cleanliness may not necessarily be the best idea for health.

Recently the excessive hygiene hypothesis has been proposed. Can we be too clean? Regular exposure to immune challenges actually keeps our immune system healthy. Being overly hygienic may, in fact, deprive the immune system of this regular workout. It may literally weaken the immune system over time or cause it to not be weaker, but to just be dysfunctional.

Recent studies show that there's an association between decreased immune system exposure—not just from washing hands, but from having a very clean environment, like a very clean house—and increased levels of bacterial proteins in the blood. There are more bacteria thriving in the body if you live in a very clean environment. It also may correlate with certain diseases which are involved with immune function like asthma or allergies. These have been on the increase recently and this is one hypothesis to possibly explain that. But, of course, a major exception to this notion that we can be too hygienic applies to anyone who is immunocompromised—a patient with the acquired immunodeficiency syndrome, who is on chemotherapy, chronically ill, or has some defect in their immune system.

While most bacteria and other microorganisms are harmless, there are still some that are harmful. We do need to take reasonable measures in order to keep hygienic and free from infection. Basic precautions are important. Knowing when to use an antibiotic is also very helpful, but also when not to use an antibiotic or another drug. While basic hygiene is good, scientists are actually considering the possibility that our modern society may in fact be too hygienic for our own good. A little exposure to germs may not be a bad thing.

Vague Symptoms and Fuzzy Diagnoses
Lecture 13

We begin to get a little suspicious when the more we investigate a questionable diagnosis or a vague diagnosis, the less we seem to understand about the pathophysiology. If the people who are promoting the notion of this problematic diagnosis use what we call special pleading, they explain away all the lack of evidence that we would predict should be there if the disease had a specific biological cause, for example.

This lecture is about diagnoses: the labels we attach to the signs and symptoms that people have. The core myth of this lecture is that all diagnoses are the same and equally valid. The truth is that we arrive at these labels in very different ways. For example, there are some diagnoses that we would call a disease, like diabetes. It's a pathological disorder we can identify. A disorder does not necessarily have a pathological change in any cells, but there is some problem with functioning that is identifiable; an example of this is attention deficit hyperactivity disorder. There are also syndromes, which are lists of signs and symptoms that tend to occur together. A clinical syndrome may not be one specific disease. ALS is actually a clinical syndrome, not a specific diagnosis.

It also is important to recognize that there are categories of diseases. Sometimes we may identify that a disease belongs to a certain category—for example, inflammatory versus nutritional versus degenerative—even though we can't get more specific than that. This all relates to how doctors make diagnoses in the first place. What do they mean? How do we understand and use them in medical practice? Ultimately, the goal of understanding the illness is to come up with treatments that are effective.

We don't want to wait until we understand every last thing about a disease or a disorder before we treat it. There are multiple ways to treat a syndrome or a disorder before we completely understand its cause. People often think only in terms of curing a disease, but mostly physicians simply treat various aspects of a disease. For example, we may reduce the risk of developing a disease. We may slow its progression or even stop it from progressing. We may reverse some of the damage or disability that has resulted from the disease. We may alleviate symptoms and improve quality of life, prevent complications of the disease, or prolong survival with it. None of those things would be considered a cure, but they are all tremendously useful.

There are multiple ways to treat a syndrome or a disorder before we completely understand its cause.

Let's continue to examine how doctors make diagnoses. There are different types of diagnoses: There are clinical diagnoses, which are based on having a certain set of signs and symptoms. (Symptoms are something the patient experiences; a sign is something you see when you examine a patient.) There also are laboratory methods, like blood tests and X-rays, of making or confirming a diagnosis. And when a diagnosis is made entirely by biopsy, we call that a pathological diagnosis.

Doctors also sometimes make what we call a diagnosis of exclusion. You have an appropriate clinical syndrome, and we rule out everything else that can cause that syndrome. What you're left with is the diagnosis of exclusion—something we know can cause those symptoms, even though we may not have any laboratory test to confirm it.

There are many problematic diagnoses, however, that are out there. They are less clearly established, more ambiguous, and more controversial. What are some of the warning signs of these problematic diagnoses? They tend to be a clinical syndrome, not something that is tied to a specific laboratory finding. They tend to have common, nonspecific symptoms, such as pain and fatigue. Problematic diagnoses also tend to be highly variable in their presentation. The symptoms and signs that get attached to that diagnosis don't suggest one cohesive, coherent underlying cause.

Another problem is diagnosis creep. Once you have a label—a questionable label based on nonspecific symptoms without anything very objective to verify it—it tends to apply to an ever-expanding list of presentations, with a broader and broader scope. In addition, there's diagnosis expansion, which means applying the diagnosis to milder and milder versions.

Treating these problematic illnesses—when we have only a vague syndrome without anything specific to hang our hat on—is also, of course, problematic. They tend to be resistant to specific biological interventions and to benefit only temporarily from treatments that are likely to have a placebo effect.

I think we've covered a lot of information about what doctors think about when they're making a diagnosis. There are a lot of pitfalls and it can often be very tricky to make an adequate diagnosis. The approach that we often take is to look for things that we know how to diagnose and how to treat. If we make a diagnosis, then we treat based on the diagnosis that we make. We find any contributing factors and essentially treat what we find.

But sometimes we rule out all of the known pathological contributors or causes of a disease. We're left with a syndrome of symptoms without a clear biological cause, but we have ruled out anything serious or treatable. In that case, it's most effective to then shift our emphasis to treating the patient to improve their quality of life. That is very important and should not be neglected. We shouldn't get distracted from treating quality of life because of a search for a diagnosis that may not be there or just for the false comfort of having a label to attach to symptoms. ■

Suggested Reading

Barbour, *Lyme Disease.*

Lipson, "Fake Diseases, False Compassion."

Questions to Consider

1. Do you think chronic fatigue syndrome is a genuine disorder?

2. What makes one diagnosis useful and another problematic?

3. Do you think we overmedicalize everyday symptoms?

Vague Symptoms and Fuzzy Diagnoses
Lecture 13—Transcript

Do you have any of these following symptoms: fatigue, headaches, hair loss, irritability, depression, decreased memory or poor concentration, low sex drive, easy weight gain, backache, joint aches, or poor sleep? Then you may have Syndrome X, a potentially medical illness that only I can diagnose or treat. Seriously, Syndrome X doesn't exist. What we're going to talk about in this lecture are diagnoses themselves, the labels that we attach to signs and symptoms to people with certain complaints.

The core myth of this lecture is that all diagnoses are the same and equally valid. The truth is that we arrive at these labels in very different ways. For example, there are some diagnoses which we would call a disease, like diabetes. It's a pathological disorder we can identify. There is something specific malfunctioning in some specific part of the body that is leading directly to these signs and symptoms that make up the diagnosis.

We also may use the term disorder. A disorder does not necessarily have a pathological change in any cells, but there is some problem with functioning that is identifiable. An example of a disorder would be Attention Deficit and Hyperactivity Disorder. There are also syndromes. A syndrome is a list of signs and symptoms that tend to occur together. It's a clinical syndrome, but it may not be one specific disease. It may be multiple things. For example, amyotrophic lateral sclerosis or ALS, Lou Gehrig's disease—something that I treat—is actually a clinical syndrome, not a specific diagnosis.

It also is important to recognize that there are categories of diseases. Sometimes we may identify that a disease belongs to a certain category. For example, this is inflammatory versus nutritional versus degenerative, even though we can't get more specific than that. This all relates to how doctors make diagnoses in the first place. What do they mean? How do we understand and use them in medical practice?

Diseases tend to have a certain history over the course of our understanding of them. They generally begin as an identified clinical syndrome. We notice that different patients present with the same signs and symptoms that tend to have the same natural history. This means that they develop in the same way and they last for the same amount of time. This leads to the search for potential causes and risk factors. Risk factors will make somebody more likely to get it than someone else, like maybe particularly vulnerable populations or patterns of occurrence. This is epidemiological data that gives us a lot of clues about what might be causing an identified syndrome. For example, if it's spreading like an infection, maybe it's an infectious organism that's causing it.

Then, of course, we want to treat people. Ultimately, the goal of understanding the illness is to come up with treatments that are effective. We don't want to wait until we understand every last things about a disease or a disorder before we treat it. We try to treat it based upon sometimes just luck, just observing that some people do better with certain kinds of treatments. Alternatively, we try to understand based upon treatment trials. You may try different treatments to see if they work. Let's try antibiotics; if it is an infection, then that should work. It will also tell us something about what is causing it.

There are multiple different ways also to treat a syndrome or a disorder even before we completely understand its cause. Often, people think only in terms of curing a disease as if you can either only cure it or do nothing useful. In fact, most of what physicians do is not directly geared towards curing a disease or disorder. It is simply treating various aspects of it. For example, we may reduce the risk of developing a disease. We may slow its progression or even stop it from progressing. We may reverse some of the damage or disability that has resulted from the disease. We may alleviate symptoms and improve quality of life, prevent complications of the disease, or prolong survival with it. None of those things would be considered a cure, but they are all tremendously useful.

But, of course, we always want to understand as much as we can about the cause. We use the technical term "pathophysiology." That means everything about biologically that's happening with the disease. For example, in diabetes, we know there are certain cells in the pancreas that produce insulin and in type I diabetes, those cells are dying off. We know it's an autoimmune process that's killing off those cells. That's all the pathophysiology of type I diabetes.

Understanding pathophysiology is not all or nothing; it's not as if we know everything or we know nothing. Oftentimes, we deepen our understanding of a disease over time. We may at first realize that this is autoimmune. Then, we may understand what part of the immune system is malfunctioning and then what cells are being targeted. The knowledge can get deeper and deeper. We need to think of our knowledge about a disease as a spectrum, not an all or nothing thing. Further, one clinical syndrome may turn out to be many pathophysiological diseases, like the example of ALS that I gave before. It's almost certainly not one disease; it's probably two, three, or maybe even many.

Let me go over a little bit the types of names that we use in describing diseases. We call this the disease nomenclature. It's the way in which we classify different diseases. Nomenclatures usually start off describing just the clinical presentation. We attach a name to one version of a presentation that looks one way and another version that looks a slightly different way. As we understand, however, the true underlying cause of the disease, the nomenclature is often completely rewritten. For example, the muscular dystrophies were first named based upon clinical syndrome. But, over the years, we discovered specific genetic mutations that were causing specific muscular dystrophies. The nomenclature had to change. We renamed many of those diseases based upon the mutations as opposed to just how it was presenting clinically.

There are also different ways to make a diagnosis. There is what we call clinical diagnoses. A clinical diagnosis is based upon having a certain set of signs and symptoms. Symptoms are something the patient experiences; a sign is something you see when you examine a patient. There also are laboratory ways of either making or confirming a diagnosis. That means blood tests or x-rays, looking for anatomical or metabolic abnormalities. Oftentimes, these may make a specific diagnosis or a diagnosis may be a laboratory finding. For example, if you have vitamin B12 deficiency, it's based entirely on having low vitamin B12 levels in laboratory blood testing and that going along with having the clinical symptoms that are caused by a B12 deficiency.

There's also a special kind of laboratory test called a biopsy where we take a piece of a tissue and look at it under a microscope. When a diagnosis is made entirely by biopsy, we often call that a pathological diagnosis. With some diagnoses, the diagnosis is actually the name we give to a very specific pathological finding that you only see on a biopsy.

Doctors also sometimes make what we call a diagnosis of exclusion. You have an appropriate clinical syndrome and we rule out everything else that can cause that syndrome. What you're left with is the diagnosis of exclusion—something we know can cause those symptoms, but may not have any laboratory test to confirm it. We, for example, may diagnose patients with an Alzheimer's type dementia. That is a syndrome, not the disease Alzheimer's disease. Alzheimer's type dementia is what you have when you have dementia, chronic memory problems, and we've ruled out all the treatable causes. What you're left with is the diagnosis of exclusion, of Alzheimer's type dementia.

Also, since we're talking about these diagnostic labels that we attach to patients, it's important to recognize that treatment is not necessarily intimately tied to those labels. It often is, but often it isn't and that's important to recognize. The thresholds, if you will, for giving a treatment is not always the same as the threshold for making a specific diagnosis. The threshold could be higher or lower. In other words, I may give you a specific diagnosis, but you still don't meet the criteria for benefitting from a specific treatment. Also, I may not be able to really definitively answer the question about whether or not you have a certain diagnosis. But, you have enough findings that it's been demonstrated that you will do better long term if we give you a treatment. Thus, the treatment is often evidence-based and a different consideration from whether or not we attach a certain label to a presentation.

That's an overview of how we think about diagnoses and how we use them clinically. There are many problematic diagnoses, however, that are out there. They are different than diagnoses which are more clearly established, not controversial, and unambiguous. Here are some of the features that we have recognized to be wary of because they tend to occur with these problematic diagnoses. For example, they tend to be a clinical syndrome, not something that is tied to a specific laboratory finding.

They tend to have common symptoms. They have symptoms that we call the "symptoms of life." Anyone is likely to have them. Examples are pain, poor sleep, or the list of symptoms I went over at the beginning of this lecture. Many of the symptoms are vague or non-specific. This is a very important concept to understand. A specific symptom or sign is one that only one or a few or a narrow range of diseases will display.

At one end of the spectrum, we have signs that are what we call pathognomonic. That means that, if you have that sign or symptom, than you have that one diagnosis because it's the only thing that causes it. If you have an acute Lyme infection, for example, you're 70 percent likely to have what we call a bull's-eye or targeted rash. If you have that targeted rash, you have Lyme disease because it's the only thing that causes it. At the other end of the spectrum are maximally non-specific symptoms like fatigue. Hundreds, thousands of different things can cause you to just have low energy, to be fatigued. Therefore, having fatigue doesn't really narrow the list of possible diagnoses very much. It's very non-specific.

Problematic diagnoses also tend to be highly variable in their presentation. They don't have one very clearly identifiable natural history. The symptoms and signs that get attached to that diagnosis don't suggest one cohesive, coherent etiology. That's the fancy word for underlying cause. They have different symptoms that suggest different causes and don't all hang together. There's often also no clear pattern. Efforts to identify risk factors are not successful. They result in conflicting results or result in a pattern that is highly suggestive that these symptoms are due merely to stress or what we call a psychogenic illness.

There also tends to be what we call "diagnosis creep." Once you have a label—a questionable label based upon non-specific symptoms without anything very objective to verify it—then it tends to apply to a greater and greater expanding list of presentations, a broader and broader scope. Eventually, almost anyone or any symptom can be blamed on this broad diagnosis.

In addition, there's diagnosis expansion, which means applying it to milder and milder versions. Maybe there are some diagnoses which are legitimate when they are applied to very specific severe versions. Rather than broadening the application, it gets expanded to include milder and milder versions. Not everyone who's a little tired has chronic fatigue syndrome. Not every child who's a little overactive has ADHD. But, that, again, has a tendency to happen over time. Sometimes that does legitimately happen because it's tied to better data collection. For example, the definition of hypertension was expanded because it was found that lower levels of hypertension, high blood pressure, did increase the risk of heart attacks and strokes. It became more reasonable to include that in the definition.

Treating these problematic illnesses—when we have only a vague syndrome without anything specific to hang our hat on—is also, of course, problematic. They tend to be resistant to very specific biological interventions. They tend to benefit only temporarily from treatments that are likely to have what we call a placebo effect or placebo effects—which is something I will get into in much more detail in another lecture. They often respond to psychological interventions like stress reduction. They appear to respond to a variety of treatments that don't have a common or plausible underlying mechanism.

I mentioned before about the pathophysiology of disease. While we don't need to fully understand the pathophysiology or all the things that cause a disease biologically, the more and more we investigate a disease, the more we should learn about its pathophysiology. We begin to get a little suspicious if the more we investigate a questionable diagnosis, or a vague diagnosis, the less we seem to understand about the pathophysiology. If the people who are promoting the notion of this problematic diagnosis use what we call special pleading, they explain away all the lack of evidence that we would predict should be there if the disease had a specific biological cause, for example.

They use extreme speculation from preliminary or basic science. Basically, they take any little clue that pops up in pre-clinical or laboratory evidence and extrapolate that wildly to making clinical claims. That's another red flag to watch out for. The practitioners who make a specialty out of treating these controversial or problematic diagnoses also tend to share a few features. This should raise some red flags for you if you encounter them. One is that they often practice outside of the reach of regulation. They may have an offshore practice. Tijuana clinics are very popular because they're just across the border, but in Mexico where there are very, very lax regulations. That's always a red flag.

Often, they have to fend off attempts to bring them within the standard of care so they may be investigated by regulatory agencies for the quality of the care that they're delivering. They often will carve out special exceptions for their practices. They will sometimes use the political process in order to gain exemption from mechanisms that are meant to enforce a standard of care. They will often claim to be victims of a conspiracy, either of the medical establishment or the medical community, and that their ideas are being suppressed. They will often use unproven diagnostic techniques in order to prove their diagnoses and follow up with unproven therapeutic interventions.

With that as a background, I'm going to turn to some specific examples that will illustrate a lot of the features that I just discussed. I'm going to start with a very controversial disorder, chronic Lyme disease. Lyme disease is an infection caused by a bacterium, a spirochete, called Borrelia burgdorferi. It is not controversial. It is a well-established, pathophysiological infection. It is a real and serious illness. It was first identified in 1975. It's named after Lyme, Connecticut—my backyard—where it was first discovered. It's still endemic. However, we've now discovered several other species of Borrelia that can cause a Lyme infection syndrome. It has been recognized in different parts of North America and in Europe.

Lyme disease has several different stages to it like other spirochetes, like syphilis, for example. There is primary Lyme disease, which is the acute infection. There is also a secondary phase to Lyme disease where it's spreading throughout the body. It can go to the joints, heart, and nerves, for example. It may cause a Bell's palsy or a facial paralysis. It may cause shooting pains in different nerves that are affected. It may cause backaches, headaches, and joint stiffness. It can interfere with sleep and cause heart palpitations.

Then there's the most serious version of Lyme disease called tertiary Lyme. This is a chronic Lyme infection. Lyme has to go untreated or undertreated for a long period of time in order for this to occur. Tertiary Lyme will typically develop within two years of the initial infection. The Lyme spirochete here will set up a chronic infection in the joints or nervous system. When it's in the nervous system, we may call it a neuro-Lyme. It can have symptoms of memory loss, spinal involvement, and chronic meningitis. Because Lyme is a bacterial infection, it is treated with antibiotics. Several specific antibiotics have activity against the Borrelia spirochete and work quite well.

After a tick bite—before we even know there is an infection—there is evidence to show that a short course of oral doxycycline can reduce the risk of developing Lyme disease. That's now standard practice. When an infection is documented to occur, a course of oral doxycycline, amoxicillin, or cefuroxime—these are antibiotics that have activity against Borrelia burgdorferi—for a few weeks is effective in completely eliminating either stage I or stage II infections. If you have tertiary Lyme or neuro-Lyme, then you need intravenous antibiotics for up to six weeks with either ceftriaxone or penicillin. That's a much longer course with a more effective antibiotic that has good penetration into the nervous system in order to eradicate the infection.

How do we diagnose Lyme? It is based a lot on the clinical presentation. You have to have symptoms of an infection. The rash helps, but you don't need to have that rash. It's only present about 60 to 70 percent of the time. The confirmation is through blood tests. We look for antibodies, your immune system making antibodies against the bacteria. They take time to occur, though, so an acute infection may occur before there is time for the antibodies to occur. We may need to retest in six or eight weeks and then see the rising titers, as we call them, of the antibodies.

The initial blood test is usually what's called an ELISA test, which is a screening test. If that's positive, we can confirm it with a much more specific but involved test that's called a Western blot. Those are the two types of blood or spinal fluid tests that we would use. They have been shown to be very sensitive and specific, again, when enough time has passed. The controversy comes in with the notion of chronic Lyme disease that is either present without ever having a documented primary infection or that chronic infection that survives antibiotics. That's where we get into the controversy.

These occur in various settings. For example, the etiology is often unclear meaning that there was no documented infection. They may have non-specific symptoms. They may lack the symptoms that we ordinarily attach to Lyme disease. We can't find a chronic infection. When we look at the blood, the ELISA or the Western blot, it's not there. Oftentimes, they don't respond to treatment as we would predict either. Thus, there are many atypical features to people who present with chronic Lyme disease.

As I said, sometimes the presentation occurs or the claim is made for symptoms of chronic Lyme disease, this controversial entity, in people who never had Lyme disease. They are presenting with a syndrome of non-specific or vague symptoms. Sometimes, it follows a documented Lyme infection where someone is infected and they're treated. The infection itself is eradicated, but they have chronic symptoms following it.

In some cases, this may be due to—again, maybe legitimate—the fact that there are chronic problems with immune activity. Sometimes the immune system can be activated from an infection. You can have what's called a post-infectious syndrome. Sometimes the infection itself may have done damage. If it did get into the nervous system, then it may have caused damage to the nervous system and those symptoms are chronic. The notion of having chronic symptoms after having had Lyme disease is not controversial. That does sometimes occur. The real controversy is the notion that there's a chronic infection, an active infection that evades detection and treatment.

In essence, you have to believe in an atypical Lyme disease that's seronegative, meaning the blood work is negative, and that's treatment resistance. That is a lot of what we call special pleading. What does the evidence show? If we look at the evidence, it does not support the notion that there's a chronic Lyme infection that survives adequate antibiotic treatment. We have looked at several studies of antibiotics in patients who are often diagnosed as having chronic Lyme. In this case, we're not asking the question, do people have chronic Lyme infection? We're just asking, do they get better if we treat them with antibiotics? There, the answer is clearly no. There have been several studies which show no benefit.

Let's move on to another very controversial syndrome, chronic fatigue syndrome. In order to make the diagnosis of chronic fatigue syndrome or CFS, you need to have chronic fatigue that lasts for more than six months without another documented cause like Multiple Sclerosis or lupus—which are chronic diseases which can cause chronic fatigue by themselves. In many cases, it's therefore a diagnosis of exclusion. You have fatigue and we've ruled out all other causes so you're left with just this chronic fatigue.

In some, a chronic infection with a virus has been documented. We do have here a pathophysiological disease in some cases. The Epstein-Barr virus and other viruses have been implicated in some cases. However, in many cases the diagnosis is questionable because there's no documented infection or patients don't meet the strict criteria for the diagnosis. The risk here, if we prematurely apply the label of chronic fatigue syndrome to patients who have fatigue, is that we'll miss the real underlying cause. The Centers for Disease Control, the CDC, estimates that as many as 40 percent of the people who are diagnosed with chronic fatigue syndrome actually have a serious and treatable underlying disease that's being missed. That's the danger of prematurely applying a label to someone.

At times, the true underlying diagnosis may be socially or personally undesirable. For example, people may be chronically fatigued because they have a sleep disorder or they may have a psychiatric disorder like depression and anxiety. Rather than accept that diagnosis, they search for another diagnosis that they would find more acceptable.

Let's move to fibromyalgia. I encounter a lot of patients who walk into my office with the diagnosis of fibromyalgia, but what is it really? It does remain somewhat controversial. However, like chronic fatigue syndrome, there appears to be a vaguely, but probably genuine, pathophysiological disease that involves a chronic low level of inflammation in the muscles and the fascia. The fascia is the connective tissue that surrounds the muscles. But, in order to make the diagnosis, you have to have symptoms that last for three or more months and you need to have specific tender points.

There are 18 identified tender points on the body and you need to have 11 of them. When you meet those full criteria, then it's reasonable to apply the diagnosis of fibromyalgia. It's still a clinical syndrome without a really well understood pathophysiology, but at least there are strict criteria so we can talk about it as an entity. However, most people who are walking around with the diagnosis of fibromyalgia don't meet those strict criteria. The diagnosis is often applied to anyone who has chronic unexplained muscle pain or aches while the underlying cause is often not adequately assessed. That means that, like with chronic fatigue syndrome, it can lead to missed diagnoses. For example, many people who are diagnosed with fibromyalgia have chronic sleep deprivation. That diagnosis is missed because they're prematurely labeled with a vague or non-specific diagnosis. They may also have chronic depression. They may have something else, a less specific diagnosis than fibromyalgia—just a myofascial pain syndrome. We're beginning to get a handle on some of the underlying changes to the tissue that are causing those.

But, again, if you don't look for it because you've already settled prematurely on a vague diagnosis, you'll miss the opportunity to make a more useful diagnosis. Still, it exists as a syndrome and for that reason, it has been studied therapeutically. There are actually two drugs on the market that are approved in the United States by the FDA for the treatment of fibromyalgia. They are Cymbalta and Lyrica.

Another syndrome that I don't think has a kernel of legitimacy to it is multiple chemical sensitivity. This is alleged to be a cumulative effect of exposure to toxins and chemicals in the environment. Symptoms do not follow any clear pathophysiology, however. There's no documented pathology. There's none of the effects that you would expect from any specific toxin or chemical. This goes as far, in some patients, as alleging sensitivity to electromagnetic waves. However, studies have failed to find any consistent pattern or effect to either electromagnetic waves or again, just a cumulative effect of chemicals in the environment.

Another diagnosis similar to multiple chemical sensitivity is candida hypersensitivity. Candida albicans is a fungus. It's very common. Many of us colonized with it. It exists on our bodies, but not causing an infection. It can cause infection and usually crops up in the immunocompromised or people who are on antibiotics. However, there are those who think that chronic undiagnosed, mysterious candida infections can be responsible for an epidemic of symptoms such as fatigue, irritability, constipation, diarrhea, and the list goes on. Again, they are all of the non-specific and vague symptoms of life that tend to get attached to these vague syndromes.

Candida hypersensitivity exists in the absence of the expected signs of candida infection or allergy. The signs we expect to be there are not there. There's a claimed connection by some to multiple chemical sensitivity and also to causing diseases such as Multiple Sclerosis and chronic fatigue syndrome. But, there's no evidence to support any of these connections. The notion of chronic candida hypersensitivity was started largely by a Dr. C. Orian Truss in 1978 when he published his findings in a fringe journal followed by a popular book. However, there was no evidence or research trail to back up his claims. It was really nothing more than pure speculation on the part of a single individual.

The American Academy of Allergy, Asthma, and Immunology have come to their conclusion after reviewing all of the evidence regarding chronic candida. They concluded that it is speculative and unproven. Its supposed symptoms are essentially universal, the symptoms of life. It results in the overuse of oral antifungal agents and while adverse effects from oral antifungal agents are rare, they are inevitable. The anecdotal experience is often misleading.

In conclusion, I think we've covered a lot of information about what doctors think about when they're making a diagnosis. There are a lot of pitfalls and it can often be very tricky to make an adequate diagnosis. The approach that we often take is to look for things that we know to treat, know how to treat, and know how to diagnose. These are all of the biological or serious entities that could plausibly cause the symptoms that a patient or a client is presenting with. If we make a diagnosis, then we treat based upon the diagnosis that we make. We find any contributing factors and we essentially treat what we find.

But, maybe we will rule out—we'll whittle away—all of the known pathological contributors or causes of a disease. We're left with a syndrome of symptoms without a clear biological cause, but we have ruled out anything serious or treatable. In that case, it's most effective to then shift our emphasis to treating the patient to improve their quality of life. That is very, very important and should not be neglected. We shouldn't get distracted from treating quality of life because of a search for a diagnosis that may not be there or just for the false comfort of having a label to attach to symptoms.

Herbalism and Herbal Medicines
Lecture 14

The history of herbalism goes back farther than the human species itself. Many animals will chew on different plants when they have symptoms or infections.

Herbalism is the appealing notion of using plants to strengthen our health and treat medical symptoms, but what does science tell us about modern herbalism? You may be surprised to learn that modern herbalism is scientific. In fact, the core myth of this lecture is that there's something fundamentally different between herbalism and modern pharmacology. They are both part of the same science, which is identifying useful substances that have some biochemical effect in the body that can be exploited. Herbalism, or phytotherapy, simply restricts its range to plant-derived substances.

Pharmacognosy is the study of drugs or drug substances of natural origin as well as the search for new drugs from natural sources. A lot of modern pharmacology derives from the study of the health effects of plants or things that are derived from plants. Many modern drugs, for example, themselves are plant components. Modern pharmacology, which includes studying plants and other natural sources, has a specific definition. Essentially, a pharmacological agent or drug is any substance that has a biochemical effect on the body, including the microbes in the body, beyond its purely nutritional value.

In short, herbs are drugs. But in some countries, like the United States, herbs are marketed as if they were supplements. They are regulated as if they were food or vitamins. Herbs often have many active ingredients. The justification for this is the notion of synergy: that different substances individually might not have much of an effect but when taken together have a useful clinical effect. There can be synergistic effects in herbs; however, we can't assume that that's the case. We need to base any such determination on actual scientific evidence.

It also needs to be noted that chemical substances in plants or herbs—which are taken for their pharmacological activity—have the same range of side effects and toxicities that other drugs do. We should not fall into the false dichotomy of thinking that herbs are fundamentally different from drugs.

What about dosing? One of the primary advantages to the drug development process is that we isolate a specific chemical. We can then deliver it in amounts that are very precisely measured. When herbs are studied, it turns out that many have tremendous variations in the amount of active ingredients they contain. Part of the reason for this is the variation from plant to plant. It's very hard to control for the amount of active ingredients just by using a certain amount of the plant itself.

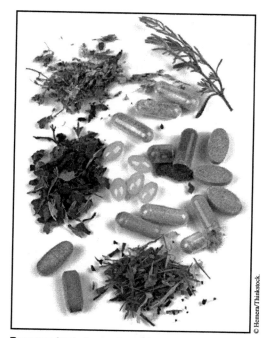

© Hemera/Thinkstock.

Because herbal supplements are not regulated, their purity and dosing are not guaranteed.

One thing we've learned in the last hundred years or so of doing scientific experiments for medical treatments is that, for every hundred or so treatments that look very promising in the laboratory, very few of them actually make it all the way through clinical research and are shown to be safe and effective in people. Sometimes there are in vitro or preclinical data that suggest a potential role for an herb, but it isn't appropriate to extrapolate from these preclinical studies to clinical claims.

Another area of concern is that recently it's come to light that many herbal products are contaminated. Some of them contain other herbs that are not on the label. A 2009 study of herbal remedies that were purchased over the Internet found that about 20% of them were contaminated with heavy metals above safe limits. This included lead, mercury, and arsenic—some as much as 10,000 times the safe limits. This raises the notion that we need better quality control.

We should not fall into the false dichotomy of thinking that herbs are fundamentally different from drugs.

Plants are legitimate sources of safe and effective drugs. We have explored them to discover many useful chemicals. Much of the low-hanging fruit has already been picked, but there is still a lot of research that can be done. There may be very effective drugs, treatments, and even herbal preparations out there waiting to be discovered by careful research. But herbal remedies today are poorly regulated. Herbs need to be recognized as the drugs they are and regulated appropriately so that they can be used safely and effectively. ■

Suggested Reading

ICON Group International, *Pharmacognosy.*

Samuelsson and Bohlin, *Drugs of Natural Origin.*

Questions to Consider

1. Should herbs be regulated as food supplements or as drugs?

2. What does the scientific evidence say about the most popular herbal remedies?

Herbalism and Herbal Medicines
Lecture 14—Transcript

In Tanzania, a young female suffering from intestinal parasites chews on the succulent shoots of a small tree called Vernonia amygdalina. Within a day, her symptoms are relieved. Even more interesting is that this is a young female chimpanzee. Herbalism is a very appealing notion of using plants in order to treat our symptoms and for health. But, what does science really tell us about modern herbalism?

The history of herbalism goes back farther than the human species itself. Many animals will chew on different plants when they have symptoms or infections, for example. Every culture has managed, through mostly trial and error, to identify many local plants that have useful medicinal and even recreational purposes. For example, many ancient cultures identified that caraway can be used for indigestion. There are an estimated 400,000 known plant species around the world, likely even more. This is a vast natural chemical laboratory.

A lot of the older notions that are bound up with herbalism tend to be mystical in nature, like many beliefs that originated thousands of years ago. The notion that some plants contain a mixture of substances that are specifically designed to be useful medically for people is a mystical one—not one that is in line with modern science. It also tends to be a very anthropocentric view of nature. It is certainly incompatible with an evolutionary view, which tells us that plants, like other things, evolve for their own survival. There's no particular reason to think that any individual plant will have a special combination of many substances which are designed to be beneficial for human health.

Despite these mystical roots, it would be silly to ignore the vast potential of science-based herbalism. Again, this vast chemical laboratory out there is just waiting for us to explore it. Modern herbalism is scientific. It has the same kind of relationship to mystical herbalism as does say modern chemistry does to alchemy or modern astronomy does to astrology. We don't ignore or minimize these sciences because of their pre-scientific roots.

In fact, the core myth, if you will, of this lecture is that there's something fundamentally different between herbalism and modern pharmacology. In fact, they're all part of the same science which is identifying useful substances that have some biochemical effect in the body that can be exploited. Herbalism, or phytotherapy as it's sometimes called, simply restricts its range to using plant-derived substances rather than anything.

There's also a term called "pharmacognosy." That is the study of drugs or drug substances of natural origin as well as the search for new drugs from natural sources. A lot of modern pharmacology derives from the study of the health effects of plants or things that are derived from plants. Many modern drugs, for example, themselves are plant components. For example, quinine was originally derived from the cinchona bark. Poppy or opium is a source for morphine and all opiates, which is an important class of pain relieving drugs. Digitalis was originally purified from foxglove, a pretty flower. I actually have one in my backyard. Digitalis is used for many heart conditions that basically can affect heart electrical function. This is still a very active area of research.

Modern pharmacology, which includes studying plants and other natural sources, has a specific definition. Essentially, a pharmacological agent or drug is any substance that has a biochemical effect on the body, including the microbes in the body, beyond its purely nutritional value. Thus, things that are just nutrients are not drugs by their nature. It alters the biochemistry or function of some or all of the cells in the body. When herbs are taken to have a biochemical effect on the body, they are being used like drugs. Again, I want to dispel that false dichotomy that something fundamentally different is going on.

How do drugs work? What do we mean by "effect the biochemistry of the body?" Pharmacology is largely an attempt to understand all the different ways that we can interact with the body in order to affect function and health—treating symptoms and altering the course of diseases, for example.

Let me run through the types of mechanisms of drugs so we can better understand them. One thing that drugs do is they bind to receptors on cells. Cells communicate with each other. They read their environment by having chemical signals bind to receptors on or even inside cells. A substance that binds to those receptors and either activates them or blocks or inactivates them is one pharmacological mechanism of some drugs.

Drugs may also alter the effects of enzymes. An enzyme is a protein that will make a biochemical reaction go faster. By interacting with them, a drug may either increase or decrease the rate of a biochemical reaction. Drugs may also activate, inhibit, or mimic the effect of hormones, which are a specific class of substances which do signal throughout the body. They're part of the endocrine system.

Drugs may have antimicrobial activity. They may alter the activity of neurotransmitters which are core to nervous system functioning. They may affect brain or nerve function by increasing or decreasing the activity of neurotransmitters. They may alter ion channels. These are protein channels on the surface of cells that affect and control the flow of charged ions into and out of the cell. They are very important for cell function. They may also alter transcription, the rate at which transfer RNA is transcribed into proteins or it increase or decrease proteins.

There are other mechanisms still. There are osmotic agents which alter fluid inside the body. They may cause fluid to go from one part of the body or compartment to another. Other drugs may interfere with cell division or important steps in synthesis such as chemotherapeutic agents used to treat cancer. There are still other drugs with other functions.

In addition to the actual pharmacological activity that a drug has, we like to know as much about how a drug interacts with the body as possible. They are very important and powerful tools in medicine so therefore, we like to understand them as much as possible. These other aspects of drug are broken down into two broad categories. Those categories are pharmacodynamics—ways in which the drug affects the body, like many of the things that I just mentioned—and pharmacokinetics.

Pharmacokinetics you can think of as the ways in which the body affects the drug. Pharmacokinetics includes things like how the drug is eliminated from the body. Is it through the liver, kidney, or some other way? How is it metabolized? Is it detoxified by the liver or maybe there are active metabolites—the drug is turned into other drugs that have other functions. We also like to know what the half life of a drug is. How long does it hang around inside the body and where does it go? Which parts of the body does it have access to? Is it protein bound? Many substances are bound by proteins in our blood and protein binding may inactivate part or all of a drug in our blood.

Another very important aspect of drugs is bioavailability. This essentially means how much of a substance we take by a certain route gets into our body and gets to the site where it has its activity. Bioavailability is critical to understanding what the ultimate effect of a drug is going to be in the body. It also determines how a drug can be taken—internally or orally, you can eat it; intravenously; injected into a muscle; or given rectally and absorbed through the rectal mucosa. Those are the common ways in which drugs are given.

It also involves how much is metabolized. When you take a drug orally, it gets absorbed in the intestines. The blood that absorbs the things from the intestines passes through the liver, through the portal system. This gives the liver an opportunity to get a first crack at any substance which gets absorbed into our system through the intestines. It may detoxify, it may metabolize a drug before it has a chance to really get distributed to the rest of the body. Even when a drug's getting into the body, the first pass through the liver inactivate most of it. Essentially, this determines how effective or how potent a drug is going to be in terms of how much is going to get to the target tissue.

Drug development is largely the process of identifying and isolating very specific active ingredients, a specific molecule. This often does start with identifying the effects of a plant. Then, it's looking at the dozens, sometimes hundreds of individual chemicals or molecules in the parts of that plant. Next, it's isolating individual ones and then seeing what their bioavailability, pharmacokinetics, and pharmacodynamics are. At that point, chemists may get involved. They may tweak or alter the chemical structure of that molecule in order to increase bioavailability or to make it less toxic, for example.

Once the chemists have identified and altered, if necessary, a molecule, it needs to go into actual testing. This breaks down into two basic phases or categories. There is preclinical research which is everything before we give it to people. This includes in vitro studies. In vitro literally translates to "in glass," and is done in test tubes or Petri dishes. Then, there are in vivo studies, "in life," which are studies in animals. Once we've learned as much as we can from in vitro and animal studies—and if a new candida drug appears to be basically safe and may have some interesting effects that we want to exploit—then we move on to the second type of research called clinical trials.

Clinical trials have four phases. The first phase is giving small doses to healthy people just to make sure it doesn't have any unanticipated side effects and to learn more about its pharmacodynamics and pharmacokinetics. Phase II trials are small, preliminary studies in target patients, patients with a symptom or a disease that we would be interested in treating. If a drug is safe and shows promise at that point in time, then it goes on to phase III trials. These are large, definitive clinical trials. Those are the trials that determine if a drug is going to get approved for the marketplace. Once a drug is on the market, we do what are sometimes called phase IV studies which is post-marketing research. Essentially, we continue to follow a drug and look for any rare side effects that were not seen during the actual experimental research.

In light of all of that, we want to think about what herbs actually are. Herbs have pharmacological effects. They have substances which have pharmacokinetics and pharmacodynamics. They are taken so that they can have some kind of biochemical effect similar to what I described. In short, herbs are drugs. But, in some countries, like in the United States for example, they're actually marketed as if they were supplements. They are regulated as food or as if they were vitamins.

However, they're generally not taken for their nutritional value. They are taken as pharmacologically active ingredients—drugs. Herbs, in fact, often have many active ingredients because they're not purified. The justification for this is the notion of synergy; that different substances maybe individually don't have much of an effect, but when taken together they have an important useful clinical effect.

There is, again, a kernel of truth to that as there often is to misconceptions. There are some times where we would combine two or three substances together because they have some synergistic quality. Maybe they have the same effect but with different side effects so we can get the same ultimate clinical effect while minimizing side effects. Maybe one substance increases the bioavailability of another, the one that actually has the pharmacological effect that we're going for.

But, these kinds of synergistic effects can only be discovered after doing careful research and combining substances in a way that makes sense. It would be an awful coincidence if they occurred together in the same plant through chance alone. There's no particular reason to think that evolution would select for such combinations. It can still occur. There can be synergistic effects in herbs; however, we can't assume that that's the case. We would hopefully want to base any such determination on actual scientific evidence.

It also needs to be noted that these chemical substances in plants or herbs— which are taken for their pharmacological activity—have the same range of side effects and toxicities that any other drugs do. Again, we don't want to fall into the false dichotomy of thinking that herbs are fundamentally different than drugs.

What about dosing? One of the primary advantages to the drug development process is that we isolate a specific chemical. We can then deliver it in amounts that are very precisely measured. We have some idea about what the bioavailability is, how much is going to get into the blood, what the blood levels are going to be, and what the half-life is or how long they're going to stay there. With herbs we often don't have all or even any of this information. In fact, when herbs are studied for their likely active ingredients, it turns out that many products have tremendous variations in the amount of active ingredients in various products.

For example, a 2003 study of St. John's Wort shows a 17-fold difference when looking at markers for how much St. John's Wort is actually in the tablet from one pill to the next pill—even in the same bottle. One brand was compared to another brand and compared to the labeled dose. The amount that researchers found in the pills in the bottle varied from 0 percent—meaning that the label was accurate—to 109 percent, meaning that there could be twice as much or half as much in the pills as was on the label. Therefore, it makes it very challenging to give a precise dose when you don't even know how much of the active ingredients are in the products that you're giving.

Part of the reason for this variability is that there is a tremendous amount of variation from plant to plant. The amount of different chemicals in a St. John's Wort plant, for example, can differ from season to season, from plant to plant, from one part of the plant to another, and from year to year based upon environmental conditions. It's very hard to control for the amount of active ingredients just by giving a certain amount of the plant itself.

There are also issues that come up with quality control. Often, there is the lack of standardization beyond the notion of dose. Claims for different types of popular herbal remedies are often based upon folklore, pure marketing, or at best, anecdotal or uncontrolled experience—not hard, scientific evidence. Sometimes there are in vitro or pre-clinical data, which is interesting. It may suggest a potential role for an herb, but then those findings are extrapolated to clinical claims.

One thing we've learned in the last hundred years or so of doing scientific experiments for medical treatments is that, for every hundred or so treatments that look very promising in the laboratory, very few of them actually make it all the way through clinical research and are shown to be safe and effective in people. It really isn't appropriate to extrapolate from these preclinical studies to clinical claims.

There is also the issue of bioavailability. A substance that's part of an herb or an entire herb may have very interesting effects when you look at what they're doing to cells in a Petri dish, but that doesn't mean that those constituents are going to get to those cells in your body. Most drugs fail because they lack adequate bioavailability. Any particular plant at random is statistically unlikely to have adequate bioavailability for the putative active ingredients.

Recently it's come to our attention also that many herbal products are contaminated. They may have other herbs in them that are not on the label. Sometimes, Chinese herbal remedy names may refer to several different plant species. There have been some cases where the wrong herb was given because of this confusion leading to significant toxicity. A 2009 study of herbal remedies that were purchased over the Internet found that about 20 percent of them were contaminated with heavy metals above safe limits. This included lead, mercury, and arsenic, some as much as 10,000 times the safe limits. Again, this raises the notion that we need better quality control.

I'm going to talk about some of the most popular herbal remedies that are on the market in light of what we have said up to this point. Starting with echinacea, in the middle of the 2000 aughts, if you will, echinacea was the most popular herbal remedy on the market. Echinacea is also called purple coneflower. It comes in various plant species, most commonly promoted for the prevention or the treatment of the common cold.

This was first popularized by a German-American, H. C. F. Meyer, in the late 1800s. He claimed he discovered the remedy from the Plains Indians. The Plains Indians did use echinacea for many things including snake bites and toxicity, but it was never specifically used by them for the common cold. Meyer simply made this up and used the Plains Indians as a popular marketing ploy for the time.

Of course, American Indians also used many other plants for many reasons. They used tobacco, for example, as an herbal remedy. The fact that an indigenous population used an herb at all, let alone for a particular purpose, doesn't necessarily mean that it would hold up to modern scientific investigation as to its safety or effectiveness. However, this does become a very popular marketing strategy. Meyer himself marketed echinacea as a cure-all. He even claimed that it would cure cancer. In Europe, it really became most popularly recommended for the common cold. But, this was not based upon any preexisting evidence or the actual history of use of echinacea. Like with all of these claims, the history is interesting in how the claims came about. But, at the end of the day, the scientific evidence trumps everything else.

Initially, what we see with herbal remedies—as with many things in medicine—there are many small, preliminary studies. Usually, the results of such small and preliminary studies are mixed. They're all over the place. Some show benefit; some don't show benefit. In essence, we're asking, is there any even potential here to justify doing more involved, rigorous, and large clinical trials?

The largest and best controlled clinical trials that were eventually done in echinacea showed that it had no benefit in the prevention or treatment of the common cold. The biggest one was an NIH study published in the *New England Journal of Medicine* in 2005. They compared three preparations of echinacea versus placebo—a null or inactive substance—in 437 healthy adults. They found, unequivocally, no effect, no benefit from echinacea.

Those who are selling echinacea for claims that it cured the common cold criticize this research. They said that there are different species of echinacea and therefore, the one that was used in the study wasn't the correct one. They said that different parts of the plant are used. The root, herb, flower, or the whole plant can be used. Therefore, studying one part doesn't tell you anything about the other parts. There are various preparation methods—dried herbs, extracts, or fresh-pressed juice. Therefore, again, testing one doesn't tell you about the others. Also, preparations contain combinations of species or plant parts and only purified ones or extracts were used in the study.

However, this amounts to nothing more than special pleading, an excuse for why these studies turned out to be negative. If what they're saying is true, then how could you know that any particular preparation of echinacea in fact worked? The results of the published research by the NIH did have an effect on the popularity on this remedy. At one time, it was a $300 million per year market in the United States alone. It represented about 10 percent of the herbal market. But, after this, it dropped to about half of that. That still means that, even in the wake of pretty negative evidence, there is still a multi-million dollar industry for echinacea as an herbal remedy for the common cold.

Let's go on to ginkgo biloba, another very common herb that is claimed to have benefit for memory, mental function, and maybe even Alzheimer's disease itself, a degenerative form of chronic dementia. The proposed mechanism for ginkgo biloba is that it is a blood thinner. It thins the blood a little bit. This may lead to improved circulation including improved blood flow to the brain.

However, on close examination, this is not a very plausible mechanism of action. Blood flow to the brain is actually already quite carefully regulated. Unless you have end-stage vascular disease, disease of the blood vessels in your brain, a slight thinning of the blood is not going to improve blood flow and oxygen deliver to your brain. For most people, it doesn't make any sense that a mild blood thinner would have benefits. In some people with vascular disease, it could make sense. However, if that is the case, we have other blood thinning agents like aspirin, which is much more effective actually than ginkgo biloba. If ginkgo works by that putative mechanism for dementia, then aspirin should work much better. But, as always, we could talk endlessly about mechanism and putative mechanism. At the end of the day, that needs to be put in the context of actual clinical research. Does it work?

A 2008 study published in the *Journal of the American Medical Association* showed: "In this study, G biloba at 120 mg twice a day was not effective in reducing either the overall incidence rate of dementia or Alzheimer's disease incidence in elderly individuals with normal cognition or those with minimal symptoms of dementia or minimal cognitive impairment." That's a long way of saying that ginkgo biloba doesn't work for memory or dementia.

How about St. John's Wort, the one that I've mentioned previously? This comes from the plant Hypericum perforatum. It is claimed to be beneficial for mild depression. The clinical evidence, again, shows mixed results. Perhaps there is some benefit for mild depression, but not for serious depression. A large trial in major depression was negative. But again, the evidence shows that there may be some benefit for mild depression.

Interestingly, St. John's Wort contains several potential active ingredients including a monoamine oxidase inhibitor. This has already been identified as a class of drugs that is effective for treating depression. What more evidence is there that St. John's Wort is a drug? It actually contains previously identified drugs that are active in depression so it certainly is plausible that it can have some effectiveness. But, is it a good strategy for treating depression? We have all the old problems that I mentioned about dosing and purity. In addition, because it is a drug, recent evidence has shown us that St. John's Wort has all of the drug-drug interactions that you would expect a drug to have.

Most notably, it reduces the effectiveness of anti-HIV drugs—a population of patients for which St. John's Wort was being specifically recommended to treat mild depression. It also induces enzymes in a liver system that we call the P450 enzyme system. This is a very common enzyme system that metabolizes drugs. When you induce or increase the activity of these enzymes, it can decrease the effectiveness of other drugs that are also metabolized by the P450 system. St. John's Wort may contribute to serotonin syndrome, a side effect of antidepressants.

Let's turn now to saw palmetto. This comes from the fruit of the Serenoa repens plant. It is used for benign prostatic hypertrophy or enlargement of the prostate which is very common in men. Most men will develop some degree of BPH by the time they get into their 70s. A 2009 Cochrane review of clinical trials concluded: "Serenoa repens was not more effective than placebo for treatment of urinary symptoms consistent with BPH." Unfortunately, there is no effect.

Another one is black cohosh. It is used for symptoms of menopause like hot flashes, mood disturbances, diaphoresis, palpitations, and vaginal dryness. The mechanism is not clear, but we do know that there are no clear estrogen receptor effects. That's the most common mechanism that you would think about it. If it does improve those symptoms, then maybe it's working through estrogen receptors. That's been pretty much ruled out, but it may work through some other mechanism. Again, biology is complex. We can't always reach definitive opinions based upon mechanism alone.

The clinical data, unfortunately, is scanty. It's only short-term and the results are mixed. At this point in time, we simply cannot say if black cohosh is effective in treating symptoms of menopause. But, there is a special caution in women with a history of breast cancer. This is because some drugs that are used to treat the same symptoms can increase the risk of recurrence from breast cancer. Therefore, it's reasonable to assume the same precautions until we understand more about this particular herb.

In conclusion, plants are legitimate sources of safe and effective drugs. Again, it is a very useful natural laboratory of chemicals. We have already explored a lot of it in order to discover many useful chemicals. Much of the low-hanging fruit, in fact, has already been picked—the very effective drugs that are in common plants that we know about. But, there is still a lot of research that can be done. There may be very effective drugs, treatments, and even herbal preparations out there waiting to be discovered by careful research.

However, herbal remedies today are poorly regulated. They're mainly regulated as if they were food or supplements; they are not regulated as drugs, which they clearly are. In fact, they are drugs that have highly variable dosing and poor quality control. While I have nothing against the concept of using plant-derived substances or even straight herbs for health benefits, I think it's important to avoid the false dichotomy of thinking that herbs are acting somehow differently than drugs. I think they should be recognized as the drugs they are and regulated appropriately so that they can be used safely and effectively.

Homeopathy—One Giant Myth
Lecture 15

Homeopathy ... is even more popular in Europe than in the United States. In Europe, it is a $1.4 billion a year market, according to *Business Week*. It is popular with the British Royal family and is currently supported by the NHS [National Health Service].

There are a lot of misconceptions about what homeopathy is. Many people think that homeopathy means herbal medicine or natural medicine, but this is not true. Homeopathy, in fact, is a 200-year-old philosophy-based system. It's based on the notion of vitalism, the idea that living creatures have an essence or vital force that animates them. Homeopathy survives today due to cultural inertia and despite a complete lack of scientific evidence.

Homeopathy was developed by Christian Friedrich Samuel Hahnemann (1755–1843), a German medical doctor. In the 1790s, Hahnemann came up with several laws that govern the actions of homeopathic remedies. The first law of homeopathy is called the law of similars. He claimed to discover this principle when he noted that the cinchona bark, which is used to treat malaria, caused him to have symptoms very similar to those of malaria. He therefore generalized this one observation to this law, which became one of the cornerstones of homeopathy.

Hahnemann's next law is the law of infinitesimals. He believed that substances transferred their essence to water in which they were diluted. The greater the dilution, the greater this transference of essence was. The law of the individual remedy states that each person's totality of symptoms has a single underlying cause. Therefore, homeopathic remedies are intended to treat all of those symptoms at once with a single remedy. Homeopathic remedies also include the notion of potentiation. Between each dilution, homeopathic remedies are potentiated by succussing them. That means shaking them in a certain way; this is more of a ritual than science or chemistry.

What does the clinical evidence show? There have actually been hundreds of clinical studies of homeopathic remedies. After reviewing all of the evidence for homeopathy, the scientific community has come to the conclusion that there is no evidence to support homeopathy for any indication. Also, homeopathic remedies are no different than placebos.

The scientific community has come to the conclusion that there is no evidence to support homeopathy for any indication.

There are many homeopathic products on the market, however. They are marketed because of loose regulations without evidence for either safety or effectiveness. Homeopathic remedies are generally safe, because they're usually just water. There is no active ingredient, so they don't really have the potential to cause direct harm. But this is not universally true of homeopathic remedies. Some homeopathic products cheat the system by including measurable levels of active ingredients but using the homeopathic label to skirt regulations.

One example is Zicam. This is a product that was marketed as homeopathic. Some preparations of it have measureable and meaningful amounts of zinc oxide, which is shown to treat and reduce the symptoms of a cold. However, zinc oxide is also known to cause anosmia, a sometimes permanent loss of the ability to smell. Several people who were using Zicam had permanent anosmia as a side effect. That caused regulatory agencies to take a second look at it and to temporarily suspend it from the market.

One justification for the ultradilutions of homeopathic remedies that's often given is the analogy to vaccines or allergy shots. This is a myth and not an apt analogy. A vaccine contains a measurable, if small, amount of antigen meant to stimulate the immune system. Allergy shots give a small amount of a substance to which one is allergic in order to provoke the immune system to make blocking antibodies. They make antibodies to the substance to help prevent an allergic reaction. In order for allergy shots to work, you have to give a small dose and then build it up to increasingly larger doses. Eventually, you're giving a fairly significant dose in order to provoke a sufficient immune response. Therefore, there is no analogy whatsoever to a preparation that has no measurable amount of anything in it.

Testimonials and anecdotes tend to support what people want to believe. There are also placebo effects, which can make anything seem to work. There's also often a failure to recognize the harm that could be done with these types of interventions. I mentioned that homeopathy mostly is a completely inactive substance; it's just water without any active ingredient. Some people will say if it does nothing, how could it possibly do any harm? The harm often comes in preventing effective treatment. There are many cases of harm occurring to people relying upon homeopathic remedies who could have easily been treated with modern medicine.

There's a broader intellectual conflict that's represented by homeopathy. It's between science-based medicine—what we recognize today as the modern scientific approach to biology, healing, and disease—and what we would now think of as magical thinking. Over the last 200 years, the scientific approach has clearly won out. It has produced all of modern medicine, whereas homeopathy is stuck in the 200-year-old ideas of its founder. Completely inert treatment may have actually been an advantage to what was passing for standard medicine 200 years ago. But today, science-based medicine has brought us a host of effective treatments. ■

Suggested Reading

Barrett, "Homeopathy."

Ernst, *Homeopathy*.

House of Commons Science and Technology Committee, "Evidence Check 2."

Science-Based Medicine (blog), "Homeopathy."

Questions to Consider

1. Do you know what the central claims of homeopathy really are?

2. Why has homeopathy survived as long as it has, despite a complete lack of scientific validation?

Homeopathy—One Giant Myth
Lecture 15—Transcript

In this lecture, I'm going to talk all about homeopathy. There are a lot of misconceptions about what homeopathy actually is. Most people I speak with think that homeopathy means herbal medicine or natural medicine, but this is not true at all. Homeopathy, in fact, is a 200-year-old philosophy-based system. It's based upon the notion that we call "vitalism." It's the notion that living creatures have an essence, a living energy, or vital force that animates them. It survives today due to cultural inertia; cultural beliefs tend to last for a long time. It survives despite a complete lack of scientific evidence.

Interestingly, homeopathy is very loosely regulated in many countries. In 1938, the Food, Drug, and Cosmetic Act created an inclusion for homeopathic remedies so that they did not require any testing for safety or effectiveness. They essentially were grandfathered in or automatically included as approved substances. Items listed in the homeopathic material medica and its supplements are automatically approved according to the FDA rules from this act. This resulted from one man, Senator Royal Copeland, a senator from New York. He was a homeopath and he sponsored the 1938 FDA bill. He added in the exemption for homeopathic products.

Homeopathy, however, is even more popular in Europe than in the United States. In Europe, it is a $1.4 billion a year market, according to *Business Week*. It is popular with the British Royal family and is currently supported by the NHS. It's not regulated at all in countries like Germany and Austria although other countries in Europe do require some licensing in order to prescribe homeopathic treatments.

Let's go back to homeopathy's roots. I think that will give us a more thorough understanding of what it actually is. Christian Friedrich Samuel Hahnemann, 1755 to 1843, was a German medical doctor who gave up his medical practice and developed the principles of homeopathy in the 1790s. These were first published in a paper describing homeopathy in 1796. Hahnemann came up with the term "homeopathy." He also came up with the term "allopathy." That describes his thinking about the medicine of the time.

Allopathy, which means "against the symptoms" was a term that he used to describe bloodletting, purging, and leaches—the kind of treatments that medical doctors were doing at the time. Treating the imbalances in the four humors is an example. He came up with the term homeopathy to describe his system of working with symptoms. It refers to his intent—that working with the symptoms was the way to restore wellness.

Hahnemann came up with several laws, what he considered to be scientific laws that govern the actions of homeopathic remedies. The first law of homeopathy is called the Law of Similars or like cures like. This is partly based upon the more ancient notion of sympathetic magic. In many cultures, there were many beliefs that, for example, rhino horns would be a treatment for impotence because it resembles a certain body part. That was sympathetic magic and Hahnemann's ideas flowed naturally from that ancient idea.

He claimed to discover this principle when he noted that the cinchona bark, which is used to treat malaria, caused him to have symptoms which are very similar to malaria. He therefore generalized this one observation to this Law of Similars, which became one of the cornerstones of homeopathy.

Hahnemann believed that symptoms were the body's way of fighting off illness. Therefore, those symptoms should not be opposed, but should be supported. Homeopathic remedies are supposed to create symptoms similar to the disease, ailment, or symptoms that are being treated to aid the body in using those symptoms to fight off the underlying problem. Therefore, from his point of view, medicine that treats the symptoms in order to reduce or suppress them is likely to make an illness worse.

Hahnemann's next law is the Law of Infinitesimals. He believed that substances transferred their essence to water in which they were diluted. The greater the dilution, the greater this transference of essence was. Homeopathic dilutions are described as either factors of 1/10 dilution, which is called an X dilution or C, which stands for a 1/100 dilution.

It's not uncommon for 10x, 100x, or, let's say, 30C dilutions to be made in homeopathic remedies. For example, a 10C homeopathic dilution is diluted 1×10^{20}. A 30C dilution is 1×10^{60}. Even 200C dilutions are not uncommon.

This often exceeds what we now refer to as the dilutional limit. Avagadro's number, which was known at the time of Hahnemann, is 6.02×10^{23}. That describes the number of molecules in a mole or a specific amount of its substance. That gives you an idea of how many molecules of a substance there are in a small amount of something.

For example, 10^{23}—if you're diluting something to the 60th power, that's many, many, many orders of magnitude more dilute. What that means is that there is an insignificant chance of there being even a single molecule of active ingredient remaining once you get past that dilutional limit. In order to have a 50 percent chance of a single molecule, for example, with a 30C dilution, you would need a volume of water equal to 10 million kilometers in radius. Imagine a sphere of water 10 million kilometers large. That's how much water you would need to drink in order to have a 50/50 chance of getting a single molecule of a 30C remedy.

This notion that you can dilute something far past the point where there's likely to be any actual substance left actually violates a well-established law of thermodynamics. The laws of thermodynamics tell you that you can't get energy from nothing. If Hahnemann's Law of Infinitesimals were correct, then it would actually violate these laws of thermodynamics. The Law of Infinitesimals, like the Law of Similars—or the notion that like cures like—have not been established by science. There's nothing in the 200 years of science since Hahnemann came up with his ideas that tells us that either of these ideas have any validity.

In an attempt to rescue this notion that you can have these super dilutions that still have some biological activity, modern homeopaths have come up with the notion that water has memory. What they claim is that maybe the molecules of what you're diluting in a homeopathic remedy aren't there, but it has imparted the memory of that chemical substance to the water. The water remembers what was diluted in it. However, water is water. Evidence shows that it's a fluid, the molecules do not hold onto any complex chemical structure beyond a fleeting moment.

In order for homeopathy to work through a mechanism like water having memory, the water would have to hold on to the memory of what was diluted in it even through serial dilutions—again, long past there being any molecules left. Often the water or alcohol that the remedy was diluted in is either taken as a liquid or it's sometimes put on a sugar pill. It's dissolved in sugar. That water memory would have to persist even when it's ingested and absorbed through the intestines into the blood. It would still have to persist while the water is diluted in the blood and then transfer through the body to whatever the biological target is, wherever in the body it's supposed to have its effect.

This is beyond implausible. The studies which show this microsecond fleeting ultrastructure to water in no way provides any scientific support for the notion that homeopathic remedies can contain anything active. Further, this notion of water memory doesn't explain how a homeopathic remedy is supposed to know what it's supposed to remember. Water is never absolutely pure. Any water that you drink or that you use is going to have had other things diluted in it or it will have been exposed to many substances in the past. Why doesn't homeopathic water remember many things that it was exposed to in the past? How does it know the one thing that it's supposed to remember?

Hahnemann also came up with the Law of the Individual Remedy. He believed that each person's totality of symptoms, all of their symptoms taken together, had a single underlying common cause. Therefore, homeopathic remedies are intended to treat all of those symptoms at once with a single remedy. Of course, this creates an impossible complexity. If you think about all of the permutations of even a few symptoms that can exist, simple mathematics very quickly tells you that you get to an incredibly high number of possible different combinations of symptoms.

Yet Hahnemann believed that he could come up with the individual remedy for each one of these billions or trillions of different possible combinations of symptoms. There's also no basic medical or scientific reason to assume that a person can only have one illness at a time and that every symptom somebody has has one single common underlying cause. As physicians, we recognize that, while we don't like to make unnecessary diagnoses—we like to make as few diagnoses as possible—people often present to us with multiple chronic illnesses. Maybe there's an acute problem superimposed on top of that. People often have multiple things going on. Assuming that every patient has one and only one ailment is certainly not a scientific or logical approach.

Homeopathic remedies also include the notion of potentiation. Between each dilution, homeopathic remedies are potentiated by succussing them. That means shaking them in a certain way. This is more of a ritual than science or chemistry. You have to shake it a certain number of times in certain directions, again, without any scientific justification for that. Even in the cleanest conditions, there will be many more contaminants in that alleged remedy than the active ingredient that is being succussed at the particular time.

Hahnemann also believed in an idea that he called "miasms." Miasms are underlying disorders of the vital force, the life energy that he believed was important to health. He thought it was disorders of this underlying vital force that actually produced the symptoms. Homeopathic treatments, therefore, are addressing the underlying miasm. As you can see, Hahnemann had a completely alternate notion of biology, health, and disease, separate from what we now understand to be the case 200 years later.

What Hahnemann did and what homeopaths still do in order to know which remedy to give for which totality of symptoms or underlying miasm is called a homeopathic proving. These were conducted in the 1800s and early 1900s, most of the provings that support homeopathic remedies today. These were essentially designed to establish which substances cause which symptoms. These tests were essentially anecdotal. They were not designed scientifically.

One common myth that is often promoted by homeopaths is that these provings are evidence for the effectiveness of homeopathy. But, it's important to recognize that homeopathic provings are not scientific tests to show that homeopathic remedies have any particular effect—or that they are effective in treating any symptom, ailment, or disease.

Another concept that is fundamental to homeopathy is that of constitutional symptoms or constitutional remedies. Hahnemann and homeopaths believe that people have certain personality types, which have an affinity for certain remedies. So there are these astrology-like personality profiles, such as the Ignatia type personality profile. That is somebody who is nervous, tearful, and dislikes tobacco smoke. The Pulsatilla personality type is a young woman with light hair and blue eyes who is gentle, fearful, romantic, emotional, and friendly, but also shy. The sulfur type likes to be independent. If you're somebody who has blue eyes and is a little shy, a homeopath might interpret that as meaning that you need Pulsatilla as a homeopathic remedy to treat your symptoms.

What about the clinical evidence? Up to this point, I've been largely talking about the underlying concepts of homeopathy—ideas that may have made sense or resonated 200 years ago before we understood things like anatomy, physiology, and biochemistry. They sound a little bit like magical thinking probably to modern ears. In any case, it's always good to independently investigate the question of does something work. Forget about the plausibility of the mechanism—not to say that that's not important, it's very important to put clinical evidence into context—but we also do want that clinical evidence.

There have actually been hundreds of clinical studies of homeopathic remedies. There have been systematic reviews to try to pull all of that evidence together and to see what it actually tells us. After reviewing all of the evidence for homeopathy, the scientific community has come to the conclusion that there is no evidence to support homeopathy for any indication. Also, homeopathic remedies are no different than placebos or inactive substances. Finally, there's a general pattern we see which is very typical. This pattern is that the better designed the study, the larger it is, the more rigorous it is, and the better controlled it is, the more likely it is to be negative. The best studies all show no effect. They are negative. When we see this pattern—the better the study becomes, the more likely it is to be negative—that is very indicative of a treatment which doesn't work.

The person who has probably spent the most time reviewing homeopathic remedies is Dr. Edzard Ernst. He started his career actually as a homeopath. Though he is a medical doctor, he did use homeopathy and many other so-called alternative treatments. But, he was interested in becoming rigorously evidence-based in the treatments that he uses. He published what he called a systematic review of systematic reviews of homeopathy. Here is his conclusion after reviewing all of that evidence. He writes:

> There was no condition which responds convincingly better to homeopathic treatment than to placebo or other control interventions. Similarly, there was no homeopathic remedy that was demonstrated to yield clinical effects that are convincingly different from placebo. It is concluded that the best clinical evidence for homeopathy available to date does not warrant positive recommendations for its use in clinical practices.

That is a long and careful way of saying that homeopathy doesn't work.

There are many homeopathic products on the market, however. They are all marketed because of loose regulations without evidence for either safety or effectiveness. The claims are essentially not regulated. Homeopathic remedies are generally safe because they're usually just water. There is no active ingredient, so they don't really have the potential to cause direct harm. That's not universally true of homeopathic remedies. This is because some homeopathic products sort of cheat by including actual measurable levels of active ingredients yet using the homeopathic label in order to skirt regulations.

If a product is marketed as homeopathic, in many countries, it's not regulated; it doesn't need to provide evidence of safety and effectiveness. But, the manufacturers may include an ingredient that has some known medicinal benefit in measurable amounts. The definition of what is a homeopathic remedy then becomes very loose and vague.

One example is that Zicam. This is a product that was marketed as homeopathic. Some preparations of it have measureable and meaningful amounts of zinc oxide. Zinc oxide actually is shown to treat and reduce the symptoms of a cold. Zicam was marketed as a homeopathic cold remedy with an active ingredient that is known to reduce symptoms of a cold. However, zinc oxide is also known to cause anosmia, a sometimes permanent loss of the ability to smell. Several patients or people who were using Zicam had permanent anosmia as a side effect. That caused regulatory agencies to take a second look at it and to temporarily suspend it from the market.

There is one particular homeopathic remedy that deserves a little bit of a closer look because it has an interesting history and that's oscillococcinum. This is actually a very common homeopathic ingredient. The term was coined in 1925 by the French physician Joseph Roy. On examining the blood of flu victims, he thought he saw an oscillating bacterium. He called it the oscillococcinum, the name for this oscillating bacterium.

It turns out, however, that this was just an illusion, an artifact of bad microscopy. The oscillococcinum doesn't even exist. Despite the fact that it doesn't exist, you can buy preparations of oscillococcinum on the market. It is a common remedy used by homeopaths. It is prepared from duck liver and often provided in a 200C dilution. It is most frequently used for the flu, but again, will be used for many indications.

One justification for the ultra-dilutions of homeopathic remedies that's often given—which is a complete myth—is the analogy to either vaccines or allergy shots. However, this is not an apt analogy. A vaccine contains a measurable if small amount of antigen meant to stimulate the immune system. Allergy shots give a small amount of a substance to which one is allergic in order to provoke the immune system to make blocking antibodies. They make antibodies to the substance which does not provoke an allergy. But, it will bind to the substance to which someone is allergic and prevent an allergic reaction. In order for allergy shots to work, you have to give a small dose and then build it up to increasingly larger and larger doses. Eventually, you're giving a fairly significant dose in order to provoke a sufficient immune response. Therefore, there is no analogy whatsoever to a preparation that has no measurable amount of anything in it.

Some homeopaths incorporate other types of techniques into their diagnostic approach. For example, there is something called electrodiagnosis. This is basing a remedy upon the electroacupuncture according to Voll or EAV. This is a technique that was developed by Reinhold Voll in the 1950s. It is based on a galvanometer, which is a device that detects electrical conductance. Essentially, it's just measuring skin conductance which will vary based upon how much you press it against the skin and how much sweat there is on the skin. You can actually get it to say pretty much whatever you want if you move it around a little bit. It doesn't have any relationship to anything biological that's happening inside the person's body.

Despite homeopathy's popularity, in recent times there has been somewhat of a backlash. Scientists who are critical of homeopathy have been quite successful by just describing to the public what homeopathy actually is. They dispelled myths and misconceptions about homeopathy. In 2009, some of these critics staged a mass homeopathic suicide. They took massive doses of homeopathic preparations as a stunt to show that they had no biological activity. They were all perfectly fine and without any symptoms or side effects after taking these massive doses.

In 2010, the House of Commons Science and Technology Committee in the UK released a report called *Evidence Check 2: Homeopathy*. Their goal was to review very thoroughly and systematically all the evidence for homeopathy, to speak with proponents and scientists of all opinions, and come up with a recommendation for policymakers in the UK. They concluded—and were very clear in their conclusion—that homeopathy cannot work based upon what we know about science. It does not work when you look at the clinical evidence. They recommended that all UK support for homeopathy be pulled including doing no further research as it was no longer warranted. In addition to that, a separate report in 2010 by the British Medical Association declared that homeopathy was witchcraft and likewise recommended that all support for homeopathy be pulled.

Homeopathy isn't the only philosophy-based and old notion of healing or medicine that has survived until modern times. There are many medical techniques that are still around today that have a similar history and pattern of promotion and that lack plausibility and evidence. To name just a few, for example, there is phrenology. That's the notion that your personality will affect the shape of your brain, which then affects the shape of the skull over the brain. Also, by reading the bumps on your skull, you can not only detect ailments, but you can also tell someone's personality. Phrenology was disproven in the middle of the 19th century and completely fell out of favor by the early 20th century.

Applied kinesiology, however, is still around today. This is the notion that you can diagnose the sensitivity to a substance or you can find a treatment that will work for somebody by testing their muscle strength. Essentially, a person is told to hold out their arm while they hold a substance or maybe a potential treatment. The practitioner will then push down on the arm to measure the person's strength. If they get weaker, that means that the substance causes an allergy or a bad reaction. If it makes them stronger, that means it's something that could potentially treat them.

However, in blinded tests, applied kinesiology is shown to be all just illusion and what we call the ideomotor effect. When you think you're supposed to be stronger, you try a little harder. When the practitioner wants to break the muscle strength of the person he's testing, they can do it. But, when they're blinded and they don't know what the results are supposed to be, they do no better than chance.

Another very interesting one is iridology. Like homeopathy, this was a philosophy that was generated based upon a single observation by a single person. This is the notion that the iris of the eye contains a detailed map of your entire body—a homunculus if you will, a representation of the body. By looking at the flecks and colors in the iris, you can make statements or conclusions about the general health of somebody and even diagnose specific problems. Iridology, although not very popular, is still around today.

All of these modalities were mostly promoted by single individuals. They have also been progressively out of touch with the progression of science. Most of them are also single systems promoted as a panacea. They are either a treatment for every kind of symptom and illness that can be or a way to diagnose any problem with a single method. Why do some of these modalities persist while others don't? That's a really interesting question that I have thought about and I don't think there's any simple answer. I do think that those that tend to persist rely heavily on testimonials, meaning anecdotal evidence or uncontrolled evidence like people saying they took a remedy and it helped them.

Testimonials and anecdotes tend to support what people already want to believe. They're not rigorous or controlled so it's not really a way to tell if something is effective or not. There are also many placebo effects, which I will talk about in more detail in another lecture. Placebo effects can make anything seems to work. There's also often a failure to recognize the harm that could be done with these types of interventions. I mentioned that homeopathy mostly is a completely inactive substance; it's just water without any active ingredient. Some people will say, well, what's the harm? If it does nothing, how could it possibly do any harm?

The harm often comes in preventing effective treatment. There are many cases of harm occurring to people relying upon homeopathic remedies. For example, in Australia, a couple years ago, there was a nine-month-old girl whose father relied entirely on homeopathy to treat her severe eczema. At any point in the course of this eczema, this severe skin rash, she could've been treated and cured by modern medicine. But, the parents relied entirely on homeopathy until the child became so sick that she unfortunately died.

There's also a recent case of a doctor of homeopathy whose wife had colon cancer. She decided also to rely completely on homeopathy—along with the philosophy of her husband—for treatment, forgoing surgery or any other proven or efficacious treatment. Unfortunately, she died very unpleasantly from her illness. Therefore, there is harm even from treatments which are not directly toxic.

These systems, I think, also persist because they cater to the hopes of people who are chronically ill and are looking for a treatment. Sometimes that can even get to desperation and a willing to try anything that might work. Oftentimes, there's a lack of appreciation for the underlying science. For example, many people don't know what the claims of homeopathy actually are and how out of touch with modern science they are. Also, they're allowed to persist due to inadequate regulation.

But, I also think that just historical contingency, plain old luck, plays a role. Why is homeopathy around today and not so much phrenology or similar systems? Sometimes the marketing is better. If you have a famous person who supports your treatment, it's likely to go farther. It's just plain luck and historical contingency in many cases.

There's a broader intellectual conflict that's represented by homeopathy. It's between science-based medicine—what we recognize today as the modern scientific approach to biology, healing, and disease—and what we would now think of as magical thinking. Hahnemann rejected attempts to understand disease through studying anatomy, physiology, pathology, and chemistry. He wanted to replace those burgeoning scientific notions that were just getting underway 200 years ago with the notion that most illness, as he claimed, was caused by the vital essence or vital force being out of harmony with nature.

Over the last 200 years, the scientific approach has clearly won out. It has produced all of modern medicine whereas homeopathy is stuck in the 200-year-old ideas of its founder. At the time of Hahnemann, that conflict may have been reasonable based upon what was known at the time. Completely inert treatment may have actually been an advantage to what was passing for standard medicine 200 years ago. But, today, science-based medicine has brought us a host of effective treatments. Homeopathy or other worthless, even though directly harmless, treatments can interfere with effective treatment.

Facts about Toxins and Myths about Detox
Lecture 16

Have you ever considered having your colon cleansed? How about ear candling or having the toxins leached out of the bottom of your feet or squeezed out of your muscles? Are the fears over toxins and their treatments real medicine, or just more marketing hype? You can probably guess where I'm going to go with this one.

This lecture is about toxins in the environment; fears of these toxins; and alleged treatments for toxins, such as detoxification or "detox." Technically, a toxin is a poison that is produced by a living organism, such as a protein. Colloquially, it refers to any substance that is poisonous to a living organism. In reality, everything can be a toxin or can be completely safe, depending on the dose. Even water and oxygen can be toxic at high enough doses.

Our bodies have mechanisms for dealing with toxins. One of the most significant is the liver, which produces enzymes to metabolize toxins in order to neutralize them. Other organs are also involved: The kidneys continuously filter the blood, removing harmful waste products or toxins and then excreting them in the urine. The skin also excretes toxins through sweat.

So are there any real toxins that you need to worry about? Yes, toxicity is a real potential health hazard. For example, there are risks of overdose. One of the most common overdoses is multivitamins or supplements, particularly of iron in children. Overdoses can happen with just about any prescription or recreational drug. Even common ones like alcohol can cause toxicity due to excessive use.

Food is another source of toxins or potentially harmful chemicals. For example, pathogenic bacteria can contaminate food. There may also be contaminants in food production, and fresh fruits and vegetables may contain small amounts of pesticides. Other environmental toxins include lead and cigarette smoke.

Yes, there are toxins in our environment. But does this mean that the claims made for detox treatments are legitimate, that they can remove toxins from the body? There is no evidence for the need for routine or nonspecific detox. This is just marketing hype, a marketing strategy playing off fears of toxins in the environment. In case of genuine toxicity or genuine overdose, targeted medical diagnosis and treatment is necessary, not some nonspecific detox product.

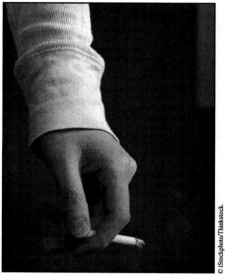

© iStockphoto/Thinkstock.

First- and secondhand tobacco smoke are common sources of toxins in our environment.

Let's look now at some of the popular detox treatments that don't have medical legitimacy. For example, there is the colon cleanse—cleaning toxins out of your colon or out of intestinal walls. One version of this is the coffee enema, which claims to clean out toxins that are collecting and gunking up the intestinal wall. There is no evidence for toxins or anything clogging up the walls of the intestines. The intestines continuously move waste through, and everything eventually comes out. There is no theoretical reason for coffee enemas or other colon cleanses. This is also not a risk-free procedure. Enemas carry the small but real risk of perforating the colon.

Another entirely different type of treatment with the same claims of detoxification is rolfing. This is a deep, often painful, muscle massage. The idea is that by squeezing the muscles very strenuously, you will squeeze out the toxins into the blood, and then they'll be removed by the liver and kidneys. There's no proven health benefit to rolfing, and it actually contains a small risk of nerve or muscle damage.

Next we have ear candling. The procedure is to put a wax candle in your ear with your head down on its side. The claim is that burning this candle in your ear will draw out the wax, and toxins, from inside your ear. This has been studied in several different ways. First of all, there's no negative pressure created, no sucking action. In addition, the wax that collects on the plate at the base of the candle has been shown to be entirely composed of wax from the candle itself; it's not earwax. The black sooty material that proponents often say is the toxins drawn out of the body is nothing more than ash from the wick of the candle. The procedure also carries the risk of burning or damaging the eardrum.

There are also many herbal or diet detox products—too many to name. This is a very common type of supplement on the market today. These are usually harmless mixes of vitamins, herbs, or some food regimen. They are alleged to give your body a break from toxins or to augment your liver and kidneys' ability to remove toxins from your body. There is no basic science or any clinical evidence to support any of these claims.

Ultimately, dealing with the notions of toxins and human health is about balance. Yes, there are toxins, and you do need to be reasonably aware of them. However, it is easy to spread unreasonable fears that are not based in science. Sometimes these unreasonable fears are used to sell products that make nonspecific claims not backed by science. The bottom line is not to get scammed by fear. Beware of products that make claims that have not been verified by science. Let's end with a quote from some colleagues of mine, Simon Singh and Edzard Ernst, who said about detox products, "The only substance that is being removed from a patient is usually money." ∎

Suggested Reading

Australian Skeptics, "Debunking the Detox Myth."

Karasov and Martinez del Rio, *Physiological Ecology*.

Novella, "The Detox Scam."

1. What are the most common toxins to be aware of?

2. Which detox products, if any, are legitimate? Why?

Facts about Toxins and Myths about Detox
Lecture 16—Transcript

Have you ever considered having your colon cleansed? How about ear candling or having the toxins leached out of the bottom of your feet or squeezed out of your muscles? Are the fears over toxins and their treatments real medicine, or just more marketing hype? You can probably guess where I'm going to go with this one. This lecture is about toxins in the environment, fears of these toxins, and alleged treatments for toxins, such as detoxification or "detox," as it's often called.

First, let's start with what the definition of a toxin is now. As the word is used, it refers to any substance that is poisonous to a living organism. Technically, a toxin is a poison that is produced by a living organism, such as a protein. Colloquially, it's used to mean any poison. In reality, everything is a toxin, or can be a toxin, or it can be completely safe, depending on the dose. Toxicity is all about dose. Even water and oxygen can be toxic at high enough doses.

Toxins are everywhere in our environment, not just a product of our industrial world. Nature itself produces millions of toxins. In fact all drugs—all prescription drugs or recreational drugs—are toxins that have a dose range in which they have some property that can be exploited to have a desired health effect while being safe in terms of other effects, like side effects. But, at higher doses, all drugs will have toxicity and some have very, very significant toxicity.

We all evolved an emotion known as disgust. That is a specific emotion. The reason why we have this inherent tendency to experience that is putatively to protect us from exposure to things in our environment that could be harmful to us. This is aided by a strong memory reaction when we have an exposure to a taste or an odor that is followed by any kind of nausea or negative health experience. This creates a strong memory and an aversive conditioning. We learn very quickly what things in our environment will make us feel sick. We learn to be disgusted by them and to avoid them.

Nausea itself is also a protective sensation. It causes you to vomit up and to expel things that are toxic that you maybe have recently put into your body.

What about products that promise to "detoxify" or detox programs? These play upon this inherent notion of disgust or this emotion that we have. But, our bodies have their own mechanisms for dealing with toxins. This is no surprise. We are swimming in a sea of toxins, if you will. We evolved in an environment that is loaded with potential hazards, harmful substances, and toxins.

Of course it makes sense that we evolved some natural biological functions that will help protect us from these toxins. One of the most significant natural detoxification systems in our body is the liver. The liver is often referred to as the chemical factory of our bodies. It produces enzymes which metabolize toxins in order to neutralize them. There is also what we call the portal system. It's a separate blood supply or blood flow that goes from the intestine to the liver.

The reason for this is to give the liver an opportunity to metabolize or detoxify things that we absorb from our intestines. When you eat food, it goes into your intestines. This food may have chemicals, drugs, or toxins in it that get absorbed into your blood system. That then goes directly to the liver so that it can be metabolized and detoxified before it gets passed on to the rest of the body.

This is referred to as the first pass effect. When studying drugs to see their bioavailability—how much of the drug will get into the blood and body—we have to account for the fact that the liver is going to be able to metabolize much of it, if it is a liver-metabolized drug, before it will get to its target. Many metabolized toxins by the liver are then secreted in bile and excreted in the stool.

Other organs, however, are also involved in freeing our body or removing toxins from our body. The kidneys, for example, continuously filter the blood, removing any harmful waste products or toxins from the blood and then excreting them in the urine. The skin also secretes or excretes toxins through sweat. We eliminate some toxins through our breath. For example, carbon dioxide, which it a waste product, is exhaled in our breath.

Are there any real toxins that you need to worry about? Sure, toxicity is a real potential health hazard. There are some toxins that you need to be reasonably concerned about. For example, there are risks in our environment of overdose. One of the most common overdoses is multivitamins or supplements largely because people don't realize the overdose potential. One of the most common specific substances is just iron. Iron in supplements can cause a lot of harm if taken in overdoses. This often happens in children who think that chewable vitamins are candy and eat too many of them.

Overdoses can happen with just about any prescription drug. Therefore, any prescription drugs you have in your house should be kept safe and away from children with protective caps, for example. The same is true with recreational drugs. Even common ones like alcohol can frequently cause toxicity due to excessive use. There may also be contaminants. Heavy metals can contaminate supplements or any product that has been improperly manufactured. It's not uncommon for street drugs to have very serious contaminants in them. One example is MPTP, which is a frequent chemical contaminant of street drugs that can cause rapid serious permanent neurological injury.

Food is another source of toxins or potentially harmful chemicals. For example, pathogenic bacteria can contaminate food. These can not only cause direct infection causing symptoms from the infection itself, but some bacteria release what are called endotoxins. Most of the harm that they do to a person that they infect is through these endotoxins. In fact, some of the most toxic chemicals in nature are bacterial endotoxins. These include the tetanus toxin, botulinum toxin, and others.

It's important to note that, even if cooking kills the bacteria, if the bacteria has already had an opportunity to release endotoxin, cooking may not destroy the toxin itself. This often happens when food is reheated. For example, when the food is cooked, the bacteria may not be completely killed. The food is then left to be stored for awhile. The endotoxins may build up and is not inactivated by subsequent heating, even if that subsequent heating or cooking kills any remaining bacteria.

There may also be contaminants in food production. There was a recent case of melamine, a plastic, that found its way into baby food in China. That is a dramatic example, but less dramatic examples occur also. Fresh fruits and vegetables may contain small amounts of pesticides. This can largely be helped through thorough washing, for example. Washing vegetables for 30 seconds or so has been shown to significantly reduce pesticides on those fruits and vegetables. Still, we can get exposed to them and sometimes and not in insignificant amounts from eating just our food. Seafood may also be contaminated with methylmercury. This also can be a significant health concern.

There are many toxins in our environment as well. For example, there is lead. Lead is a heavy metal that causes neurological and other damage. It exists in old paint. Although lead is no longer used in paint on homes or other things people will come in contact with, there are still in existence old buildings or other structures that may have old lead paint on them, which will then flake off and can cause contamination for animals or small children. Lead paint chips actually have a sweet taste to them and that may cause a small child to put them in their mouth.

There is also environmental mercury, not just mercury from seafood. You can get mercury in the environment from coal burning plants. Small amounts of mercury contaminants in the coal are released into the air when the coal is burned. Many types of manufacturing also involve mercury. For example, the felt used in some hat manufacturing used to contain significant amounts of mercury. This is the origin of the term mad as a hatter. Hatters will often get chronically contaminated with mercury which would cause neurological damage. That led to the notion that hatters may have psychological disease or be mad if you will.

Thermometers used to contain elemental mercury, which is very, very toxic, although this is no longer used because of the extreme toxicity. However, not all mercury that is in the environment is necessarily a health hazard. For example, there is mercury amalgam. That is a combination of metals that are used by dentists to fill cavities. There are many concerns. A somewhat popular belief among a subset of people is that mercury amalgam can leach mercury into the bloodstream and cause chronic mercury toxicity.

However, this has been studied for years and it's been shown that the amalgam in these fillings is not a significant source of mercury. They do not cause any demonstrated toxicity. The exception to that are the dentists themselves because they have a long-term occupational exposure to mercury amalgam. That long-term exposure may result in toxicity if they don't use proper technique.

Another very common source of toxins in our environment is smoking. Both firsthand and secondhand tobacco smoke contain tar, nicotine, and many other things that are harmful or potentially toxic to people. The workplace is also a very significant potential source of exposure to toxins and harmful chemicals. That is a place where, depending on the job and what work is being done—for example, certain kinds of manufacturing—there may be routine handling of chemicals, fumes, gas or exposure to heavy metals. There may also be silicates or other fine products in the air that can be breathed in.

For this reason, there are usually, in most countries, tight regulations to minimize human exposure to these potential toxins. This includes wearing face masks or gloves or working only under a hood with good circulation of air to avoid excessive exposure. This is particularly important because exposure to these chemicals or toxins can occur over many years or even decades.

Yes, there are toxins in our environment, but our bodies evolved generally to deal with them. We do need to be concerned about genuine overdosing or genuine toxicity. But, does that mean that the claims made for detox treatments are legitimate, that they can remove toxins from the body? This is the claim that is made. However, rarely are specific toxins mentioned. Toxins are referred to in just a vague sense. They largely ignore the body's inherent ability to remove toxins or they claim that this is insufficient, that the body needs help in removing these toxins.

There is no evidence for the need for routine or non-specific "detox." This is just marketing hype, a marketing strategy playing off fears of toxins in the environment. In case of genuine toxicity or genuine overdose, targeted medical diagnosis and treatment is necessary, not some non-specific detox product. What does this medical detoxification consist of? It consists of many things. It depends on what the toxicity is. Most people know that if you have a poisoning or exposure to toxicity and you don't know what to do, there are toxicology centers or poison control centers that you can call to get advice about what to do with a specific exposure.

To give you some examples of serious medical interventions that would be used, chelation therapy is used to bind to heavy metals. It brings those heavy metals out of the body through the stool or through the urine mostly. If someone does get a mercury or a lead toxicity for example, either oral or intravenous chelation is one of the things that would be used in order to treat that toxicity. For things that are consumed by mouth, activated charcoal can also be put into the stomach. Activated charcoal binds to many substances and will then inactivate it so that it can be withdrawn from the body or it will pass harmlessly through the intestines.

For venom such as from snakebites for example, there are often, but not always, anti-venoms. These are the specific antidotes that will reverse the causes of the negative health effects of those venoms and can in fact save lives if given in a timely fashion. Drug overdoses can sometimes be counteracted by other drugs which will have the opposite effect. For example, atropine is a drug that has the opposite effect as the effects of the poison gas sarin. Soldiers who may be at risk of being exposed to this poison gas are often given vials of atropine that they can autoinject in order to immediately counteract that toxin.

Let's look now at some of the popular detox treatments that don't have medical legitimacy. For example, there is the colon cleanse—cleaning toxins out of your colon or out of intestinal walls. One version of this is the coffee enema, which claims to clean out toxins that are collecting and gunking up the intestinal wall. There is no evidence for toxins or anything clogging up the walls of the intestines. The intestines continuously move waste through and everything eventually comes out. It doesn't get backed up. There is no theoretical reason for coffee enemas or other colon cleanses. Again, there are no specific toxins that anyone can point to as getting backed up in the colon.

This is also not a risk-free procedure. By doing an enema, there is a small but real risk of perforation, of making a hole in the colon. If that occurs, that becomes a serious risk of infection in the perineal cavity where the intestines are. That could be very serious even life threatening. Oral colon cleanses don't have that risk. They involve eating or drinking some type of gummy material or other substance which passes entirely through the GI system without being absorbed. This gummy type substance will then harden. It may harden inside the intestine and form what's called an endocast. It looks like a long stringy thing with bumps that resemble the inside of the intestine.

The people who buy these products are being told that that endocast is made of things that were blocking up or gunking up the intestine itself; those are the toxins. That is the backed-up material that you are cleaning out. But, that's not true. In fact, studies have clearly shown that the only thing that comes out is the gum that was taken in the first place without any toxins or any other material that was being left in the intestine.

Another entirely different type of treatment, but with the same claims of a detoxification is called rolfing. This is a type of deep, often painful, muscle massage. The notion here is that, by squeezing the muscles very strenuously, you will squeeze out the toxins that can then be cleared from the body. They'll get into the blood, out of the tissues, and then they'll be removed by the liver and the kidney. However, again, no specific toxins are mentioned. No specific increase in the excretion of toxin is measured.

There's no proven health benefit to getting rolfing, as a onetime treatment or for ongoing health maintenance. This is one that, again, contains a small risk with no proven benefit. The risk is from actual nerve or muscle damage. I've actually seen at least one patient who had a permanent and significant nerve injury from getting rolfing performed upon them.

There is also something called ear candling. This one seemed strange to me from the first time that I heard about it. The procedure is to put a wax candle in your ear with your head down on its side. The candle sticks inside the ear and there is a plate at the base of the candle. Inside the candle is a paper or other kind of wick which you then light. You allow the candle to burn down. The claim is that, by burning this candle in your ear, the burning wax will draw out the wax from inside your ear. It will suck and draw out toxins along with it. This is another method of clearing out the toxins from your body.

This has been studied in several different ways. First of all, the basic underlying notion that ear candling, the burning of the candle, is sucking or drawing anything out from inside the ear has been shown not to be true. There's no negative pressure created, no sucking action. In addition, the wax that collects on the plate at the base of the candle has been examined. It's been shown to be entirely composed of wax from the candle itself; it's not earwax. It's all candle wax. The black sooty material that proponents often say is the toxins that were drawn out of your body is nothing more than ash from the wick of the candle itself. This one is simply an entire scam.

It's also not entirely safe. A1996 survey of 144 ENT physicians, for example, showed that 14 had seen patients who had been directly harmed by ear candling. This is mostly due to accidental burning, but also may include damage or rupture to the eardrum.

In addition to the products mentioned already, there are many herbal or diet detox products—too many specifically to name. This is a very common type of supplement on the market today. These are usually harmless mixes of vitamins, herbs, or some food regimen. They are alleged to give your body a break from toxins or to help or augment your liver and kidneys' ability to remove toxins from your body. There is no basic science or any clinical evidence to support any of these claims.

Some of these regimens can be rather tedious and even risky. They have no effect on the body's natural ability to detoxify itself. They do not undo months or years of an unhealthy lifestyle. You can't overeat, eat too much salt, not exercise, and eat too much fat and then think that you can take a detox program and undo that damage.

Many consumer protection agencies have gotten involved with trying to at least educate the public about the fact that these frequent or common detox programs or products are of no specific benefit. For example, in 2005, Australia's consumer watchdog Choice conducted a study of seven popular detox kits. Their conclusion is as follows:

> Detox supplements provide little or no known benefit over a healthy diet. A week or two on a detox program won't absolve you from a

year of unhealthy eating, smoking, or drinking too much alcohol. We suggest you save your money.

A UK consumer group called Sense about Science, investigated detox products in the UK and found that they were not backed by any science. Additionally, they found that many companies admitted to taking mundane products that they already had on the market like basic cleansers or bath products and simply renamed them as "detox" products—purely as a marketing ploy.

Often, a component of these detox treatments or detox programs is hydration. Sometimes hydration is given just as hydration therapy, as a detox program all by itself. The notion here is that, by drinking a lot of water while avoiding eating or other things, that this will give your system a chance to "flush out" the toxins. All this water will just flush out all of the toxins getting backed up in your body. This, of course, is not true as you might guess by now.

Also, there are significant risks to pushing fluids to this degree on the belief that you will flush out these toxins. There is a risk of what we call hyponatremia, which is a low sodium level in the blood. What happens is that the kidneys' ability to hold on to and regulate different ions like sodium, chloride, and potassium is overwhelmed by the continuous drinking of water. Your kidneys can only concentrate your urine so much. You have to lose some water. Therefore, what happens is once the kidneys are overwhelmed, the levels of sodium begin to drop and other things. But, sodium is usually the first one that causes problems. When the sodium level gets too low, it can cause delirium. It can even lead to serious neurological conditions like seizures.

In fact, in 2008, a UK court awarded 800,000 pounds to a woman who suffered brain injury from a seizure from a detox program. The program recommended both decreased food intake and extremely high water intake. She was drinking as much as five liters in one day.

There are also skin cleansers, products that claim to remove toxins through the skin. One common type of these skin cleansing detox products are foot pads. You are meant to put these pads on your feet and then, often sleep overnight. When you wake in the morning, you will find that there is a black substance on these pads. They have turned black. The consumer is told that that black stuff is the toxins that were removed from your body. In fact, examination of these foot pad detox products show that the black stuff on them is just dirt and oil removed superficially from the skin. There is no documented removal of any toxins.

I mentioned previously that chelation therapy is a legitimate FDA approved treatment for poisoning from heavy metals, like mercury, lead, or cadmium. However, since the 1950s, it has also been used by a small minority of fringe practitioners. It is used for additional indications for which it is not indicated—additional uses that are not FDA approved and for which there is no science. This includes detoxing the body from alleged substances which are causing heart disease or problems with circulation. Oftentimes, it is alleged that heavy metal poisoning diseases like autism, which is not the case. Therefore, chelation therapy is offered to treat these disorders, which are allegedly but incorrectly tied to heavy metal poisoning.

There have been many studies of chelation over the years. Again, this has been a controversy since the 1950s, mostly in cardiovascular disease but also in claudication. Claudication is pain in the calves resulting from insufficient blood flow to the muscles. There was, for example, a double blind study in 1992 in Denmark of 153 patients. It showed no benefit from chelation therapy for claudication. Also, there have been multiple studies looking at cardiovascular disease or heart disease showing no benefit from chelation therapy.

However, proponents refuse to give up on their claims and are continually pushing for further study. The ethics of doing further studies on chelation therapy for heart disease have been questioned by many on the basis that this is not a risk-free procedure. Also, there's already sufficient evidence to conclude that this is not a theoretically sound use of chelation therapy. The clinical evidence shows that there is simply no benefit.

Again, as I mentioned, it is not a risk-free procedure. Chelation therapy can also lead to decreased levels of ions in the blood, specifically calcium. Decreased calcium can lead to cardiac arrhythmias; tetany, which is an involuntary contraction of the muscles; and kidney damage, even in healthy individuals. It can also decrease zinc levels, which can lead to immune dysfunction. It can decrease the blood's ability to clot leading to bleeding disorders. In the extreme, chelation therapy can even lead to death. For example, in 2005, a five-year-old boy with autism, Tariq Nadama, died while receiving chelation therapy for his autism.

Other people claim that the microwave oven can put toxins in food, for example, plastics. If you microwave food in plastics, the claim often goes, that will leach toxins, specifically cancer causing toxins like dioxin into the food. If you have email or are on the Internet, you may have seen an email warning people not to cook food or store food in plastics because of this dioxin risk. It turns out that this email and this claim is nothing more than an Internet hoax. It is not based upon any legitimate research or any science. However, it is important to note that not all plastics are easily safe in the microwave.

The most reliable method for determining whether or not a plastic product is safe for the microwave is simply to read the product itself. See whether or not it is labeled as safe for microwave use. Some plastics will be able to keep their form and will not melt even under the high temperatures of a microwave. Other plastics are too fragile; they will deform or melt and should not be put into the microwave. Always look for the microwave safe indication if you want to be sure that plastics are safe for the microwave.

To give you some rules of thumb, generally speaking, thin plastics like the kind of plastic bags you would get from the grocery store are not safe for the microwave. They shouldn't be put in them. However, thin plastics like saran wrap are meant to be used in the microwave. They are strong enough and safe for the microwave. Containers that whipping cream or butter may come in, these thin "throw away" plastic containers are not intended for use in the microwave. They are generally not safe, so you should not use them for the microwave. It also should be noted that even when you do use microwave safe thin plastics like saran wrap, you should not let them come in direct contact with the food. The food generally gets much hotter than the plastics themselves. Therefore, that can heat up the wrap and cause it to melt if it is lying on top of the food itself.

Another plastic toxin fear is BPA or bisphenol A. This is an estrogen analog that is used in making clear, hard plastic. There have been concerns for many years that this estrogen analog, BPA, can leach out of plastic containers into water or food. Also, there is concern that it can have biological activity in humans and therefore poses a risk. What does the evidence show? There have been many animal studies. The animal data, however, is somewhat mixed. There are some studies showing that BPA can produce harmful effects in animals, others show that they don't. So far, there hasn't been any consistent replicated effect.

A 2004 report from the Harvard Center for Risk Analysis found "no consistent affirmative evidence for low-dose BPA effects." However, some scientists claim that even small doses may have a hormonal effect and we haven't entirely ruled out that there's any safety concern here. In addition, the NIH, the National Institutes of Health, are urging that there should be some caution in the industry using plastics with BPA.

Health Canada has banned BPA entirely from baby bottles based upon similar concerns. Some European regulatory agencies are considering similar bans. The bottom line with BPA is that at present, the science is equivocal. This probably means that, if there is any effect, it is probably small. But, if you want to be on the safe side, you can follow the more strict recommendations of the NIH or Health Canada.

Ultimately, dealing with the notions of toxins and human health is about balance. Yes, there are toxins. They can adversely affect you. You do need to be reasonably aware of them. However, it is easy to spread unreasonable fears that are not science-based. Sometimes these unreasonable fears are used in order to sell products which make very non-specific claims that are not themselves backed by science. All alleged risks or real risks from toxins need to be put into perspective. There's no such thing in science as zero risk. We can only say that a risk is too small to worry about.

Meanwhile, the bottom line of this lecture is not to get scammed by fear. Beware of products that make claims that have not be verified by science; where toxins are not specifically named; where toxins are not specifically measured so that you can confirm they're actually being removed from your body; where there are no clinical studies in people to show that it's safe and there are health benefits; or where there are serious health concerns like with chelation therapy or with colonic enemas. I'm going to end with a quote from some colleagues of mine, Simon Singh and Edzard Ernst, who said about detox products, "The only substance that is being removed from a patient is usually money."

Myths about Acupuncture's Past and Benefits
Lecture 17

> The notion that acupuncture is ancient has led to what some call the argument from antiquity. If the idea's been around for thousands of years, then it must have some merit. But, on closer inspection, this is simply not true.

Acupuncture is perhaps the most misunderstood of the so-called alternative treatments. The history of acupuncture is different from what many people might suppose. The first myth of the acupuncture history that I'd like to debunk is the notion that it is uniquely Eastern. In fact, the ideas behind acupuncture were common to most ancient cultures, East and West.

A concept that you may think of as Western—and that is also common among many cultures—is the use of bloodletting. There are significant historical records that show that traditional acupuncture points were very similar to the bloodletting or lancing locations that were being used in the West. Chinese acupuncturists were largely peasant healers who practiced minor surgery, bloodletting, and needling. All of these practices were mixed together in one cohesive system.

But in China in the 1930s, there was a period of acupuncture reform. Chinese pediatrician Cheng Dan'an moved the traditional acupuncture points from over veins to over nerves. He distanced the practice of acupuncture from bloodletting; he changed the concept to using fine needles to affect nerve function. This is the modern concept of acupuncture, which is taught in the West.

The modern practice of acupuncture involves sticking a very thin needle into one of thousands of acupuncture points to a certain depth. The needle is then rotated in order to elicit what's called the *de qi*, which is a vibrational sensation. It's that sensation that is thought to represent the unblocking of the flow of the vitalistic energy.

There are many different claims made for the modern incarnation of acupuncture. The most common claim is pain relief, but it's also used to treat nausea, addiction, and back pain. There is also something called medical acupuncture that is used to treat diseases, including serious illnesses such as cancer, and to enhance the chances of becoming pregnant. There are also claims made for acupuncture anesthesia, the ability to perform invasive surgery with nothing but acupuncture for pain relief.

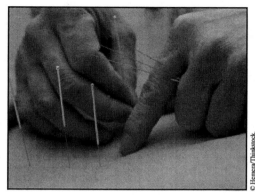

Some scientists have sought a modern, physiologically based explanation for how acupuncture may be producing the effects that are attributed to it. These, so far, are mostly speculation. There have also been published studies looking at other biochemical effects. In

The perceived benefits of acupuncture may actually be placebo effects.

2010, a study was published in *Nature Neuroscience* that found that needling with an acupuncture needle caused the local release of a chemical known as adenosine. In response to this, local pain and inflammation decreased. But there are significant limitations to this study: It was done in mice, and there were no controls in this study. All we can really say, based upon this study, is that there is a local tissue response to minor trauma. This then inhibits the inflammation and pain that results from that trauma—not surprising when you really think about it. But, the specific mechanism that was identified may lead in the future to treatments that will help address both pain and inflammation.

What about the clinical research for acupuncture? Acupuncture is one of the most studied of the alternative modalities. The main challenge in designing acupuncture trials has been properly blinding both the acupuncturist and the subject. It's hard not to know if a needle is being stuck into some part of your body or if you are doing the sticking. However, this technology has evolved quite nicely. There are several kinds of controls that are used in high quality research. These controls include sham acupuncture and placebo acupuncture.

The results of this research are very informative. Sham acupuncture studies have shown that it doesn't seem to matter where the acupuncture needles are placed. Placebo acupuncture shows that it doesn't matter whether you stick the needles at all—the needles don't have to be stuck through the skin in order to get the same effect. An example of this is a 2009 large back pain study published in the *Archives of Internal Medicine*. That study compared individualized acupuncture, cookbook acupuncture, and placebo acupuncture. All 3 groups had exactly the same response. It doesn't matter where you stick the needles, and it doesn't matter whether you stick the needles.

Acupuncture is one of the most studied of the alternative modalities.

What does this mean? How do we interpret this research? It means that the perceived benefits come from the other aspects of acupuncture, not sticking needles into specific locations. Some of these effects may be placebo effects—the expectation of benefit, the desire for benefit. They may also be nonspecific effects from the ritual that surrounds acupuncture. While receiving acupuncture, you may be lying down on a table for 30 to 60 minutes. There may be pleasant music playing in the background. The acupuncturist may palpate the acupuncture points, maybe even providing a little massage. There's the positive interaction with a therapeutic person. All of these contribute to having a perceived benefit, especially for subjective symptoms like pain.

There have been many systematic reviews of clinical trials for acupuncture. Reviews of acupuncture for back pain, in vitro fertilization, chemotherapy side effects, and addiction have all been completely negative. They conclude that either it doesn't work at all or for some indications. There's no evidence to show that it works, but there hasn't been enough research to completely close the door. The one exception to this is nausea. There is weak evidence for a mild effect in treating nausea. But, again, this is preliminary evidence that is not yet definitive. ■

Suggested Reading

Eckman, *In the Footsteps of the Yellow Emperor.*

Kavoussi, "Astrology with Needles."

Science-Based Medicine (blog), Archive for the "Acupuncture" Category.

Taub, "Acupuncture."

Questions to Consider

1. How have the concept and practice of acupuncture changed over the centuries?

2. Can modern science provide a plausible mechanism for the alleged effects of acupuncture?

3. What does the clinical evidence tell us about the effectiveness of acupuncture?

Myths about Acupuncture's Past and Benefits
Lecture 17—Transcript

Acupuncture has garnered a great deal of attention in recent years, both scientific and public. Although surveys show that a minority of Americans have ever tried acupuncture, only about 6 percent per year with only 1 to 2 percent in recent years. Use is similar in Europe, although acupuncture use in Europe goes back to as early as the 17th century. It is perhaps, however, the most misunderstood of the so-called "alternative" treatments.

The higstory of acupuncture is different than what many people might suppose. The first myth of the acupuncture history that I'd like to debunk is the notion that it is uniquely Eastern or Chinese. In fact, the ideas behind acupuncture were common to most ancient cultures, East and West. These ancient ideas were interwoven and shared among these cultures. They did have their unique cultural manifestation. But, the underlying ideas were actually mainly the same.

How old is acupuncture itself? Interestingly, there was a frozen Neolithic man recovered from the Alps, whimsically called the Iceman. The Iceman is about 5300 years old. He was tattooed. He had tattoos in 57 different places on his body with both dots and lines. These dots, the locations on his body where the tattoos are, correspond to traditional acupuncture points. They likely reflect "therapeutic tattooing;" the tattoos themselves were meant to be therapeutic. This was, as I said, found in the Alps, not in China or in the East. That shows that the notion of acupuncture points were in that part of the world as far as 5300 years ago.

The Chinese have a concept for life energy which is called chi. This includes the concept of yin and yang, which are essentially positive and negative energies or two different versions of this life energy. This energy is alleged to flow through the body, sometimes through rivers or channels called meridians. This notion of a life energy is not unique to China or to Eastern cultures. In Sanskrit, there is mention of a life energy called *prana*. The Greeks had a notion of life energy that they called *pneuma*, which is also the same word for breath. The Romans had *spiritus*. All of these words are also tied to the concept of "breath" and that is the origin of these words in their respective languages.

Life energy is an interesting concept. It's often referred to as vitalism or the vitalistic force, the force that makes living things different from nonliving things. This is one of those concepts that is universal to most ancient cultures, again, not specific to Eastern or Chinese culture. However, this notion of vitalism was eliminated from the science of biology about 150 years ago. Essentially, vitalistic explanations were used to explain aspects of biology that we didn't currently understand.

Whatever process we didn't understand invoked vitalism as the explanation. Eventually, that simply became unnecessary—once we had anatomy, physiology, and biochemistry to explain the functions of life. Life energy simply became superfluous. It always was little more than a placeholder. There was no evidence for life energy; it simply was the default explanation that was used until biological sciences advanced sufficiently.

Astrological concepts were also very common in many ancient cultures. This is the notion that events on Earth—our lives, faith, perhaps our personalities, health, and illness—were somehow controlled or influenced by the heavens. Again, it was a very common ancient notion. In a book called the *Yellow Emperor's Canon of Medicine*, the oldest version of which comes from 111 C.E., there is the following quote: "Heaven is covered with constellations, Earth with waterways, and man with channels." This refers to channels of chi—again, making this implicit connection between human health and what happens in the heavens.

The original map of acupuncture points, in fact, was based largely upon astrological charts. The sun moving through the ecliptic, the plane of the solar system, corresponds with the Chinese Zodiac and further, the flow of chi. Both were thought to influence health. In the West, it was thought that the zodiac was a microcosm for the different parts of the body, again, making a connection between what was being observed in the skies and human health and biology.

Another concept that you may think of as a Western, or particularly European, concept that also is very common among many cultures is the use of bloodletting as a treatment. It turns out that there are significant historical records that show that traditional acupuncture points were very similar to the bloodletting or lancing locations that were being used in the West. European bloodletting points correspond to Eastern acupuncture points.

Chinese acupuncturists were largely peasant healers who practiced minor surgery, bloodletting, and needling. All of these practices were sort of mixed together in one cohesive system. There is also this overlap of the concept of "balance." Acupuncturists used needling in order to balance the yin and yang of chi. That's similar to the notion of Western practitioners using bloodletting in order to balance the four humors.

Another ancient text we can look to as evidence of this intermingling of the notions of acupuncture, needling, and bloodletting comes from an ancient Chinese medical text called the *Su Wen*. In chapter 16, we find the following quote:

> The *chi* of the body flows in accordance with heaven and earth, during the spring you may bloodlet the *shu* points, during the summer you may bloodlet the *luo* connecting points. After bloodletting allow the bleeding to stop on its own accord and then press on the acupuncture point waiting for the energy to make one complete circulation around the body.

What we see in this quote was that acupuncture points were being used for bloodletting and that the notion of blood was intimately tied with the notion of energy in the body. Life energy, acupuncture, bloodletting, and the heavens and the Earth—all the concepts come together, mixing Eastern and Western concepts around these ideas. Even today, there are practices that intermingle these ideas.

There is a practice in Japan called Shiraku, which is the word for bloodletting. It is still practiced today. It intermingles the ideas of *ki*, their word for chi, and acupuncture. The treatment is used to treat blood stasis. This is based upon the concept that the flow of blood gets blocked, may become static, and this extra blood that's backing up needs to be removed from the body. This is exactly the same concept that Galen came up with when he formulated the notion of the four humors, the dominant humor being blood.

Galen was actually an experimentalist, as close to a scientist as there was 1700 years ago. He made significant advances in our understanding of biology. Before Galen, it was believed that the veins that we can see poking up through our skin were filled with air. Galen figured out that the veins are filled with blood although he didn't know about circulation. He didn't know the blood circulated through the body. He thought blood was produced locally in the tissue where it was then later consumed. But, when the blood got backed up in this cycle, that caused illness and the blood needed to be removed through bloodletting.

Again, we see a connection from this concept, this Galenic concept of blood stasis, and bloodletting surviving in modern Japanese Shiraku mixed with ideas of acupuncture. Modern Shiraku practitioners will also use a technique called cupping. With cupping, a cup—a literal cup—is placed over the skin, over an area where there is believed to be blood stasis. Sometimes with cupping techniques, you may burn herbs on top of the cup. This creates heat, which is believed to then draw out the blood. Cupping exists today in other manifestations; the same technique, essentially, is used to draw toxins out of the blood.

We see, in the evolution of many of these ideas, that you have a technique which is very old. However, the underlying philosophy behind the technique evolves over time as cultures and thinking change. Needling was used initially as a form of bloodletting and then as a form of altering the flow of chi. Cupping was used initially to draw out blood, but now the notion is that it's drawing out toxins. The techniques themselves have not changed very much.

However, in China, there was a period of acupuncture reform. The medical practice of combining astrology, bloodletting, and other manipulations to balance energies was falling out of favor in China. Acupuncture was opposed in China and the East over the last few centuries. It was outright banned in 1919. In the 1930s, however Chinese pediatrician Cheng Dan'an brought back acupuncture. He moved the traditional acupuncture points from being over veins to being over nerves. He changed to using much finer needles rather than the more cutting needles that were used previously. He distanced—quite deliberately—the practice of acupuncture from bloodletting, from lancing the veins. He changed the concept to using fine needles to affect nerve function.

This modern concept of acupuncture—what most people think of as acupuncture today—was promoted in the 1950s and 1960s by Maoist China. It became part of the "barefoot doctor" movement, which was used to meet the healthcare needs of the very large population in China. Out of this came the modern institutions of acupuncture that were then later exported to the West especially the United States.

Modern acupuncture points, what we think of as the acupuncture points, actually have their history in bloodletting. Originally there were 365 acupuncture points, one for every day of the year. However, over the centuries, the number has increased dramatically. Today, there are thousands of acupuncture points. In fact, it's hard to find a place on the body that isn't on or near an acupuncture point. The modern practice of acupuncture involves sticking very thin needles into these points to a certain depth. The needle is then rotated in order to elicit what's called the *de chi*, or the *de qi*, which is a vibrational sensation. It's that sensation which is thought to represent the unblocking of the flow of the vitalistic chi energy.

There are some variations on the way acupuncture is practiced today. What I described is the standard acupuncture. But, there are those who practice what they call electroacupuncture. Essentially, that entails putting a needle through an acupuncture point, attaching an electrode to it, and sending an electrical current through the needle. It's often combined with what is called moxibustion, which is the burning of herbs on the needle. Again, this is meant to affect the flow of life energy or perhaps to draw out toxins. Also, some people practice acupressure, which applies pressure to acupuncture points, but doesn't use a needle. There is no penetration through the skin.

There are many different claims made for the modern incarnation of acupuncture. The most common claim is pain relief, but it's also used to treat nausea, addiction, and back pain. There is also something which is called medical acupuncture where it's used to treat diseases, including serious illnesses such as cancer. It's used commonly to enhance the chances of becoming pregnant, including combining it with in vitro fertilization. There are claims that are made for acupuncture anesthesia, the ability to even perform invasive surgery with nothing but acupuncture for pain relief.

Modern proponents of acupuncture and modern scientists reject the notion of chi, these ancient notions of life energy, of a connection to the heavens, for example. Some scientists have searched for a modern, physiologically-based explanation for how acupuncture may be producing the effects that are attributed to it. These, so far, are mostly speculation. They include things like reducing inflammation in the tissue or counter-irritation, which is the notion that, if you stimulate one sensory pathway, it reduces nearby sensory pathways. You may have noticed that if you bang your elbow, for example, and it hurts, you may rub it. Rubbing the elbow creates a non-painful stimulation or conduction of sensation that will inhibit the more painful sensation.

Others have speculated that perhaps the needle insertion causes the local release of endorphins. Endorphins are natural chemicals in our body that act like morphine. They bind to the same receptors, inhibiting the conduction of pain. Others claim that it may have affects on blood flow or direct effects on nerve function.

There have also been published studies looking at other biochemical effects. In 2010, a study was published in *Nature Neuroscience* that found that needling with an acupuncture needle caused the local release of a chemical known as adenosine. They found that adenosine was binding to the adenosine A1 receptor. In response to this binding, local pain and inflammation decreased. This study, of course, doesn't necessarily tell us that that's how acupuncture, as otherwise practiced, works. There are significant limitations to this study. First, it was done in mice. Mice are much smaller than people. It's hard to extrapolate the effects of a needle being stuck into the knee of a mouse to that being stuck into a human.

There were also no controls in this study. It was an uncontrolled study. They made no comparison to other forms of minor trauma or to trauma in places that do not correspond to acupuncture points. All we can really say, based upon this study, is that there is a local tissue response to minor trauma. This then inhibits the inflammation and pain that results from that trauma—not surprising when you really think about it. But, the specific mechanism that was identified may interestingly lead in the future to treatments that will help in addressing both pain and inflammation.

What role do these possible mechanisms play in acupuncture itself? To put this into perspective, it's very important for scientists and physicians—who are trying to understand what really works in our treatments—to separate out non-specific effects from specific effects. What the research shows is that acupuncture may have some non-specific effects, but there are no specific effects that are directly attributable to those factors which are specific to acupuncture.

For example, there may be some effects that will result from local stimulation of minor trauma. However, these local effects that have been documented are not only not specific—any local trauma can cause them, for example—but also, they wouldn't explain anything other than a short-term, local pain relief. They wouldn't explain any of the other myriad claims that are made for acupuncture. This point, I think, needs to be made very clear—that, in science, we need clear definitions. We need to separate out the non-specific effects or sometimes the rituals that surround treatments—especially those treatments that have evolved over years and centuries—from what's really happening, the specific components of them that are having the actual biological effect.

What about the clinical research for acupuncture? Acupuncture is one of the most studied of the alternative modalities. There are, in fact, hundreds of clinical trials with acupuncture. There is a long and complex history of research that has evolved and become quite rigorous. Most studies of acupuncture, like most studies of anything in medicine, are preliminary, small, and poorly controlled. They're what we might call pilot studies or preliminary studies. They are trying to get an idea of whether acupuncture has any chance of being safe and effective before resources are committed to a larger, more rigorous, and definitive trial.

The main challenge in designing acupuncture trials has been properly blinding both the acupuncturist and the subject. It's hard not to know if a needle is being stuck into some part of your body or if you are doing the sticking. However, this technology has evolved quite nicely. There are several kinds of controls that are used in high quality research. These controls include what's called sham acupuncture.

Sham acupuncture uses acupuncture needles. It inserts them through the skin, but not at acupuncture points and specifically not at the points that are supposed to produce the clinical effect that's being studied. You can also do individualized versus so-called "cookbook" acupuncture. Cookbook acupuncture involves sticking a needle or sticking acupuncture needles into predetermined points. Individualized acupuncture involves an acupuncturist using the traditional methods of traditional Chinese medicine to decide which acupuncture points the patient requires for their symptoms.

There is also placebo acupuncture. Placebo acupuncture uses an opaque sheath so neither the acupuncturist nor the patient knows what's inside that sheath. The acupuncturist depresses a plunger and that will do one of two things. It will either stick a real acupuncture needle down to an appropriate depth through the skin or it will just poke the skin. This is done with either a dull needle that doesn't penetrate the skin or, in some studies, toothpicks are used—things that have no chance of penetrating the skin. Therefore, the acupuncturist doing the study doesn't know if they're actually penetrating the skin. Also, the person who's receiving the treatment doesn't know if their skin was poked with a toothpick or a needle.

The studies do show that people really cannot tell the difference. They still get a very local sensation that they cannot tell apart. The results of this research are very informative. This high-quality research shows that, first of all, it doesn't seem to matter where the acupuncture needles are placed. Therefore, high quality studies that compare sham acupuncture versus so-called verum or true acupuncture show no difference. It doesn't matter where you stick the needles.

The placebo acupuncture shows that it doesn't matter *if* you stick the needles—the needles don't have to be stuck through the skin in order to get the same effect. An example of this is a 2009 large back pain study published in the *Archives of Internal Medicine*. There, they compared individualized acupuncture, cookbook acupuncture, and placebo acupuncture. All three of those groups had exactly the same response with no difference. It doesn't matter where you stick the needles and it doesn't matter if you stick the needles.

What does this mean? How do we interpret this research? It means that the perceived benefits come from the other aspects of acupuncture, not sticking needles into specific locations. Some of these effects may be placebo effects—the expectation of benefit, the desire for benefit. They may also be non-specific effects from the ritual that surrounds acupuncture.

While receiving acupuncture, you may be lying down on a table for 30 to 60 minutes. There may be pleasant music playing in the background. The acupuncturist may palpate, which means touch or feel, where the acupuncture points are, providing a little bit of sensory feedback and maybe even a little massage. There's just the positive interaction or attention from a therapeutic person. All of these contribute to having a perceived benefit, especially for subjective symptoms like pain. Apparently, all of the benefit that comes from acupuncture for pain comes from these non-specific effects, not sticking the needles through the skin. In fact, an acupuncturist who is a colleague of mine told me that, in his personal experience, all of the benefit from acupuncture comes before you even stick the needles through the skin. It's just from the interaction with the patient.

There's also been systematic reviews of published, rigorous study. A 2010 such review published in *Chinese Medicine* could find no evidence for the existence of acupuncture points. Acupuncture points don't appear to have any physiological reality. This makes sense when you understand the history of acupuncture. The invention of where the acupuncture points are located was not based upon any underlying biological concept or certainly, any modern understanding of anatomy or physiology.

There have been many systematic reviews of clinical trials for acupuncture. Systematic reviews of acupuncture for back pain, in vitro fertilization, chemotherapy side effects, and addiction have all been completely negative. They conclude that either it doesn't work at all or for some indications, there's no evidence to show that it works, but there hasn't been enough research to completely close the door. The one exception to this is nausea. There is weak evidence for perhaps a mild effect in treating nausea. But, again, this is preliminary evidence that is not yet definitive.

I think the research and public understanding of acupuncture is further confused by using terms non-specifically. Various interventions are often called acupuncture, even though they have different mechanisms of action. The most notable on in my opinion is electroacupuncture. Oftentimes, I see reports of an acupuncture study that shows a beneficial effect in pain. Therefore, acupuncture works. However, when you read the study, you may find that, in some cases, the study was actually a study of electroacupuncture.

This is important because using electrical stimulation across the skin is a proven treatment for pain. In fact, it's called TENS, or transcutaneous electrical nerve stimulation. We already know that stimulating the nerves or stimulating the skin can produce a decrease in chronic pain. Combining that with acupuncture, however, is just sloppy science. It doesn't get us to the final point of understanding what is it about the intervention that's actually working. Saying that acupuncture works because electroacupuncture works is similar to saying that injecting morphine through a hollow needle reduces pain, therefore acupuncture works. The variable that is consistently associated with an effect is the electricity. It's not anything to do with the acupuncture needle.

What about acupuncture anesthesia? Many people have hard claims that people have undergone surgery with only acupuncture. If that's true, there must be something important happening physiologically from acupuncture. In the West, these claims date back to New York Times' columnist James Reston's appendectomy in China during the summer of 1971. Reston reported that he had local anesthetic and an epidural during the surgery and post-op injections for pain. However, when he reported this story, the story evolved or was misinterpreted as him getting only acupuncture for the surgery itself when that was not the case.

In response to these claims and these beliefs, several investigative teams have been sent from the West to China to see firsthand the reality of acupuncture anesthesia. However, all of these investigative teams have failed to confirm that acupuncture anesthesia is a reality. In some cases, they found that morphine was being administered in the IV fluid. Morphine, of course, is a very powerful painkiller. Therefore, you can't separate out any pain relieving effect from the morphine from what is allegedly occurring with the acupuncture. In other cases, patients were found to be complaining of pain but were pressured by the surgical staff to keep quiet about their pain.

What about brain surgery? There are cases where people have undergone brain surgery with acupuncture anesthesia and still other cases. However, this is true, but misleading. The brain actually does not feel pain. The brain, ironically, is numb. In fact, during neurosurgery—brain surgery—patients are routinely kept awake because they need to assess their neurological function to make sure that nothing is going wrong with the surgery. In short, there are no cases where acupuncture is clearly adding a significant anesthetic effect or an effect that is sufficient to do surgery that would otherwise require significant or general anesthesia.

How do we put all of this information together? The perspective of history I find to be very informative. None of the claims or beliefs surrounding modern acupuncture are supported by historical facts or by scientific research. In fact, what is called acupuncture today bears very little resemblance to what is documented to have been acupuncture in the past. It is a modern invention largely involving swapping out older ideas like chi and bloodletting with newer ideas such as nerve function and removing toxins.

However, the notion that acupuncture is ancient has led to what some call the "argument from antiquity." If the idea's been around for thousands of years, then it must have some merit. But, on closer inspection, this is simply not true. Despite its origins, acupuncture may tell us something useful about the perception and the treatment of symptoms like pain. Patients who undergo acupuncture often feel better. Trying to explore why that's the case may help us treat pain patients more effectively. We can exploit these non-specific benefits. We may be able to exploit physiological studies, like the adenosine research I mentioned, in order to develop more effective treatments for pain—as long as we separate them from the historical roots of the rituals that surround acupuncture.

Myths about Magnets, Microwaves, Cell Phones
Lecture 18

For centuries, magnets have fascinated people. This has contributed to widespread use in many dubious devices and also fraudulent health claims. At the same time, magnetism and electromagnetism are legitimate, real forces of nature that are biologically effective and are used in legitimate scientific research.

Electromagnetism is a fundamental force of nature. In essence, we are all electromagnetic creatures: The processes and chemical reactions that all living cells use to carry out the processes of life are electromagnetic at their core. Therefore, it is no wonder that the connection between healing and magnetism is as old as knowledge of magnets themselves. But this has also led to many myths about healing and magnetism.

Magnetic fields are involved with biology in that cells use electrical currents as part of their basic functions. The nervous system is essentially an electrical system. It is true that focused, powerful, dynamic magnetic fields can alter brain function. In fact, we use a device called a transcranial magnetic stimulation with diagnostic and therapeutic effects. For example, this device uses a dynamic magnet—which uses an alternating magnetic field—at a very specific frequency or different frequencies to turn on or off certain parts of the brain.

This is an important new device in neuroscience research because activating or inhibiting parts of the brain allows us to figure out what those parts of the brain do. It's important to recognize that medical devices that use electromagnetic fields are largely dynamic magnets. They are not only fairly powerful, but they also involve a rapidly alternating polarity or strength with a certain frequency. Most of the magnetic devices on the market, however, are static magnetic fields. Static magnetic fields do not cause any change in conduction. They do not induce an electrical current and are essentially biologically inert.

What are the proposed mechanisms for typical magnetic healing devices that are on the market? One claim is that these magnetic fields will attract the iron in your blood. But this is not plausible: The form of iron in your hemoglobin is not ferromagnetic; it does not respond to a magnetic field. Other claims include increase in immune activity or decrease in immune activity, to reduce inflammation. Neither of these has been supported by research.

Using cell phones for a short period of time, less than 10 to 15 years, has not demonstrated increased association with brain tumors or other health risks.

It's interesting to note, to put this into perspective, that we routinely expose patients to very powerful magnetic fields. Magnetic resonance imaging (MRI) is a technology we use to look inside the brain or other parts of the body. Patients go inside a very large and powerful magnet, somewhere between 2 to 4 Tesla. This is literally millions of times more powerful than the magnetic devices you can buy at the drugstore. Over years of using MRI scans and studying them quite extensively, we have found that putting someone in a powerful static magnetic field doesn't have any biological effects beyond the ones that we're exploiting to create the images.

What about negative biological effects of electromagnetism? In the 1980s, several studies suggested a possible link between power lines and the electromagnetic fields that they generate and leukemia. Power lines do generate magnetic fields. However, in the wake of these preliminary studies, larger epidemiological studies failed to show any correlation. The concerns were essentially laid to rest by larger, better studies, but with this type of evidence, a small correlation can never be completely ruled out.

What about microwaves; do they pose a threat to us or the food that we eat? Microwaves are simply a frequency of electromagnetic waves that are in the microwave frequency. While microwaves do alter the chemical composition of food, they do so in a way that's really no different from just cooking food, so there are no specific concerns about that.

But there is the concern about radiation leakage from the microwaves themselves. If microwaves are properly constructed, any radiation leakage is insignificant and poses no health risk. The only risk would be from having a faulty microwave oven: one that was not well constructed—which regulations should prevent from happening—or one that is failing in some way. However, it is true that you shouldn't stand immediately next to a microwave while it's operating. Doing that very briefly is fine. But because there may be a small amount of radiation close to the microwave, you shouldn't stand next to it for long periods of time.

Cell phones present another source of radiation, an increasingly ubiquitous form of exposure to nonionizing radiation. After all, we often hold cell phones close to our heads. Is it possible that our brains are getting exposed to this nonionizing radiation and this may cause an increased risk of cancer or other health problems?

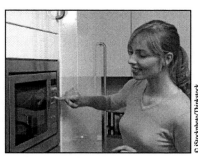

The plausibility of this claim is actually quite low in that the electromagnetic fields produced by cell phones are very weak. Also, it is nonionizing radiation, which has a very weak effect on biological tissue. Ionizing radiation, like the kind you would get from radioactivity, does cause DNA and other types of cell damage. This question of whether there any health risks from cell

Microwaves do not alter the chemical composition of food any more than cooking does.

phones has been studied for years. At present, what we can say is that there is no clear-cut risk from using cell phones. Using cell phones for a short period of time, less than 10 to 15 years, has not demonstrated increased association with brain tumors or other health risks.

However, the literature is still a bit mixed and not definitive for long-term exposure: that greater than 15 years or in children who begin to have exposure to cell phones at a young age. There still may be a reason for a small amount of caution there. ∎

Suggested Reading

Flamm, "Magnet Therapy."

Mesmer, *Mesmerism.*

Questions to Consider

1. What effects do magnets have on the human body?

2. Why do you think magnets are such a common target for dubious remedies?

Myths about Magnets, Microwaves, Cell Phones
Lecture 18—Transcript

I have always been fascinated with magnets. Maybe you have been, too. They seem almost magical with their ability to exert a mysterious force over distance. Imagine how magical they must have seemed when magnets were first discovered. Electromagnetism is a fundamental force of nature. In essence, we are all electromagnetic creatures. The processes and chemical reactions that all living cells use to carry out the processes of life are electromagnetic at their core. If anything can be said to be the real force of life, it's electromagnetism.

Therefore, it is no wonder that the connection between healing and magnetism is as old as knowledge of magnets themselves. But, this has also led to many myths about healing and magnetism. Before the physics of magnetism was even understood, various ancient cultures discovered magnetic stones—some calling them lodestones—and used them for healing. The Yellow Emperor's healing text, which is a 1st century B.C.E. medical text from China, is the first mention of using magnets to heal.

The effects of electromagnetic fields on living tissue have been studied since Paracelsus, a physician and scientist. After him, William Gilbert, who lived from 1544 to 1603 and was a physician to Queen Elizabeth I, wrote *De Magnete* in 1600, describing hundreds of experiments on electricity and magnetism, and debunking many of the quack medical devices using magnets of his day. Following him, there was Thomas Browne, who lived from 1605 to 1682. He continued the academic attacks on popular magnetic remedies.

Interest in magnets and healing, however, really took off with Franz Anton Mesmer. He is credited as being responsible for much of the modern fascination with healing magnets and the rise of magnetic quackery. He was a physician practicing in the late 18th and early 19th century. He combined the notion of "animal magnetism," a term that he coined—which he believed was a magnetic fluid that flowed through all animals—with hypnotism. This is why he also gets a mention in my lecture on hypnotism.

He capitalized on the increasing scientific research into electricity and magnetism that was going on in his day. This theme is often repeated—the notion that the public is fascinated with, understandably, the latest scientific research, the latest discoveries, but they haven't had time yet to really understand the true nature of this new scientific discipline. That situation is ripe for exploitation by those who want to market a new device or a claim that's very sexy and that is easy to fool people about what the real nature of it is.

For example, at the turn of the 20th century, radioactivity was recently discovered and was all the rage. There was a plethora of radioactive tonics and snake oil products selling radioactivity for health. Later in the 20th century, radio wave devices were common. Today, many promoters of questionable health claims may invoke quantum mechanics. This is something that sounds very cutting edge, but it's something not much of the public understands. Even legitimate medical biological research such as stem cells can be exploited in this way. While stem cells are a very legitimate and promising form of medical research, there are today many clinics promising stem cell therapies which are going way beyond the evidence and are not supported by science.

Electromedicine continued to exist after Mesmer. Elisha Perkins. In 1795, following the fame of Mesmer, developed his "magnetic attractors," which was the first patented magnetic device. He claimed that these magnetic attractors could draw off electric fluid that was causing disease. However, he could not cure himself of yellow fever and he died of the disease in 1799.

Electrical and magnetic healing were popular through the 19th and into the 20th century. James Clerk Maxwell, in 1873, wrote his *Treatise on Electricity and Magnetism*, in which he first described the notion that electricity and magnetism are actually both parts of the same underlying fundamental force which we now know as electromagnetism. The rise of magnetic healing in the 19th century was closely tied to the spiritualist movement. These two movements came together in D. D. Palmer. D. D. Palmer is most famous as being the founder of chiropractic. He was both a magnetic healer and a spiritualist.

Let me give you a little bit of a background on the origins of chiropractic. This is too big a field to cover in any detail, chiropractic medicine itself. In terms of the origins, D. D. Palmer first published his book *The Magnetic Cure* in 1896. The following year, in 1897, he published his work on chiropractic. A lot of the founding ideas for chiropractic evolved out of his magnetic and vitalistic beliefs. His notions were that there is a vitalistic living force—not electromagnetism—but something more mysterious that was responsible for health and disease.

Eventually, these ideas evolved into the notion that subluxations were blocking the flow of a life force that D. D. Palmer called "innate" or "innate intelligence"—a spiritual, vitalistic force. This also led to the notion that cells and specifically nerves have a "vibrational" frequency. When these vibrational frequencies were out of harmony, this led to both heat building up in the nerves and to inflammation. By manipulating the spine, you can alter the pressure on the nerves, change their vibrational frequency, and eliminate or reduce this heat and inflammation.

Today, a hundred years after D. D. Palmer, chiropractic has evolved into a very diverse profession. In fact, a lot of different practices are carried out under this very broad banner of chiropractic, which I don't really have time to get into in any detail. Suffice it to say, along this spectrum, we have at one end some chiropractors who cling pretty closely to the original vitalistic ideas of D. D. Palmer. At the other end of the spectrum, there are chiropractors who are very evidence-based and whose practice is almost indistinguishable from a physical therapist or a sports medicine physician.

Let's get into the 20th century now. In the early 20th century, electromagnetic medicine was capitalizing on growing knowledge about these forces. Also, at this time in history, there was a general belief that science would solve all problems. There was a lot of faith in the power of science to do many things. A doctor by the name of Albert Abrams developed his "radionic" theory of physiologic frequency manipulation based largely on radio frequencies, which are just one frequency of electromagnetic radiation.

He developed a device called the Abrams Dynamizer, which he could use to diagnose any illness. You simply take a drop of blood, put it on a little slide, insert it into his device, and then the device would spit out a ticker-tape type diagnosis. He later developed a follow-up device called the Abrams Oscilloclast, which used radio frequencies to then heal whatever disease was diagnosed by the Dynamizer. Essentially, he claimed that the radio frequencies of the body were out of tune or out of harmony. By using radio emissions, he could realign those radio vibrations or those living vibrations in the cells to cure the underlying disease.

Abrams' fame did not last for long. But, it did last for many years in which his devices became extremely popular. There were thousands of them sold to many physicians and other practitioners throughout the United States. There were literally millions of patients treated with Abrams' devices. This led to millions of anecdotes of tremendous healing, everything from high blood pressure to diabetes to many other ailments.

However, Abrams never let anyone examine his devices. They were sealed boxes. He claimed that they were proprietary and therefore, he would not let anyone actually investigate the machinery inside his boxes. When he died in 1924, however, a team from Scientific American was finally able to crack open one of his devices. What they found inside was loose and useless machine parts, not even a functioning device. In essence, the Abrams Dynamizer and Oscilloclast was a scam within a scam. The underlying principle of using radio waves to diagnose and heal disease was not supported by science.

Now, 80 plus years later, we can say with more scientific rigor and confidence that his claims were not based upon anything scientific. Also, his devices didn't even work as he claimed. This is a very important lesson in history. This is because we still have to account for the fact that there were millions of people who believed that their symptoms and diseases were healed by devices that we now know for sure were completely useless.

What about magnetic devices today? Fascination with magnetic healing has waxed and waned over the years. It tends to follow a pattern of increasing interest. After a while, people realize that it's not a panacea. Maybe some research is done which is not very encouraging and interest may wane for awhile. Then, another generation comes along and this cycle of fascination and disappointment follows all over again. But, there's always a background level of interest in magnetic healing devices.

They are largely allowed to perpetuate through loose regulations, but also just interest in magnets as a healing modality. There are a plethora of magnetic products with equally widespread academic skepticism. Reading the historical accounts of scientists and academics and their relationship to the magnetic claims and devices of their time, I've found them remarkably similar to what's happening today.

Magnetic fields are involved with biology in that cells use electrical currents as part of their basic functions. The nervous system is essentially an electrical system. It conducts electricity along axons and to neurons. It is true that focused, powerful, dynamic magnetic fields can alter brain function. In fact, we use a device called a transcranial magnetic stimulation with diagnostic and therapeutic effects. This is a device that uses a dynamic magnet—which uses an alternating magnetic field—at a very specific frequency or different frequencies in order to turn on or off certain parts of the brain, for example.

This is an important new device in neuroscience research because, by activating or inhibiting certain parts of the brain, we can find out what those parts of the brain do. It's important to recognize that these legitimate medical devices that use electromagnetic fields are largely dynamic magnets. This means that they're not only fairly powerful, they also involve a rapidly alternating polarity—a north/south pole—or strength with a certain frequency.

Most of the magnetic devices on the market, however, are static magnetic fields. It's a magnetic field that is not changing. Static magnetic fields do not cause any change in conduction. They do not induce an electrical current the way a dynamic magnetic field does. Static magnetic fields are essentially biologically inert.

What are the proposed mechanisms for the typical kinds of magnetic healing devices that are on the market? One claim that is often put forward is that these magnetic fields will attract the iron in your blood. Every hemoglobin molecule in your blood has an iron atom in the middle of it, that's what it holds on to and releases the oxygen. Is this claim plausible? It turns out that the form of iron in your hemoglobin is not what we call ferromagnetic. It does not respond to a magnetic field. No magnets, whether static or dynamic, attract the hemoglobin in your blood; they do not alter blood flow.

Other claims include increase in immune activity, which has not been demonstrated to occur. Others claim a decrease in immune activity, to reduce inflammation, which has also not been supported by research. None of the proposed mechanisms for static magnetic fields have been demonstrated experimentally.

It's also interesting to note, in order to put this into perspective, that we routinely expose patients to very powerful magnetic fields. MRI scans, or magnetic resonance imaging, is a technology we use to make images of the body, to look inside the brain or other parts of the body. Patients need to go inside a very large and powerful magnet, somewhere between 2 to 4 Tesla. This is literally millions of times more powerful than the magnetic devices you can buy at the drugstore. Over years of using MRI scans and studying them quite extensively, putting someone in a powerful static magnetic field doesn't have any biological effects beyond the ones that we're exploiting in order to create the images. These don't have any healing or harmful effects either.

There are many different types of devices on the market. Mainly they are small, not very powerful static magnets. They can be, for example, bracelets that you are meant to wear that might have affects either locally or even remotely on the body. Maybe static magnets are inserted into braces or wraps that you're meant to wrap around the part of the body that is having symptoms. Claims for such devices include reducing pain, treating arthritis, and improving athletic performance. Even serious illnesses such as cancer are sometimes claimed.

Studies with these devices are generally negative, but as expected, there is the occasional positive study. This means that, by just random chance and statistics alone, if you do enough small studies, you're going to see a scatter of results—some positive, some negative, some neutral—even for something that doesn't work. That's the pattern that we see for these magnetic devices.

What we are not seeing are well-designed, replicated studies showing a consistent beneficial effect.

To review some of this research—and there actually has been quite a bit of it—the New York College of Podiatric Medicine found that magnets did not have any effect on healing heel pain. Over a 4-week period, 19 patients wore a molded insole containing a magnetic foil, while 15 patients wore the same type of insole with no magnetic foil. In both groups, there was a 60 percent reported improvement. That means that there was a non-specific placebo response to either treatment, but the magnet didn't make any difference.

In 1982, Hong et al. found that magnetic necklaces produced no relief of neck or shoulder pain. In 2002, a small study of about 30 subjects found that the use of a magnet for reducing pain attributed to carpal tunnel syndrome—compression of the median nerve at the wrist—was no more effective than use of a placebo device. Other studies have shown no effect using magnets to treat back pain. A study out of the University of Virginia that tested magnets on sufferers of fibromyalgia found little reason to be enthusiastic about these treatments.

A review of the worldwide scientific literature regarding magnet therapy found and I quote:

> The scientific evidence to support the success of this therapy is lacking. More scientifically sound studies are needed in order to fully understand the effects that magnets can have on the body and the possible benefit or dangers that could result from their use.

Again, this is a long way of saying that the evidence doesn't support their use. There's always room for doing more research, however.

Another systematic review concluded: "The evidence does not support the use of static magnets for pain relief, and therefore magnets cannot be recommended as an effective treatment. For osteoarthritis"—that's a degenerative form of arthritis—"the evidence is insufficient to exclude a clinically important benefit, which creates an opportunity for further investigation." Again, further research is reasonable. But, there's still, at the end of the day, no evidence to support any clinical claims made for existing magnetic devices.

Commercial devices are often comprised of fairly weak static magnets. Sometimes these magnets are designed deliberately to be like refrigerator magnets. That means they use strips of magnets with alternating north and south poles. This accomplishes two things. It does make the overall magnetic field a little bit stronger, but it also makes it much shallower. The magnetic field does not extend very far. You can see this yourself if you take a refrigerator magnet and try to pull it off of the refrigerator. There is a sizable magnetic field when it gets very close, but if you get even a little bit away from the refrigerator, you cannot feel any magnetic field.

Sometimes these static magnets, even if they're stronger than the typical refrigerator magnet, are wrapped in cloth. This then gets in between the magnet and the tissue. Again, if you test these devices for yourself, you can see that there really isn't much of a perceptible magnetic field if you get even a few millimeters or centimeters away from something ferromagnetic like a refrigerator.

This is very significant. These magnets are alleged to have a biological effect at tissue depth, down in your shoulder, down in your knee joint, or even just below the skin. The magnetic fields are dropping off so quickly that there is unlikely to be a significant magnetic field where you think the magnetic device is supposed to be having its effect.

What about negative biological effects? If something is affecting living tissue, it can have a positive effect or it can have unwanted negative side effects. At the same time that claims for beneficial effects for magnets are being made, there are fears over negative effects of electromagnetism. In the 1980s, several studies suggested a possible link between power lines and the electromagnetic fields that they generate and the blood cancer leukemia, a very serious illness.

Power lines do generate magnetic fields. This was the discovery of Maxwell. If you have current flowing through a wire, around that flowing current would be a magnetic field. The opposite is also true. A magnetic field can induce electrical current in a wire. Concerns were raised about the magnetic fields that would be generated by current flowing through power lines near homes where people lived, especially homes that were near the high voltage power lines—the ones that would be carrying much higher voltage and more current.

However, in the wake of these preliminary studies that raised a great deal of concern about a possible link between power lines and leukemia, larger epidemiological studies were done. They failed to show any correlation. Therefore, the concerns were essentially laid to rest by larger, better studies. However, with this type of evidence a small correlation can never be completely 100 percent ruled out. All you can say is that the evidence shows no correlation. Also, any correlation that might exist must be very small, smaller than the power of the studies that we've done to detect.

What about microwaves? Microwaves are just a frequency of electromagnetic waves in the microwave frequency. Since microwave ovens have been around, there have also been fears about possible direct harm to people or maybe harmful effects on food. However, with regard to food, while microwaves do alter the chemical composition of food, they do so in a way that's really no different than just cooking food. Cooking food also changes the chemical structure of parts of the food. Therefore, microwaving is no different and there are no specific concerns.

However, concerns that microwaves may have unintended, unhealthy effects on food and water increased after a 2006 YouTube video showing a girl's science fair project. It purported to show damaging effects of microwaved water on plants. There were claims on many websites in the wake of this science fair project that microwaves change the molecular structure of water causing it to have harmful effects. This science fair project, however, was simply comparing two plants and it was not blinded at all.

This is what we call poor scientific or experimental design. There were many, many variables at play here which were not controlled for. The fact that the water was microwaved for one plant and boiled for the other plant cannot be isolated as the variable that resulted in one plant withering away and dying and the other plant thriving. This experiment has been replicated by others with more rigorous controls. They found that boiling, microwaving, or not heating water at all—always allowing the water to cool down to room temperature—has no effect whatsoever on the health of plants. This was just bad science that was perpetrated and replicated through the Internet, spreading fears about microwaves.

Changes to food from microwaves only have minor differences from regular cooking, as I've stated, with no documented risk. But, there is the other concern about radiation leakage from the microwaves themselves. If microwaves are properly constructed, any radiation leakage is insignificant and poses no health risk. The only risk would be from having a faulty microwave oven, either one that was not well constructed—which regulations should prevent from happening—or one that is failing in some way.

It is interesting that microwave ovens were banned in 1976 in Russia. This again becomes an idea that is used to spread fears about microwave ovens. Why did they do this? It turns out that they were banned because of bad shielding. However, when the technical problems were worked out, the ban was removed. Microwave ovens are currently in broad use in Russia.

However, it is true that you shouldn't stand immediately next to a microwave while it's operating. I know microwaves often have those little windows in them and you may be tempted to peak through that window and look at how your food is doing. Doing that very briefly is fine. But, the recommendations are—since there may be a small amount of radiation getting close to the microwave—that you shouldn't stand next to it for long periods of time, looking in.

There is also a real risk of water rapidly boiling in a microwave. This can happen because microwaves do not cook very evenly. Therefore, parts of the water may be heated greater than other parts of the water. Also, the bubbling action of boiling water may not get going if there's nothing to get it started. Therefore, when you open the door and then jostle a cup of superheated water that you had in the microwave, that may suddenly cause it to boil over which can present a real scalding risk. Be careful when you heat up fluids to a high degree in the microwave.

Cell phones present another source of radiation, an increasingly ubiquitous form of radiation exposure. This has raised a lot of concerns about the potential risks of non-ionizing radiation from cell phones. After all, we often will hold cell phones close to our heads, up to our ears. Maybe our brains are getting exposed to this non-ionizing radiation and over years, this may cause an increased risk of cancer or other changes, other health problems.

The plausibility of this claim is actually quite low in that the electromagnetic fields produced by cell phones are very weak. Also, it is non-ionizing radiation, which has a very weak affect on biological tissue. Ionizing radiation, like the kind you would get from actual radioactivity, does cause DNA and other types of cell damage. This question of whether there any health risks from cell phones has been studied for years. At the present time, what we can say about this evidence is that there is no clear-cut risk from using cell phones. Using cell phones for a short period of time, like less than 10 to 15 years, has no demonstrated increased association with brain tumors or other health risks.

However, the literature is still a bit mixed, unclear, and not definitive for long-term exposure, greater than 15 years, or in children who begin having exposure to cell phones at a young age. There still may be a reason for a small amount of caution there. However, again, because the literature hasn't shown any adverse effect, any effect is probably small, especially since the plausibility is quite low.

Fears about the health risks of cell phones were spread, again, by Internet videos. One in particular was the so-called popcorn video. There is a YouTube video showing cell phones surrounding popcorn kernels. After turning the cell phones on for just a short period of time, the popcorn kernels start to pop—as if the radiation from the cell phones were combining together to heat up those kernels. Imagine, you are suggested to do, what it must be doing to your brain.

There are other videos which show cell phones cooking eggs. This has done a great deal to stoke fears about cell phones. However, these videos were admitted to be a hoax. The 2008 popcorn video was a publicity stunt for a Bluetooth manufacturer. There was actually a hot plate underneath the popcorn. That's what heated them up and caused them to pop. There was also a 2005 UK science show called Brainiac, which placed an egg under 100 cell phones. That resulted in no cooking and no change in the egg whatsoever. These are complete myths and an actual hoax and nothing to be concerned about.

I'm going to turn now to some other devices not directly related to magnets. One common device or product that is either combined with magnets or sold alongside them is copper bracelets. Copper itself cannot be magnetic. Copper is not ferromagnetic; it can't hold on to a magnetic field. The claims for copper bracelets are that the copper will slowly be absorbed by the skin. This can have several health benefits including arthritis, reduction in pain, and improvements in your golf swing. That claim is particularly popular.

There are very, very few studies, however, of copper bracelets or other copper devices for these benefits. There was one study in 1978 showing a possible effect, but this was a very small study. There was a follow-up study in 2009 showing no effect whatsoever from copper bracelets. It should also be mentioned that there isn't much of a plausible mechanism to these claims. Again, we have low plausibility and no evidence to support any health claims—so beware.

Visible light is just another form of electromagnetic radiation or electromagnetic waves. Like other forms of electromagnetism, there are legitimate uses for light in medicine. For example, infrared lasers and lights are used legitimately to heat tissue and relax muscles. Ultraviolet light is used to treat psoriasis, a form of skin disease, a rash. This has led to knock-offs that use, or are alleged to use, light in order to heal. For example, you can download an iPhone app that produces a red light with claims as if it were an infrared laser. It may help in finding your car keys or some other situation where you need a quick flashlight, but you're not going to have the effects of infrared radiation from just a red light from your iPhone.

It needs to be mentioned that magnetism may in fact be useful in medicine. At the same time, there is extensive fraud. This fraud should not dissuade legitimate research and it hasn't. Just to give one example, there is a 2010 study that showed that transcranial magnetic stimulation—and to emphasize this, this is a powerful dynamic magnet—was effective for reducing the symptoms of a migraine attack.

For centuries, magnets have fascinated people. This has contributed to widespread use in many dubious devices and also fraudulent health claims. At the same time, magnetism and electromagnetism are legitimate, real forces of nature that are biologically effective and are used in legitimate scientific research. Increasingly, we are developing devices and techniques that can exploit electromagnetism in order to have real health effects. Real EM interventions, electromagnetic interventions, use powerful, dynamic, and specific magnetic fields in order to have their effects. Meanwhile, quack devices are little more than refrigerator magnets.

All about Hypnosis
Lecture 19

Have you ever been daydreaming while driving in the car and arrived at your location without remembering how you got there? ... Much of what happens in the brain while you're daydreaming—not paying attention to external stimuli, although still being able to process them enough to drive to your destination while imagining being somewhere else or in another situation—is very similar to what happens during hypnosis.

L ike most people, you probably know hypnosis from what you've seen on stage or on television. An ordinary person is put into a trance-like state and then starts walking around clucking like a chicken on cue because they were hypnotized to do so. What is hypnosis really? The first myth about hypnosis I'd like to put to rest is that it's a trance-like state. In fact, it isn't an altered state of consciousness or unique state of consciousness. It's actually a state of heightened alertness.

How do you hypnotize someone? It really just has to do with how you interact with the person. For example, the process might involve making someone more suggestible and encouraging them to relax, encouraging them to focus on the person who's doing the hypnotizing, giving them small suggestions to reinforce their attention, and encouraging visualization. Stage hypnosis is different from medical hypnosis; the latter is the topic for the rest of this lecture.

There is a very serious neuroscience surrounding what happens in the brain when people are being hypnotized. These effects fall under 4 broad categories: increased suggestibility; heightened imagination; a lack of attention to sensory information, even a sense of detachment from one's self or environment; and a decrease in executive function, which is the highest order of thinking.

Can hypnosis be used for beneficial medical or psychological effects? Let's turn first to memory. Can we hypnotize people who are having trouble remembering details and get them to recall an event in vivid detail, as is often portrayed on television? It turns out that we cannot. In fact, if anything, the opposite is true. Hypnosis is a condition in which a person is in a high state of imagination and can be highly suggestible. Therefore, patients are likely to make up details at the slightest suggestion.

But there are indeed some legitimate uses of hypnosis. Hypnoanesthesia is the use of hypnosis prior to a surgical or medical procedure to reduce the need for sedating medication. This usually involves self-hypnosis: The person uses techniques like meditation and imagery. This self-hypnosis has been shown to minimize, but not eliminate, the need for sedation. Local anesthesia is often still used. Very closely related to hypnoanesthesia is hypnoanalgesia. Reviews of evidence indicate that hypnoanalgesia is in fact useful for decreasing chronic pain.

Hypnoanesthesia is the use of hypnosis prior to a surgical or medical procedure to reduce the need for sedating medication.

Cognitive hypnotherapy uses hypnosis to treat depression, sleep disorders, chronic pain, and post-traumatic stress disorder. The techniques used involve meditation, cognitive therapy, and self-hypnosis. Cognitive therapy is a separate part of behavioral treatment or talk therapy for all of these conditions, and it has independently been shown to be effective. When hypnosis, mainly involving meditation, is combined with cognitive therapy, it's shown to have significant advantages.

I've mentioned several times the notion of meditation as a form of self-hypnosis. Meditation is not hypnosis exactly, but it is closely related. It is a self-induced state of relaxation. This relaxation may also involve active thinking, self-reflection, or an attempt to achieve a state of what is called mental silence—essentially thinking about nothing.

There are two basic types of meditation and various uses to which they are put. One is called concentration meditation. In concentration meditation, practitioners focus on an object or idea as an anchor to focus their thoughts. In mindfulness meditation, the awareness is not focused on one thing but is distributed as broadly as possible. Their awareness is diffused to everything in the environment, which puts them in a state similar to mental silence.

There is evidence to support medical uses for these types of meditation for pain, blood pressure, stress management, and muscle relaxation. So far, though, there is no evidence to support meditation for psychological conditions like attention deficit and hyperactivity disorder or anxiety. ■

Suggested Reading

Jamieson, *Hypnosis and Conscious States.*

Lynn and Kirsch, *Essentials of Clinical Hypnosis.*

Questions to Consider

1. Is hypnotism real? Do scientists know what is happening in the brain when someone is "hypnotized"?

2. Does hypnosis have legitimate clinical uses?

All about Hypnosis
Lecture 19—Transcript

Like most people, you probably know hypnosis from what you've seen on stage or perhaps on television. An ordinary person is put into a trance-like state, and then starts walking around the stage clucking like a chicken on cue because they were hypnotized to do so.

What is hypnosis really? The first myth about hypnosis I'd like to put to rest is that it's a trance-like state. In fact, it isn't an altered state of consciousness or unique state of consciousness at all. These altered states do exist. In fact, when you are dreaming, you are in a different state of consciousness than when you're awake. That's a true altered state, but hypnosis is not like this. Hypnosis, however, is a very real phenomenon that's studied by scientists. It may involve a relaxed or meditative state. However, it's actually a state of heightened alertness. A key component of being hypnotized is increased suggestibility.

How do you put someone in a condition that we would call hypnotized or how do you hypnotize someone? Again, you're not putting them in an altered state. You're not either entirely in the hypnotic state or out of one; it really just has to do with how you interact with someone else. For example, the process might involve making someone more suggestible and encouraging them to relax, encouraging them to focus on the person who's doing the hypnotizing, giving them small suggestions to reinforce their attention, and also encouraging visualization.

Stage hypnosis is something different than what is often studied by psychologists or used perhaps for medical indications. Stage hypnosis is about entertainment. It's an act. It involves screening and selecting people from the audience who are most susceptible to suggestion or even more importantly, are willing to play along. People are then encouraged to act as they are expected to, to go along with the expectations of the hypnosis narrative. It involves a great deal of social pressure. But, what I'm going to be talking about for the rest of this talk is more about what you can call medical hypnosis or the psychological phenomenon of hypnosis, not what magicians do on stage.

There is, in fact, a very serious neuroscience surrounding what happens in the brain when people are being hypnotized. These effects fall under one of four broad categories. One phenomenon that happens is increased suggestibility. Another is heightened imagination. A third is a lack of attention to sensory information, even a sense of detachment from one's self or the environment. A fourth is a decrease in what we call executive function. Executive function is the highest order of thinking, the thing that enables us to control and plan our behavior—critical thinking. That's also inhibited during hypnosis.

Hypnosis has actually been likened to daydreaming. Have you ever been daydreaming while driving in the car and arrived at your location without remembering how you got there? That's a very normal experience. People can daydream without being provoked to. Much of what happens in the brain while you're daydreaming—not paying attention to external stimuli, although still being able to process them enough to drive to your destination while imagining being somewhere else or in another situation—is very similar to what happens during hypnosis.

This is also not a trance-like state. While you're driving to your destination, you're not in a trance; you're normally awake. You're just activating your active imagination and filtering out distractions. It is a myth that people do not lie or that they do not make things up during hypnosis. It is a state that encourages making things up. Imagination, again, is a very important component of hypnosis.

Here's a word on the difference between being conscious versus unconscious or conscious versus unconscious processing of the brain. Actually, most of the processing of information and sensory information that our brain does is unconscious. You're not aware of most of what the brain is doing from moment to moment. Only a subset of the sensory information that you're processing, that's coming into your awareness, are you consciously aware of. Your brain handles the rest of it for you—even making decisions about what you should pay and should not pay attention to. Then, only a small subset is then presented to your conscious awareness. This can be documented experimentally with what is called inattentional blindness—missing information that we receive, but it's simply not perceived.

What then is responsible for our conscious awareness? This is an ongoing question that is central to much of modern neuroscience. There certainly is no definitive answer at this point in time. However, one of the leading candidate theories for what subset of brain function is responsible for consciousness is called the global workspace. This was first proposed by Bernard Baars in 1987. He hypothesized that conscious awareness stems from a discrete network of neurons that are widely distributed throughout the cortex. The cortex is the thinking part of our brain.

This global workspace puts it all together. It filters out any contradictory or unnecessary information, creating a unified picture of reality, a narrative, a stream of consciousness that we experience. Hypnosis is just a way of affecting this stream of consciousness. There is a process called hypnotic induction. Hypnotic induction is simply doing those things which puts somebody in that relaxed and suggestible condition that we call hypnosis.

Hypnotic induction is what happens before you give an actual suggestion to somebody. You're just preparing them for giving them a suggestion. This involves coordinated activity in various parts of the brain including the brainstem, which is the most primitive part of the brain, the part that involves lots of automatic functions. It also includes various parts of the cortex, like the anterior cingulate cortex, the right inferior frontal gyrus, and the right inferior parietal lobe. This causes a reduction in conceptual spontaneous thought—a decrease in thought—and a reduction in communication between these various areas of the brain.

One of the effects of this is what we call confabulation. Essentially, the mind is ready and open to receive suggestions, but may also not be consciously processing those suggestions. Further, the state may blur the distinction between imagination and memory. People who are being hypnotized, they may be suggested to imagine something—imagine yourself in a certain place or a certain situation. At the end of that experience, they may actually confuse what they were imagining with a memory of an actual experience. That process is called confabulation.

I mentioned previously an effect on executive function, this advanced or higher order planning or self-control that is done primarily in the frontal lobes. Studies show that, during hypnosis, there is inhibition of frontal lobe executive function. In essence, the hypnotized person may hand over their self-control, their executive function, to the hypnotist.

Interestingly, this has the same effect as is seen in response to say, a charismatic leader. When a politician or a charismatic speaker is said metaphorically to have hypnotized the crowd, psychological studies show that that's actually literally true. It's not just a metaphor. The effects on decreasing critical thinking and executive function are the same. You may experience a similar effect in response to a very slick, smooth talking salesman, in fact.

Hypnosis has also been studied in relationship to what we call the Stroop effect. This is a very interesting neurological phenomenon that has been very valuable for psychologists and neuroscientists in studying brain function. It's a standardized test of brain function. The Stroop test or the Stroop effect involves reporting the color of the ink that is being displayed to you rather than the word that is being written. For example, the word "blue" might be shown in red ink and the subject is being asked to name the color of the ink, not the color of the word.

This requires the suppression of the ability to read the word and that suppression takes time. Your brain has to go through the conduction, pathways, and circuitry to suppress your ability to read that word. That causes an unavoidable delay in brain processing and there's nothing that anyone can do to consciously make that delay go away.

For decades, many psychological studies showed that there essentially was no way to make the Stroop effect go away. So reliable was it, in fact, that it was used to flush out spies. For example, a foreign spy who was speaking English and pretending not to speak their native language could be given the Stroop test in their native language. This proved that they can speak it because it would produce a delay that they could not avoid.

A hypnotic suggestion is a suggestion given when somebody is in a state that has been made more susceptible to suggestion by hypnotic techniques. Dr. Amir Raz tested hypnotic suggestion and the Stroop effect. What he found is that, in a small subset of highly hypnotizable subjects, a suggestion that the words being presented to them were scrambled and unintelligible resulted in the Stroop effect going away. This was the first time in the scientific literature that anyone was able to reliably make the Stroop effect go away.

Therefore, this means that, in some people's brains, there must be something different about the hardwiring or the circuitry. Maybe it makes them more susceptible to hypnosis in general or enables them to actually inhibit parts of the functioning of their brain—inhibit it in a way that you cannot do consciously. Only about 1 to 2 percent of people in the population are able to make the Stroop effect go away under hypnosis. Their hardwiring may just be different than the other 98 percent of the population.

That's our understanding, at the present time, of hypnosis—what it is neurologically and psychologically. It's a very interesting phenomenon although what most people think about it tends not to be true. However, can it be used, can it be exploited for actual beneficial medical or psychological effects? The notion that hypnosis might be a medical intervention actually goes back quite a ways.

It originated with Anton Franz Mesmer, who lived from 1724 to 1815. He is considered the father of modern hypnosis. He believed that hypnosis came from the hypnotists themselves through energy, which he called animal magnetism. He actually used magnets in this process although he later dropped them when he found that they were unnecessary. He felt that animal magnetism was a type of life energy that flowed through channels and diseases were caused by blockage of the flow of this animal magnetism.

This was a controversial idea even at the time of Mesmer. Mesmer, in fact, had to flee from Vienna where he was practicing this animal magnetism after he failed to heal a blind musician. He went to Paris where he became famous as a healer, but the public was divided. Half the public thought that he was an important healer. The other half thought that he was a charlatan. He could not ever, however, convince the scientific community at the time of his ideas. He attracted many patients. His sessions involved staring in their eyes while touching their knees and hands, trying to influence the flow of animal magnetism.

Mesmer's career culminated in a famous investigation. King Louis XVI appointed four members of the Faculty of Medicine to investigate animal magnetism as it was practiced by one of Mesmer's students, a doctor by the name of d'Eslon. Antoine Lavoisier was one of the physicians on this panel as was Joseph-Ignace Guillotin and the astronomer Jean Sylvain Bailly. There was also a famous American ambassador—Benjamin Franklin.

Benjamin Franklin, who led up this commission, and the others found no evidence for the fluid of animal magnetism or any clinical effects of mesmerism. This led directly to the fall of Anton Mesmer. His fame then faded. He eventually ended his life, as they say, penniless and anonymous. However, the notion of mesmerism, to mesmerize somebody, had been created. Its popularity did not entirely go away.

It was rescued in 1843 by English physician James Braid as part of an attempt to distance the practice of hypnotism from animal magnetism or "animal spirits." James Braid coined the term hypnosis. Again, he wanted to remove the stigma of mesmerism, but he kept the techniques largely the same.

Despite these colorful roots for the medical uses of hypnotism, we can still ask ourselves the question, are there any useful medical applications for the techniques of hypnosis? Let's turn first to memory, which may be what most people think of first when they think of using hypnosis for a practical application. Can't we hypnotize people who are having trouble remembering details—for example, an eyewitness—and get them to recall an event or a past memory in vivid detail as is often portrayed in the movies or on television?

It turns out that that is simply not the case. You cannot hypnotize somebody to remember something that they don't remember or to relive an event in accurate detail. In fact, if anything, the opposite is true. Hypnosis is putting somebody in a condition in which they are in a high state of imagination and where they are highly suggestible. Therefore, they are likely to make up the details and make up the narrative at the slightest suggestion. In fact, hypnosis is a great way to create what we call false memory syndrome. That is having memories implanted that the person can no longer distinguish from their actual memories.

This is most notoriously the case with several UFO researchers, specifically Bud Hopkins and John Mack. They used hypnosis in order to question people who believe they may have been abducted by aliens. While under hypnosis, they were suggested to imagine themselves being abducted, to imagine a typical abduction scenario. That's exactly what emerged from their story. It's no surprise that the details that were suggested to them—or, in fact, just the details of a typical abduction scenario that we all just know from the culture—are eventually what emerged. After this session of hypnosis, those people confused that with an actual genuine memory.

Let's turn now to some legitimate uses of hypnosis. There is something called hypnoanesthesia. This means using hypnosis prior to a procedure, like a surgical or medical procedure, in order to reduce the need for sedating medication. This usually involves self-hypnosis. This is a person using techniques like meditation and imagery rather than somebody putting them into a hypnotic situation. This self-hypnosis has been shown to minimize, but not eliminate, the need for sedation. Local anesthesia is often still used in cases of hypnoanesthesia for procedures.

Very closely related to hypnoanesthesia is hypnoanalgesia. The word analgesia just means pain relief. Reviews of evidence indicate that it is in fact useful for decreasing chronic pain. It is not only useful in those that are thought to be highly hypnotizable, but it is useful in the population at large.

We know from multiple experiments that mood and attention play a very large role in the subjective perception of pain. Thus, it is no surprise that using techniques which alter one's mood—make one more relaxed, for example—and attention—which happens and is a significant part of hypnosis—can distract somebody, for example, from their chronic pain, and can also reduce the degree to which they notice their pain and the degree to which it bothers them.

Hypnosis has also been studied for smoking cessation, for people who want to quit smoking and are having a hard time doing it. There are many people who use hypnosis and make a specific claim that they can help you quit smoking. This too has been studied scientifically. A 2001 systematic review of 59 published studies showed that hypnotism was more effective than a wait list—meaning people who are on a wait list, waiting to be treated which is another way of saying doing nothing—or no intervention at all as controls. Therefore, hypnotism is better than nothing at all in an unblinded comparison.

However, if you do a placebo control in a blinded fashion, then hypnosis is no more effective. What that tells you is that there are non-specific benefits to thinking you're being treated with something which may be effective. But, there's nothing specific about hypnosis that aids in the process of trying to quit smoking.

There is also something we call cognitive hypnotherapy where hypnosis is used to treat depression, sleep disorders, chronic pain, and post-traumatic stress disorder. The techniques that are used here involve meditation, cognitive therapy, and self-hypnosis. Cognitive therapy is a separate part of behavioral treatment or talk therapy for all of these conditions. It has independently been shown to be effective. But, when hypnosis is combined with cognitive therapy either by another person or self-hypnosis—again, mainly involving meditation—it's shown to have significant advantages.

The clinical research is preliminary in many of these things, but it is very encouraging. Specifically with post-traumatic stress disorders, in addition to self-hypnosis, olfactory triggers are used. In other words, you associate a smell, an olfactory trigger, with a state of being calm and relaxed. At a later time, very much like a hypnotic suggestion, that smell, that olfactory trigger, can be used to reduce the symptoms of post-traumatic stress disorder.

I've mentioned several times the notion of meditation as a form of self-hypnosis. Meditation is not hypnosis exactly, but it is closely related. It is a self-induced state of relaxation. This relaxation may also involve active thinking, self-reflection, or an attempt to achieve a state of what is called "mental silence"—essentially thinking about nothing. It may also involve rhythmic chanting, although that tends to vary tremendously based upon the type of meditation that is being used.

There is actually no clear consensus on the precise definition of what meditation actually means. That is because there are so many different traditions of meditation. However, this active state of relaxation seems to be the key component. Meditation has long cultural roots. The earliest record of meditation goes back to 1500 B.C.E. in Hindu Vedantism, which is a Hindu philosophy. It's often tied to religious or spiritual practices. In fact, meditation was thought by many cultures to be a way of achieving a higher state of consciousness.

There are two basic types of meditation and various uses to which they are put. One is called concentration meditation. In concentration meditation, the person will focus on an object or idea, or one thing as an anchor to focus their thoughts. There's also mindfulness meditation where the awareness is not focused on one thing, but is distributed as broadly as possible. Their awareness is diffused to everything in the environment, which puts one in the state which is similar to the mental silence. If you're paying attention to everything, that's not dissimilar to paying attention to nothing.

There is evidence to support medical uses for these types of meditation for pain, blood pressure, stress management, and muscle relaxation. It has been studied for many other things. However, there's a lack of evidence for psychological conditions like attention deficit and hyperactivity disorder or anxiety. There is no evidence to support meditation for those indications at this time.

Biofeedback is a technique that is closely tied to meditation. It is, in essence, a way of enhancing meditation. It uses equipment to measure physiological function such as muscle tone or brainwaves, which are measured by putting electrodes on the scalp. This is called an EEG or an electroencephalogram. Heart rate can also be measured. By knowing what your heart rate is, how tight your muscles are, and the amount of activity in your EEG or your brainwaves, it gives you the feedback that you need in order to achieve an optimally relaxed state. The end result is really just meditative relaxation, but using these physiological measures in order to optimize them.

Claims that go beyond the documented benefits of relaxation, however, are not evidence-based. While biofeedback is an important component of treatments for conditions which are worsened by stress like migraines and blood pressure, there are other claims that go beyond just mere relaxation. But, they're not based upon any scientific rationale or evidence.

To summarize the role of meditation, it's most useful to consider what element of any treatment—such as meditation—is providing the actual benefit. While there are many different specific types of meditation—for example transcendental meditation or yoga—there are many components to these different types of meditation. But, what the research shows is that the one common element that seems to be providing medical benefit is relaxation—both mental relaxation and the relaxation of muscles.

In fact, there are some forms of meditation—so-called secular forms of meditation that don't have any underlying spiritual or philosophical basis— that focus primarily on muscle relaxation. The focus is on getting individuals to voluntarily get their muscles into a maximally relaxed state. If you strip away the elements that are the dressing of the meditation but don't include relaxation, you get down to the specific component that is having an actual measurable and beneficial effect.

Hypnosis turns out to be a very interesting and complicated myth. I get a lot of questions from people about hypnosis and they tend to be at both ends of the spectrum. From one point of view, hypnosis has a very sketchy past, a past that's mired in things like stage hypnosis. This makes people think that it's just for entertainment and also going back to Mesmer, a use of hypnosis for a variety of dubious purposes. What people think about hypnosis tends to be a myth whether positive or negative.

It turns out that hypnosis is not a trance-like state. It can't be used in order to enhance memory. The beneficial things that people think about hypnosis turn out not to be true. That leads many people to think that hypnosis is not legitimate at all. But, that's really also just another myth. Hypnosis is a very useful technique that is used, in fact increasingly used, as a very functional piece of psychological studies. We're actually learning a lot about how the brain is hardwired and how the different parts of the brain interact with each other by using hypnosis-like techniques on subjects and then seeing what happens to their brain.

In addition, there is an increasing list of specific medical indications for which hypnosis or forms of hypnosis are useful—especially surrounding pain and relaxation. A lot of research is being done into psychological applications, although that requires more research. But, people have a hard time seeing hypnosis as a legitimate medical modality because of this stigma. This stigma goes all the way back to Mesmer and is partly also due to hypnosis being used as a form of stage entertainment. But, it's important for physicians and scientists to separate out the reality of something from its origins or from the mythology. When you separate out hypnosis from its history and these other stigmas, it turns out to be medically and scientifically both interesting and very useful.

Myths about Coma and Consciousness
Lecture 20

There is a famous case of a man named Jean-Dominique Bauby, a French journalist, who had a stroke in 1995 at the age of 43. It left him locked in. He could only blink his left eye. However, he dictated the entire book *The Diving Bell and the Butterfly* one letter at a time by blinking.

TV and movies are full of stories in which someone is in a coma and then at some point, maybe even after years, they wake up—largely neurologically intact. The media also loves stories about people awaking from a coma. This all contributes to a lot of confusion about what coma actually is.

Coma is a disorder of consciousness or wakefulness. What are the causes of coma? One is trauma. Damage to enough neurons can impair the brain's ability to generate enough function to be awake. Another cause is diffuse anoxic/ischemic injury, in which something interrupts the blood flow to parts of or all of the brain. This causes enough damage to parts of the brain that you cannot generate consciousness.

A completely different phenomenon that can impair consciousness is a seizure. A seizure is typically a synchronized, abnormal electrical function where brain cells start to fire in unison. This can happen in one part of the brain or can spread throughout the brain. If a seizure occurs in enough of the brain, it can cause a person to be unconscious. Prolonged seizures can even make a person appear to be in a prolonged coma.

One myth about coma that I want to dispel is that coma is a specific brain state—like a switch that is either on or off. In fact, coma is a continuum. Diagnosing coma offers a lot of challenges to the neurologist. The primary problem is that a lot of the neurological exam is based upon a person being awake and being able to follow complex instructions and answer complex questions. That enables us to probe and query the different functions of the different parts of the brain. Another challenge is that consciousness may be intermittent. If you happen to examine a patient when she's asleep or when her consciousness is at a minimum, you may miss the fleeting evidence of that minimal consciousness.

There are a lot of new technologies currently being used or on the horizon. One of these is the functional MRI scan, which measures blood flow to the brain. By that, we can infer which parts of the brain are functioning and how much they're functioning. PET scans also image blood flow or metabolic activity in the brain so that we can infer brain activity.

What about the notion of waking from a coma? When somebody is in a coma, can they wake up? The short answer to that question is it depends.

By day 3 of a coma ... we can make a very accurate prediction about the probability of someone having potential to awaken.

The most significant factor that determines whether someone can wake up is whether the cause of the coma is reversible. With reversible causes of coma, you absolutely can wake up. For example, someone with a toxic or metabolic cause that's inhibiting brain function can wake up as soon as the toxin or the metabolic problem is removed.

Trauma has a very poor prognosis because trauma represents actual brain damage. Seizures are a bit of a mixed bag. A seizure in and of itself can cause somebody to be comatose. If the seizure is the primary or sole cause of the coma, then treating the seizure can cause somebody to wake up from a coma. But sometime the seizures were occurring in the first place due to a lot of underlying brain damage, which by itself is causing the coma.

How good are we at predicting whether someone has any potential to wake from a coma? There are a few things that we do know: The longer that someone is in a coma, the lower their prognosis or statistical chance that they will wake up. The deeper the coma—in other words, the less brain function that there is—and the older the age of the patient, the worse the prognosis is also. Within 48 hours of someone entering a coma, prognosis is very uncertain. But by day 3 of a coma, using the neurological exam alone or with additional tests, we can make a very accurate prediction about the probability of someone having potential to awaken.

Let's look at some other myths surrounding brain function. What about getting knocked out? This is another TV and movie cliché, where someone is hit on the back of the head, maybe by the butt of a gun. He'll be unconscious for an hour or so and then wake up with nothing more than a serious headache. Does this actually happen? You can knock somebody out by hitting him on the head, but he is unlikely to wake up with no injuries at any time after that. In fact, losing consciousness from a brain injury or from trauma is usually the threshold that will cause some permanent brain damage.

What about amnesia? Another common TV and movie myth is that somebody with a head injury will lose all memories of who she is and what her life has been like up to that point. There's a kernel of truth here in that a head injury, especially one hard enough to cause loss of consciousness, can cause loss of memory. However, it is a complete myth that people will forget who they are from a head injury or any neurological condition. If you have enough brain function to be awake, you know who you are. People who don't remember their name or their identity have a psychiatric condition, not a neurological condition.

Another brain myth that comes up often in the context of coma is the notion that we only use 10% of our brain. Unfortunately, this is a complete myth. We use 100% of our brain. There are many lines of evidence that support this—from anatomical studies to functional studies looking at PET scans, MRI scans, and functional MRI. The entire brain is functioning, and loss of 10% or 20% of the brain is actually correlated with a significant loss of cognitive function.

The brain is the most complex organ in the body—maybe the most complex thing that we're aware of in the universe. Although we don't fully understand brain function or how it generates consciousness, we understand a lot about it. We are getting an increasingly detailed picture of the different parts of the brain: how they function, how they interact together, how they contribute to consciousness, and how damage to different parts of the brain can impair consciousness. ■

Bauby, *The Diving Bell and the Butterfly.*

Parker and Parker, *The Official Patient's Sourcebook on Coma.*

Posner et al., *Plum and Posner's Diagnosis of Stupor and Coma.*

1. What do we know about the neural correlates of consciousness—how brain function causes our conscious awareness?

2. Can someone really awaken after being in a coma for years?

3. What would you say about the idea that most people use only 10% of their brain function?

Myths about Coma and Consciousness
Lecture 20—Transcript

TV and movies are full of stories in which someone is in a coma and then at some point, maybe even after years, they wake up from the coma—largely neurologically intact. The media also loves stories about people awaking from a coma. This all contributes to a lot of confusion about what coma actually is.

What is a coma? Coma is a disorder of consciousness or wakefulness. Of course, this raises the question, what is consciousness? What does it mean to be conscious? There's no clear neurological model of what causes consciousness. We do know that it results from brain function. The leading hypothesis—which I talk about in the lecture on hypnosis— is The Global Workspace. Essentially, it's a distributed network of parts of the cortex, of the thinking part of the brain, that work together to filter all of the sensory information, thoughts, and feelings into one continuous stream of consciousness.

In order to be both conscious and awake, one thing we know is that you need one of your hemispheres, one-half of the cortex, to be mostly functional. You also need your brainstem to be mostly functional. The brainstem has what we call the brainstem activating system. This is a collection of nuclei or centers in the brainstem—most notably the reticular nuclei, but also including other parts of the brainstem—that are sending a constant barrage of activating signal through the thalamus—the thalamus is like the relay center of the brain—and on to the cortex. The cortex—the thinking, awake part of your brain—is constantly being kicked and stimulated in order to keep functioning.

You could also look at this the other way. If you need one hemisphere and the brainstem in order to be awake and conscious, what kind of damage would you need to do in order to not be awake, to not be able to generate wakefulness? You would therefore need to damage either the brainstem or both hemispheres of the brain. Damaging one hemisphere alone is not enough to put somebody in a coma. We see this all the time in neurology. I see patients who may have a severe stroke, completely affecting or damaging one of their hemispheres, but they're still fully conscious and awake.

What are the causes of coma? Again, anatomically, you need to have both hemispheres and/or the brainstem involved. But, there are many different mechanisms of that injury. One is trauma. Trauma can cause what we call diffuse neuronal damage. Damage enough neurons—the conducting, working parts of the brain—and that can impair the brains ability to generate enough function to be awake.

You can also have what's called diffuse anoxic/ischemic injury. Anoxia is a lack of oxygen and ischemia is cell damage due to a lack of oxygen. This is like having a heart attack in your brain in that you have something that interrupts the blood flow, maybe to all parts of the brain or maybe to just large parts of the brain, but not the entire brain. This causes enough damage to different parts of the brain that you cannot generate consciousness.

There is also toxicity. There are many toxins that affect brain function. Of course, if you have something in your system that is adversely affecting brain function, that could affect the entire brain—every brain cell at the same time. These things include alcohol, narcotics, and barbiturates. There is also what we call metabolic disorders. Metabolic disorders are essentially biochemical problems. They are problems with the chemistry or the environment of the brain that doesn't allow the brain cells to function well enough in order to generate consciousness.

This could include increased waste products that are not being adequately cleared by the kidney. It could include ammonia from the liver because the liver is not functioning enough to remove ammonia, which is another toxin of metabolism. Probably the most common metabolic cause of people becoming unconscious is simple low blood sugar. The brain consumes a tremendous amount of sugar for energy. If it lacks sufficient blood sugar level, that alone can shut down brain function and make you become unconscious.

A completely different phenomenon that can also impair consciousness is a seizure. A seizure is abnormal electrical activity in the brain. It is typically a synchronized, abnormal electrical function where brain cells start to fire in unison. This can happen in one part of the brain or it can spread throughout the brain. If a seizure occurs in enough of the brain and especially in both hemispheres, then that in and of itself can cause somebody to be unconscious. You can have prolonged seizures, which can make somebody appear to be in a prolonged coma, in fact. Other things that can affect brain function enough to cause coma include a brain infection or inflammation.

One myth about coma that I want to dispel is that coma is a specific brain state—that you're either all in or not in at all, like flipping a switch. If the switch is off, you're in a coma; if it's on, you're awake. In fact, coma is a continuum. There is a seamless continuum from fully awake to completely unresponsive.

We sometimes use the word obtunded to refer to somebody who has a decreased level of consciousness, but is still conscious enough to interact with the environment and people. To some extent, they can still talk to you. They still know you. They still know that people are there, but they're very abnormally sleepy. You can think of being obtunded as essentially being in a mild coma. Beyond that, there is a minimally conscious state. This is where someone is not awake, but they are barely able to show that they have some signs of consciousness, that they can respond to the environment.

Beyond a minimally conscious state is what we call a persistent vegetative state. In PVS or persistent vegetative state, there needs to be, by definition, a complete absence of all responses to the environment. People in PVS cannot give any indication that they're aware of their environment or that they can respond to their environment. However, there still is brain function. Often, people mistakenly use the term brain dead to refer to people who are in a persistent vegetative state. But, this is not the case. That's another myth. Brain death is in fact death—a complete absence of brain function.

In PVS, the brain is still functioning. In fact, there may still be sleep-wake cycles. People in a PVS may appear to be awake in that they may open their eyes. They may have what's called roving eye movements where their eyes move around the room. But, they don't focus on anything to show that they're aware that something is present. They may open and close their eyes at different times as well. These unconscious, automatic movements can easily be misinterpreted by non-neurological experts as signs of consciousness.

Also, as I mentioned, the end stage of all this is brain death. Brain death is not really a coma. As I said, it's death. Clinically, it means a complete absence of all cortical and brainstem signs—no brain activity at all. In order to make the diagnosis of brain death, you need to meet certain strict criteria. We have medical definitions of brain death. But, in many areas—in specific states in the United States and in other countries—there are legal definitions of brain death. The reason why there needs to be legal definitions is because death is a state that has significant legal implications for that person.

These conditions that meet the medical and legal prerequisites for the diagnosis of brain death often include serial neurological exams. This means that two different neurologists need to examine the patient at some interval, usually 24 hours apart. They need to document with a very detailed and thorough exam that there is a complete absence of brain function.

Alternatively, you can use an electroencephalogram. You can use electrodes to measure brain wave activity. You can indicate or demonstrate with an EEG that all brain electrical activity is decreased to a minimal level. There are strict criteria about how high the gains need to be. In other words, you need to have the EEG set so that it would be sensitive to even very, very tiny brainwaves and still not be able to detect any brainwaves. You can also use tests that are designed to measure blood flow to the brain. If the brain is not receiving any blood flow at all, then the brain must be dead.

Diagnosing coma offers a lot of challenges to the neurologist or clinician. It's often very difficult to say exactly what the brain function is. The primary problem is that a lot of the neurological exam is based upon a person being awake and being able to follow complex instructions and answer complex questions. That enables us to probe and query the different functions of the different parts of the brain.

When somebody has impaired or maybe even absent responses, we lose a lot of our ability to examine brain function. There is still a neurological exam that we can do, a coma exam, but it's limited in its ability to really probe in detail a specific cortical function especially. Also, in addition, people may have focal neurological damage. For example, if somebody has a spinal cord injury, that makes them paralyzed. Therefore, they may not be moving their limbs, not because they don't understand the instructions to move their limbs, but because they're not able to. They're simply paralyzed.

Somebody may also be blind or deaf. They may not be answering questions because they can't hear them, not because they're unconscious. This focal neurological damage or focal neurological deficits can interfere with the ability to test someone's consciousness.

Another challenge is that consciousness may be intermittent. It may come and go. Maybe it's present for only a short period of time out of the day. If you happen to be examining a patient when they're asleep or when their consciousness is at a minimum, you may miss the fleeting evidence of their minimal consciousness. In fact, recent evidence shows that there are subtle signs of consciousness in patients with MCS or a minimally conscious state. These signs may be intermittent. They may be missed in as many as 40 percent of patients, who are then mistakenly diagnosed as having a persistent vegetative state.

But, there are lots of new technologies that are currently being used and are on the horizon. One of these technologies is called a functional MRI scan, or magnetic resonance imaging, which uses magnetic waves and radio signals in order to look in a very detailed way at brain tissue. Functional MRI scan is able to actually measure blood flow to the brain. By that, we can infer which parts of the brain are functioning and how much they're functioning.

There was a landmark study published in 2008 using fMRI scans. They showed that if a patient—who by clinical exam was in a persistent vegetative state—was asked to imagine themselves playing tennis, an fMRI scan would show a certain pattern of activity. If they were then asked to imagine themselves walking through their home, the fMRI showed a different and distinct pattern of activity. Most importantly, these patterns were reproducible. If at a later time, the patient was again asked to imagine themselves walking through their home, the pattern of activity which had previously been seen with that was again displayed.

This means that, to some degree, on some level, that patient must have been processing that information. Their brain activity was different based upon the words that were being said to them. That is a form of interacting with the environment. This patient who is diagnosed with PVS—or in a vegetative state by clinical exam—was actually found to be, at the very least, in a minimal conscious state based upon a more detailed fMRI examination. However, this research is still too preliminary for us to know what this really means for that patient's subjective experience of that consciousness. They may not be aware of their own consciousness even though their brain is still able to interact with the environment to some degree.

There are other tests that can also be used in addition to that exam. For example, there is a PET scan, or positron emission tomography. This is a way of imaging blood flow or metabolic activity in the brain and with that, inferring brain activity. Again, if the brain is functioning, we can see it with a PET scan. You can also use a digital EEG, which is a computer analyzing the EEG signals. Again, this infers which parts of the brain are working. There are also somatosensory evoked potentials where we can stimulate the feet or the hands and see if the brain responds.

What about the notion of waking from a coma? When somebody is in a coma, can they wake up? The short answer to that question is it depends. Not all comas are created equal. The most significant factor that determines whether or not someone can wake up from a coma is whether or not the cause of the coma is reversible or not. With reversible causes of coma, absolutely you can wake up from them. For example, if someone has a toxic or metabolic cause that's inhibiting their brain function, they can wake up as soon as the toxin or the metabolic problem is removed. For example, when somebody is picked up by an ambulance and is unconscious, they will often be given glucose. If they are unconscious because their glucose level is low, they may wake up immediately upon being given intravenous glucose.

Also, someone may be unconscious because they've overdosed with a narcotic. They could be given a drug called Narcan or naloxone, which will immediately counteract the activity of that narcotic. Again, they may immediately wake up. The point there is that the underlying brain anatomically is still intact. Its function is just being inhibited. If you remove whatever is inhibiting the brain function, the person can wake up from their coma.

What about trauma? Trauma has a very poor prognosis because trauma represents actual brain damage. However, trauma sometimes can be tricky because there is often focal damage with trauma that could make somebody seem like they have a lot more brain damage than they actually do. Anoxic ischemic damage tends to have the worst prognosis in terms of the ability to wake up from a coma. That's because there's actual damage to brain cells, not just an inhibition of function. Also, that damage is widely distributed throughout the brain. It's not just in one part of the brain that may give someone the appearance of being in a coma.

Anoxic ischemic injury is a common event in a prolonged cardiac arrest. The heart is not functioning; it's not pumping blood to the brain. It occurs in respiratory arrest, when someone is not breathing or getting oxygen in the blood. It also occurs in drowning injuries. Again, this has the worst prognosis in terms of waking from a coma.

Seizures are a bit of a mixed bag. A seizure in and of itself can cause somebody to be comatose. If the seizure is the primary or sole cause of the coma, then treating the seizure can cause somebody to wake up from a coma. Sometimes we see this. Somebody may have a continuous seizure, something that we call status epilepticus. Sometimes there isn't any manifestation of this seizure, this prolonged seizure, except for the fact that the patient is unconscious. If we give them a medication that can stop the seizure, they can indeed wake up from their coma as a response to that medication.

However, as I said, it's a mixed bag or a double edged sword. This is because subclinical seizure or status epilepticus, an ongoing chronic seizure, is often a result of underlying brain damage. Sometimes you stop the seizure, but the person doesn't wake up. This is because the seizures were occurring in the first place due to a lot of underlying brain damage, which by itself is causing the coma.

Of course, everyone wants to know what the prognosis is. How good are we at really predicting whether or not someone has any potential to wake from a coma? This has enormous ethical and medical implications in terms of how aggressive we should be in continuing to treat people based upon this prediction about whether or not they have any potential to wake up. There are a few things that we do know. The longer that someone is in a coma, the lower their prognosis or statistical chance that they will wake up from a coma.

The deeper the coma—in other words, the less brain function that there is—and the older the age of the patient, the worse the prognosis is also. Within 48 hours of someone entering a coma because of trauma or really any reason, prognosis is very uncertain. We'll rarely make predictions in the first 48 hours unless there is so much obvious damage that it's simply not possible. However, by day three of a coma, using the neurological exam alone or with additional information—from either the EEG or the somatosensory evoked potential—we can make a very accurate prediction about the probability of someone having any potential to awake from their coma.

Also, beyond a certain severity of brain damage, we can say that there is essentially an insignificant chance of meaningful recovery. Patients' exams may change a little bit. But, we could say that, once there is a certain amount of damage that's irreversible, patients are never going to wake up and lead a normal life. This is where the real myth of waking from a coma comes from. Once we've ruled out all the reversible and generally fairly short-term causes of a coma and we are left with someone who has been in a coma for months or years, the chance of waking from a coma is very, very small.

In addition, when you've been in a coma for months or years because of the kind of brain damage that can cause that to happen, it's also almost impossible to awake from that coma and be almost neurologically intact, like is sometimes seen in the movies. What may happen, however, is that a person may improve enough that they go from being just barely in a persistent vegetative state to just barely in a minimally conscious state. Therefore, their exam may improve. That's very rare. More likely, they may be in a minimally conscious state and after months or years, their brain may heal enough that they can barely be able to do things—like focus their attention on a person in the room, say a few words, or gain some function. But, they don't wake up and go home three days later to their normal life.

There are rare cases of people waking from a coma even after years. These cases receive a tremendous amount of media attention. However, the details are very important. When you look at the details of these cases, they usually involve people who were not in a persistent vegetative state, but were rather in a minimally conscious state. In this state, there is a small but very real chance of, again, passing over a threshold where you can be awake. It may also have involved a reversible cause that was missed. An example is a case of someone who had a brain tumor that is putting pressure on their brain and causing them to be in a coma. That tumor shrank over time, releasing that pressure, and allowing them to wake up.

A minimally conscious state versus a persistent vegetative state is a topic that comes up a lot because that distinction, while subtle, has a very important implication for prognosis. For a true PVS, a true persistent vegetative state, after three months, the prognosis is essentially zero for any meaningful chance of waking up. For a minimally conscious state, however, the prognosis is very poor but is not zero. Patients may improve to the point where they can interact, walk, maybe feed themselves, and do some basic things, as I said. That distinction is very important. It also highlights the importance of improving our technology so that we can better make that distinction.

Often family members and just interested people will ask me, when someone is in a coma, are they in there? Is the person and the personality there and aware, just not able to communicate with the outside world? Can they see, hear, and specifically, will they remember what's happening while they're in a coma? For a persistent vegetative state, the answer is somewhat easy in that it appears to be a definitive no. The brain is not doing anything near enough processing to generate memories or anything that the person will experience—and certainly not remember if, at any time in the future, they do wake up.

For a minimally conscious state, since patients are showing some evidence of conscious processing, they may be able to process or experience what's in their environment. They may actually be able to experience pain or the presence of another person. However, there is currently no evidence that anyone who is in this severe degree of coma, a minimally conscious state, remembered any of the experiences that they were having. At the very least, they're not forming memories when they're in this state.

Are there any treatments for people who are in a coma? Generally, the only way to treat a coma is to treat the underlying cause of the coma. If we can identify a reversible or treatable cause, then that's what we would treat. If, however, the coma is just due to brain damage, at the moment there is no specific coma treatment.

However, there are some very intriguing results from research. For example, recent studies using a sleep medication, paradoxically, called zolpidem did show that, in a small minority of patients, they do have a period of wakefulness when they are given this drug. Without it, they are in a minimally conscious state—again, not a PVS but a minimally conscious state. It's thought that a minority of these patients that are in this state, in an MCS, may really have a problem with their sleep-wake cycle. The zolpidem may in fact correct that. It may alter the sleep-wake cycle so that they can be awake.

Another syndrome that is closely related to coma and is often confusingly conflated with coma, but is really distinct, is called the locked-in syndrome. This refers to a patient who is mostly paralyzed. They're actually awake. They're conscious, but they're only able to give minimal signs of consciousness because they're mostly paralyzed. In a brainstem stroke for example, patients may be paralyzed from the eyes down. Everything below the eyes is paralyzed. They can only blink their eyelids. Maybe they can scan or move their eyes voluntarily or grimace a little bit, but they can't move their arms and legs and they can't speak.

Some of these patients do learn to communicate mainly by techniques such as blinking once for yes or twice for no. If they can move their eyes around, there are computer devices and other technologies that can enable them to use their vision in order to communicate more efficiently than just this once for yes, twice for no system.

There is a famous case of a man named Jean-Dominique Bauby, a French journalist, who had a stroke in 1995 at the age of 43. It left him locked in. He could only blink his left eye. However, he dictated the entire book *The Diving Bell and the Butterfly* one letter at a time by blinking whenever an assistant, Claude Mendibil, reached the desired letter. Claude would read through the letters in the order of most common usage to make it more efficient. When he arrived at the letter that Jean-Dominique wanted, he would blink. He wrote an entire book using that method alone.

Some people, however, try to communicate with those who are locked in and maybe even comatose using a technique known as facilitated communication. This is a very dubious method that was developed in 1977 by Rosemary Crossley. The technique involves holding the hand of someone who is physically or mentally impaired—not able to move normally—and helping them to type on a typewriter or point to letters on a board.

This became very popular in the 1980s before it was carefully researched. But, once that research was carried out, it overwhelmingly showed that the facilitator—the person who was holding the arm and helping the client—was doing all of the communication. This was largely through what we call the ideomotor effect, which is making small subconscious motor movements that you're not aware of. Facilitated communication was thoroughly discredited by this research, but it still crops up in some coma cases. For example, there was the recent case of Rom Houben who was claimed to be much more conscious than he actually was through facilitated communication.

I want to turn now to some other myths surrounding brain function. What about getting knocked out? This is another TV and movie cliché where people will be hit on the back of the head maybe by the butt of a gun. They'll be unconscious for an hour or two and then wake up with nothing more than a serious headache. Does this actually happen? You can knock somebody out by hitting them on the head, but they're unlikely to wake up with no injuries in any time after that. In fact, losing consciousness from a brain injury or from trauma is usually the threshold of trauma that also will cause some permanent brain damage. We call that traumatic brain injury.

Traumatic brain injury causes serious and often chronic, if not permanent, neurological symptoms like chronic headache, dizziness, vertigo—which is a sense of being off balance or spinning—cognitive impairment, poor memory and concentration, difficulty in learning new things, and difficulty with multi-tasking specifically. These are long-term symptoms, not just a brief headache from getting hit on the head hard enough to lose consciousness. These types of head injuries we call a concussion. Specifically, a concussion is any head injury that results in the temporary decrease in brain function. This could be just mild confusion or it could be all the way to unconsciousness.

What about amnesia? Another common TV and movie myth is that somebody with a head injury will become completely amnestic. They'll lose all their memories of who they are and what their life has been like up to that point. There's a kernel of truth here in that a head injury, especially one hard enough to cause loss of consciousness, can cause loss of memory. You get what we call retrograde amnesia, which is loss of memory for things before the trauma and anterograde amnesia, which is loss of memory for events after the injury.

However, it is a complete myth that people will forget who they are from a head injury or any neurological condition. You never forget who you are by an injury or by neurological damage. If you have enough brain function to be awake, you know who you are. People who don't remember their name or their identity have a psychiatric condition, not a neurological condition.

Repeated trauma can also cause chronic damage to the brain. There is something we call dementia pugilistica or dementia coming from being punched or getting blows to the head. This occurs most frequently with boxing. Studies have shown that after 12 to 16 years of boxing, about 15 to 20 percent of boxers will develop dementia pugilistica, a chronic dementia like Alzheimer's disease. This includes some famous boxers like Muhammad Ali and Sugar Ray Robinson.

I'm going to turn to another brain myth, however, that comes up often in the context of coma—the notion that we only use 10 percent of our brain. I've even had patients or family members say, well, the person who's in a coma can recover because you only need 10 percent of your brain anyway. All they need to do is improve up to that point.

Unfortunately, this is a complete myth. We use 100 percent of our brain. There are many lines of evidence that support this—from anatomical studies to functional studies looking at PET scans, MRI scans, and functional MRI. The entire brain is functioning and loss of 10 or 20 percent of the brain, for example, is correlated with a significant loss of cognitive function.

This also leads to the question of what the brain does. There are two broad categories of brain processing that the brain does—conscious versus unconscious. Actually, most of the processing that the brain does is unconscious, meaning that we're not aware of it. There are some interesting neurological phenomena that demonstrate this such as blind sight. People who are blind may still be able to navigate an obstacle course. They have no awareness that their brain is actually seeing the obstacles and is enabling them to negotiate around them.

The brain is the most complex organ in the body; maybe it's the most complex thing that we're aware of in the universe. Although we don't fully understand brain function or how it generates consciousness, we understand a lot about it. We are getting an increasingly detailed picture of the different parts of the brain and how they function and interact together, and how they contribute to consciousness, and how damage to different parts of the brain can impair consciousness. While we cannot fully explain exactly how brain function is translated into our conscious awareness, we do know that consciousness results from brain function. As we often summarize, consciousness is what the brain does.

What Placebos Can and Cannot Do
Lecture 21

> There's also what we call nocebo effects. If these psychological factors or some of them can lead to the false impression that there is a benefit from an inactive treatment, can there also be harm or perceived or measured harm from an inactive treatment? It turns out that there can be.

A placebo is any inactive substance or intervention given as a real treatment. Any perceived response to a medical intervention other than a physiological response to an active treatment can be considered a placebo response. There are many types of placebo effects. One category is psychological effects. These include the desire of the patient to improve, to please the person administering the treatment, and to justify the risk and expense of the treatment. Another powerful psychological effect is confirmation bias. This includes the notion that people tend to notice and remember events that confirm their beliefs, biases, and desires. They will also miss, ignore, or explain away any disconfirming evidence.

There are many other observational artifacts that contribute to placebo effects. An artifact is anything that causes an illusion in observation. One that scientists recognize is regression to the mean: In any system or any symptoms that fluctuate over time, any extreme in this fluctuation is more likely to be followed by a return to the mean, just from pure statistics. There are also observer effects. This is simply the understanding that the act of observing affects behavior and outcomes. For example, subjects in a clinical trial may be more compliant with their treatment when they're being regularly seen by a health-care provider.

There are also many nonspecific effects. That means that there are benefits of variables that are incidental to the treatment itself. For example, if you disrupt your stressful day to undergo a treatment, the treatment may be relaxing in and of itself. There's also psychological benefit from the therapeutic and caring attention of the provider.

What about expectation? There is a common belief that someone needs to have an expectation of benefit from a treatment for there to be a placebo effect. This itself is a myth. However, expectation may enhance or increase the placebo effects that are occurring.

Can there be real benefits to placebos? They are present. There are real benefits to placebos, but we have to put them in context to understand that they are very strictly limited. Placebo effects can cause a genuine reduction in stress from nonspecific and psychological aspects of the treatment. And reduction in stress does reduce risk factors for many real biological disorders like heart disease. Muscle tension also responds to psychological stress. When you're anxious or under a lot of stress, you'll tense up your muscles, which can cause a lot of very real symptoms. Therefore, placebo effects that reduce stress will improve those biological functions. The perception of pain is also highly subjective. Anything that provides improved mood or comfort or the expectation of benefit will improve or decrease this perception of pain.

There are real benefits to placebos, but we have to put them in context to understand that they are very strictly limited.

However, these limited and carefully delineated placebo effects should not be used to argue that placebos can have other effects that are not documented and not plausible. Placebos are not a panacea. In fact, systematic reviews of clinical trials have found no measurable mind over matter or biological placebo effect.

So is there anything beneficial to placebo effects? If so, is there any way to exploit them without deceiving patients and without using treatments that are harmful or contain unnecessary components? First of all, it's important to remember that real and effective medical interventions come with placebo effects. This includes things like a good therapeutic relationship between the treater and the patient, a positive mood and outlook, overall healthful behaviors, and improved compliance with a necessary treatment. However, placebo effects cannot ethically be used to promote pure placebo treatments.

Medical advances can largely be understood as progressively moving away from placebo interventions to biologically active and science-based interventions. But at the same time, ironically, we are trying to understand those aspects of placebo effects that are genuinely helpful. It may seem contradictory: We are using placebos as a very important tool for removing illusions and misdirections from our understanding of what works and what doesn't work. At the same time, we are trying to exploit beneficial aspects of placebo effects to maximize patient healing, reduce symptoms, and improve quality of life. It should be kept in mind that all of the benefits that you can get from placebo effects you will also get from treatments that are science based and actually work. ■

Suggested Reading

Benedetti, *Placebo Effects*.

Price, Finniss, and Benedetti, "A Comprehensive Review of the Placebo Effect."

Questions to Consider

1. What causes placebo effects?

2. Do you think a placebo effect is sufficient to justify a medical intervention?

3. Do physicians commonly prescribe placebos?

What Placebos Can and Cannot Do
Lecture 21—Transcript

When I was younger, I was told that rubbing a potato on a wart would make the wart shrivel up and go away. When I questioned as to how this might possibly work, I was told that it was all through the power of mind over matter. It was especially effective in children who were too innocent to know that it's implausible that a potato should kill a wart. Therefore, belief in its effectiveness was important to this mind over matter effect. Are placebo effects, so-called placebo effects, really mainly mind over matter or are there other scientific explanations?

The definition of a placebo is any inactive substance or other intervention given as a real treatment. The word placebo comes from the Latin for "I will please" or "I shall please." Any perceived response to a medical intervention other than a physiological response to an active treatment can be considered a placebo response. You can also consider a placebo response based upon a very practical application of any response to a placebo treatment in a clinical study.

This mind over matter notion of placebo effects is the biggest myth of this lecture. This started in 1955 when an author wrote an article called "The Powerful Placebo" and published it in the *Journal of Clinical Epidemiology*. In that article, it was claimed that the placebo effect is largely this "mind over matter" real biological effect. In this review of studies including 1082 patients, it was claimed that there was a 35 percent placebo response to inactive treatments.

However, in reality, there isn't one placebo effect; there are many placebo effects. It is anything that will cause the perception of benefit to an inactive treatment. In fact, a later re-analysis of that 1955 study showed that there was no evidence for any "mind over matter" biological effect. Rather, many different effects were identified as being responsible for the measured effects or benefits from inactive treatments.

These include many different types of things. One category of placebo effects is psychological effects. This includes the desire of patient to improve or to find relief from symptoms, to please the person who is treating them or perhaps a researcher who is studying a new treatment, and to justify the risk and expense of the treatment. This actually has a term in psychological literature. It's called risk justification or expense justification. People will invest time, money, emotion, effort, and maybe even some of their prestige in basically asserting that a type of treatment will be helpful for them or in carrying out or purchasing the treatment.

They therefore want to justify not only their expenditures, but also the decision that they made. This effect is supported by research. For example, it shows that more expensive pills have a greater measured placebo effect. If somebody spends $10.00 for a pill, they expect to get more of a benefit out of it than if they spent $5.00 for a pill. In addition, invasive or highly involved procedures have more of a placebo effect in clinical trials than just taking a pill. Again, the more that's invested in time, effort, or money into a treatment, the greater the measured placebo effect. Also, another psychological factor that can't be ignored is the desire of the doctor or the experimenter to be successful and also to please the patient and successfully improve their symptoms.

Another very powerful psychological effect is called confirmation bias. This includes the notion that people tend to notice and remember events that confirm their beliefs, biases, and desires. They will also miss, ignore, or explain away any disconfirming evidence. Therefore, it may seem like there is powerful subjective evidence to support something that you believe. You may not be aware of the fact that you are systematically seeking out and remembering only that evidence that supports something which you already believe. You have either ignored or dismissed lots of evidence which would have shown that belief to be false.

To give one example, when taking vitamin C in the belief that it will prevent the common cold, a person might convince themselves that they never get the cold when they take vitamin C. But, they occasionally may get just "the sniffles"—but these sniffles are not really a cold.

There are many other observational so-called artifacts that contribute to placebo effects. An artifact is anything that causes an illusion in observation, the impression that there's an effect there when there really isn't. One that scientists recognize is called regression to the mean. What this means is that, in any system or any symptoms—let's say in this case, disease symptoms—that fluctuate over time, any extreme in this fluctuation is more likely to be followed by a return or a regression to the mean, just from pure statistics.

If we apply this to somebody with chronic symptoms or a chronic illness, they're likely to have good days and bad days. When are you going to take your treatment? It's when you're having a bad day. If you're normally fluctuating from good days and bad days and you treat your symptoms whenever you have a bad day, just from statistics alone, that's likely to be followed by a regression to the mean and a reduction in those symptoms. Also, most illnesses are what we call self-limiting. A self-limiting illness is one that will go away or get better all by itself just through the body's natural healing abilities without any need for any specific intervention.

We often summarize this with the somewhat witty saying of, "Untreated, a cold will last for a week, but treat a cold and it will only last for seven days." Both of these types of illusions—regression to the mean and the fact that most illnesses that people come down with will get better on their own—fall prey to what we call the post hoc ergo propter hoc logical fallacy. People tend to assume—and this is just part of human psychology—that when one thing follows another thing, that it means it must have been caused by it. If B follows A, A must have caused B. But, this is just an assumption and is not necessarily true. When you take that treatment and then you get better, people want to assume that the treatment made the symptoms get better. But, that's not necessarily true and we cannot assume that.

There is also what we call the observer effect or observer effects. This is simply the understanding that the act of observing affects behavior and outcomes. For example, subjects in a clinical trial may be more compliant with their treatment and more likely to take it when they're supposed to when they're being regularly seen and examined by a healthcare provider. They may also engage in other healthy behaviors. Just the fact that they're now paying attention to their health and they are being followed for certain health outcomes may make them engage in more healthy behaviors. The act of observation has influenced the outcome all by itself.

This is most famously noted in what is called the Hawthorne Effect, which is just this observer effect. This is named after experiments that were conducted between 1924 and 1932 at the Hawthorne Works. What the researchers were trying to figure out is whether light levels affect worker productivity. If we increase the light in the factory or decrease it, can we get people to be more productive and work harder?

What they found was, when they increased the light levels and then observed the workers to see how productive they were, their productivity went up. When they decreased the light levels and then observed how productive the workers were, their productivity went up. When they returned the light to normal and observed how productive the workers were, their productivity went up. It turns out that observing how productive the workers were all by itself made them work harder and increase their productivity. The light levels had no effect whatsoever.

There are also many non-specific effects. That means that there are benefits of variables that are incidental to the treatment itself. For example, if you disrupt your busy, maybe hectic, and stressful day in order to undergo a treatment, the treatment may be relaxing in and of itself. It may force you to, again, break from your routine and sit or maybe even lie down for a period of time. The relaxation is what we would call a non-specific or incidental aspect of the treatment itself. It is not a physiological response of what the specifics of the treatment are.

But, there may be actual benefit from the relaxation, a non-specific benefit. If we confuse that benefit with the non-specific aspects of a treatment with benefit from the specific aspects of the actual treatment itself—taking a medicine, for example, or maybe getting a massage or something like that— then we will falsely conclude through this type of non-specific placebo effects that the specific treatment is what's working.

There's also attention from a healthcare provider, which not only may result in better health behavior, but also psychological benefit from the therapeutic and caring attention. This may increase somebody's mood. We know an improved mood does reduce the perception of pain. It reduces how much pain bothers people. It specifically will improve psychological symptoms like depression and other subjective symptoms.

What about expectation? There is this common belief that someone needs to have an expectation of benefit from a treatment in order for there to be a placebo effect. This itself is a myth. You do not need to believe in a treatment in order for all of these other things, which I have just mentioned up to this point, to have a measurable effect. However, expectation may enhance or increase the total amount of the placebo effects that are occurring. It can also improve mood, which, as I stated, can lead to health benefits in and of itself. Believing that you're going to get better from chronic symptoms which have bothered you may be reassuring and make people feel better, which in and of itself will reduce subjective symptoms.

Another myth about the placebo effect is that animals and babies cannot have a placebo effect. This is because they can't expect to gain benefit, but as I just said, expectation is not necessary. They can't even know that they're being treated. They're not the ones who are often reporting the benefit. It is the examination of someone else. This leads to the false conclusion that there can't be a measured placebo effect in studies of animals or babies who are too young to understand what's going on. However, again as I reviewed, there are many factors that contribute to placebo effects that have nothing to do with the knowledge or the expectation of the person who's receiving the treatment themselves.

In addition, you have to consider who's deciding if an animal or a baby is getting better or not. The illusion of some of the placebo effects may reside in the mind of the evaluator, the person who is doing the research, not in the animal or the person who is being treated.

There's also what we call nocebo effects. If these psychological factors or some of them can lead to the false impression that there is a benefit from an inactive treatment, can there also be harm or perceived or measured harm from an inactive treatment? It turns out that there can be. Clinical studies show that there is this negative placebo effect called nocebo effects. This is from the Latin for "I will harm" compared to placebo which means "I will please."

This is partly based on expectation and also on what we call hypervigilance towards everyday symptoms. If you tell someone that they're likely to get a headache, for example, or that they may start itching, that in and of itself may be enough to cause the sensation of itching or to cause a headache. This is partly what we call psychosomatic.

In addition, people have everyday aches, pains, and symptoms that they don't pay much attention to oftentimes. They're below our notice. But, when they take a treatment and they're on the alert for symptoms, then they may start to notice these symptoms that were there all the time. They may attribute them to what just happened or what treatment they just received.

This causes a bit of a dilemma for a physician because we are ethically obligated to give informed consent to our patients, to tell them all the possible significant side effects to a treatment that we are recommending for them or about to give them. However, at the same time, this may actually increase the occurrence of nocebo effects. We often have to walk a very fine line between giving informed consent without scaring patients into have these nocebo effects.

Can there be real benefits to placebos? They are present. There are real benefits to placebos, but we have to put them into context to understand that they are very strictly limited. Placebo effects can cause a genuine reduction in stress from non-specific and psychological aspects of the treatment—again, believing that you're going to get better and the comforting attention of a therapeutic agent like a physician or other treater. Reduction in stress does reduce risk factors for many real biological disorders like heart disease. The heart function responds quite sensitively to psychological and mental stress. Muscle tension also responds to psychological stress. When you're anxious or under a lot of stress, you'll tense up your muscles and that can cause a lot of very real symptoms. Therefore, placebo effects that reduce stress will improve those biological functions.

The perception of pain is also very highly subjective. Pain is a purely subjective experience. As I often say, we have no painometer. There is no way to objectively measure pain. We can only know about it by what patients tell us about what they are subjectively experiencing. Anything that provides improved mood or comfort or the expectation of benefit will improve or decrease this perception of pain.

However, these limited and carefully delineated effects from the placebo effect or placebo effects should not be used to argue that placebos can have other effects that are not documented and not plausible. Placebos are not a panacea. In fact, systematic reviews of clinical trials have found no measurable mind over matter or biological placebo effect. There was no placebo effect for any objective biological measure. Therefore, cancer patients do not survive longer due to placebo effects.

Stress is a risk factor and may even cause some health problems, but it's not significant for other problems. For things for which we're not measuring a subjective problem and for which stress is not a significant risk factor, we shouldn't have an expectation of—and the evidence doesn't show—any non-specific benefit from placebo effects.

Placebos are, however, a critical part of our medical research technology. Placebo effects are mostly why we need to carefully control clinical trials. We need to control all of the variables that can lead to placebo or nocebo effects. Ideally, in a well-designed—what we would call a rigorously designed—clinical trial, the treatment in question will be isolated as a lone variable. It will be isolated from all other possible effects including placebo effects. That way, any improvement in outcomes from that treatment can be separated entirely from these placebo effects. It's also the reason why anecdotes, which are uncontrolled stories or case histories, are not very compelling. They're not reliable because any possible beneficial or harmful effect of the intervention in question is mixed together with all kinds of placebo effects. They can't be separated out.

Placebos in clinical trials, in their simplest form, are just sugar pills. Some people may think that placebo is synonymous with a sugar pill when in fact sugar pills are placebos. However, there are other kinds of placebos as well.

In medication trials, when you're studying the effects of anything that could be given in pill form—whether a nutrient, supplement, or pharmacological agent—you would create a sugar pill or a placebo that looks identical to the medicine. Therefore, neither the person who is taking the pill nor the person who is prescribing it in the trial can know who's getting the placebo and who is getting the active treatment. We call these trials double-blind because both the treater and the treated are blinded to the treatment versus placebo.

For procedures, placebos are much more challenging. You have to design a sham procedure that can be used instead of the real procedure. It's difficult to do this. It's difficult to do a sham procedure where the person delivering it doesn't know if they're giving a real treatment or a fake placebo treatment and where the person receiving is not aware of whether or not something genuine is happening. Sometimes it's easier than at other times, but it can often be very, very challenging in designing a clinical trial.

For surgical procedures—where you have to actually perform surgery, cut through the skin down into some anatomical location, and make changes to the anatomy of a person—it's impossible in many cases to actually perform sham surgery. In order to do something that convincingly sham, you would have to open up the patient, but not do the actual surgery. This was actually done in years past. There were a few published studies where sham surgery was done as a placebo. However, for many decades, this has been considered to be unethical and it's no longer done.

There's also something called active placebos. These are placebos that are not completely inert. They are usually some medicine that's benign. They won't affect the disease that's being studied, but it will produce some side effect, for example maybe a little nausea. Maybe it will have a bitter taste. This is meant to convince the subjects in a study who are taking the placebo that they're getting a real medicine. Another way to put that is it's preventing them from being unblinded, from figuring out that they're getting the placebo and not a real treatment.

Depending on the side effects and the characteristics of the medicine being studied, active placebos may be a huge advantage. In addition, for placebo controlled trials, it is often a component of the study design to interview patients and the experimenters treating them as to whether or not they think that the patient or the subject was getting an active treatment or a placebo. That's a way to detect whether or not a study was properly blinded or not.

What about using placebos as a medical intervention? This has had a long history. Our thinking about this, ethically and otherwise, has certainly evolved over time. However, you may be surprised to hear that a 2009 survey found that as many as 60 percent of physicians admit to at least occasionally prescribing what they think of as a placebo treatment to a patient—a treatment that is no more effective than a placebo.

Sixty percent is a huge number. But, most of these physicians did this only occasionally or on rare occasions—not as a routine part of their practice. In addition, this doesn't mean prescribing a fake sugar pill, a literal placebo. It could mean doing something like prescribing vitamin B12 supplements for a marginal or a low vitamin B12 level in somebody with certain symptoms that don't have any other specific treatment. You're giving a real, active treatment for something that the patient may need. You don't really expect that it's going to treat their symptoms. The physician may hope that, as a side benefit, they also get a placebo benefit and the patient's headaches or some other symptoms may also go away.

The practice of prescribing actual placebos to patients was more common in the past. In decades past, physicians practiced under more of what we would call a paternalistic model. The physician knew best. They would make decisions for the patient and didn't have to explain every little thing that they were doing to the patient. However, this paternalistic model was abandoned long ago, at least in many parts of the world and certainly where I practice in the United States.

Let me give you a really interesting example of this old practice of prescribing placebos. In fact, there is a substance called methylene blue, which you can give and prescribe as a tablet. If you eat a tablet of methylene blue, it will only have one biological effect. It will turn your urine blue. Physicians actually engaged in the practice of prescribing these methylene blue tables to patients. They told them that it would cure their symptoms. They would know it's working if their urine turned blue, which of course the physician knew was going to happen. That was meant to reinforce and maximize the placebo effect.

These kinds of things are no longer considered ethical and are no longer done. In fact, today we would describe the philosophy of medicine as that of informed consent where the patient is more of a colleague with the physician. The decision making process occurs together. The physician or other healthcare provider is ethically obligated to get reasonable informed consent about the risks and benefits of any treatment that they're advising the patient to take, or procedure they're about to do, or prescription they're about to get.

Most patients would probably be unwilling to take a placebo intervention if they were told honestly that it was only a placebo with no active effect. But, the question is often raised—is there anything beneficial to placebo effects? If so, is there any way to exploit it without deceiving patients and without using treatments which are either harmful or contain unnecessary components? First of all, it's important to remember that real and effective medical interventions also come with a placebo effect—and the full range of placebo effects that I described including any beneficial effects.

You don't need to give a fake or inactive treatment in order to get placebo effects. In fact, it is okay to maximize these non-specific but beneficial effects. This includes things like a good therapeutic relationship between the treater and the patient, a positive mood and outlook, overall healthful behaviors, and improved compliance with a necessary or effective treatment. However, placebo effects cannot be used ethically to promote pure placebo treatments.

Some promoters of treatments that have been shown by science to not be effective, to be nothing more than an inactive intervention, have said that, well, they will at least still get placebo effects out of their treatments—and that that is sufficient to justify what they're doing. However, these placebo effects are mostly illusion. It's not sufficient to justify, in my opinion, a treatment which has no expectation of real biological benefit. It also violates the ethical considerations of informed consent.

Placebo effects tend to be fleeting in nature. They tend to be minor. They tend to for subjective symptoms or stress related symptoms only. It's generally considered not adequate as a medical intervention all by itself. In fact, looked at from the perspective of history, we have had thousands of years of experience with what, in retrospect, were essentially placebo interventions. Most of the medical interventions throughout human history have not been effective. Some of them have even been harmful. They perpetuated and continued to exist for decades, centuries, or even more than a thousand years, in some cases, because of placebo effects.

I often use this as an example when people ask how a treatment could have survived for so long if it didn't have any effect, any real benefit. Placebo effects explain that. In fact the placebo effects can be so compelling and convincing—if misleading—that they can cause the survival of treatments like bloodletting, for example. Bloodletting survived for over 1500 years if not longer. We now know, from our advantage of 20/20 hindsight of history, that it was not only worthless, bloodletting was actually harmful and contributed to the death of many patients.

Pain is an important exception that we really do need to carve out for placebo effects because pain is probably the thing that responds most to placebo interventions. Clinical trials show that about 30 percent of people will have a significant reduction in the amount of pain that they report in response to placebo interventions, completely inert interventions. This may be partly explained by the release of endorphins.

Endorphins are naturally occurring molecules that we make inside our bodies that bind to opiate receptors on our nerve cells—the same receptors that morphine and other powerful painkillers bind to. It's possible—and evidence actually suggests—that endorphin release and inhibiting pain through binding through endorphin receptors, these opiate receptors, does occur in response to some placebo interventions.

But, again, I must reinforce that safe, active, and effective treatments will also get this effect. However, you can avoid unnecessary, tedious, expensive, and risky treatment rituals by understanding that they are not necessary in order to achieve any beneficial effects of pain relief from this endorphin release or other placebo effects.

Another question I commonly hear and another myth about placebo treatments is what the harm is. If somebody subjectively experiences benefit and the treatment is inactive, then no harm is done and those kinds of interventions should be okay. However, this comes largely from a misinterpretation of what placebo effects largely are. Again, they are largely an illusion, an artifact of observation. But, even to the extent that they do provide a real subjective improvement, a placebo effect that does provide such an effect may be misinterpreted. This may lead somebody into believing that an inactive treatment or maybe even entire system of medicine or intervention has real biological effects when they don't. When you take a placebo treatment for that self-limited subjective complaint, that may lead you to believe that that treatment is reliable for more serious, even life threatening illnesses.

To summarize, there are many placebo effects, not one placebo effect. Mind over matter is a very persistent myth about placebos, but does not contribute significantly to what we measure as placebo effects. However, understanding the placebo is important to understanding the complexities of the therapeutic relationship of how people respond to various kinds of treatments. Harboring myths about placebos, however, can lead to belief in other medical myths. In fact, myths about the placebo are a gateway myth that leads to many, many medical myths and false beliefs. It can also hamper effective informed consent and decision making on the part of patients.

Medical advance can largely be understood as progressively moving away from placebo interventions to biologically active and scientifically based interventions. But, at the same time, and ironically, we are trying to understand those aspects of placebo effects which are genuinely helpful. It may seem contradictory. We are using placebos as a very important tool to removing illusions and misdirections from our understanding of what works and what doesn't work. At the same time, we are trying to exploit beneficial aspects of placebo effects to maximize patient healing and reduce symptoms and improve quality of life. However, it should be emphasized that all of the benefits that you can get from these placebo effects you will get from treatments that are science based and actually work.

Myths about Pregnancy
Lecture 22

It's expected that mothers who are pregnant will gain weight from the pregnancy itself. But how much weight gain is healthy or appropriate? It's not necessary actually for a woman to significantly increase her intake of food. An additional 300 calories per day is the average need of a pregnant woman in order to get all the nutrition that she needs.

P regnancy is a powerfully emotional event in our lives, for the women who become pregnant, but also for every family member. It's no surprise that when pregnancy comes up, friends and relatives come out of the woodwork with medical advice. But is this advice true, or is much of it myth?

Many beliefs and advice center on how to get pregnant in the first place. The reality of getting pregnant is that timing is everything. The egg and the sperm have to be in the same place at the same time. If you achieve this, fertilization occurs with a 30% success rate.

There are some other variables, however, that people consider to increase the odds of getting pregnant. Does position matter? The bottom line is no, at least not to the probability of getting pregnant. Should you save up sperm? It turns out that maximum sperm counts occur at about 48 hours, so there is no point in saving up beyond a 48-hour time period. There's also no evidence that moving around after sex reduces the chances of conception. You may have heard that if the man sits in a hot tub, that will reduce the chance of conception. That is true; heat does reduce the sperm count slightly.

Once a woman is pregnant, we often want to predict the sex of the child. There are scientific ways to do this. An example is ultrasound, which allows us to determine the sex with about 93% accuracy. But there is a lot of folklore that pretends to be able to determine what the sex of the child will be. For example, carrying low is supposed to indicate a boy, and carrying high is supposed to predict a girl. Actually, how a woman carries is determined by muscle tone and baby position; it has nothing to do with the gender of the fetus.

Another myth is that if the mother is craving sweets, she will have a girl. If she is craving salty foods, she will have a boy. Most pregnant women report that they do have cravings. This is due to altered taste and smell, though there may be other factors like nutritional needs that are not completely clear in the research. However, these cravings bear no relationship to the sex of the child.

What about choosing the sex? Some couples may not want to just predict what sex of child they're going to have; they may want to actually determine whether they have a boy or a girl. There are many folklore beliefs about this. Many of them involve timing, such as whether conception occurs during the day or at night. There are myths about conceiving during a full moon or in a particular position. Other myths involve foods that the mother eats at or around the time of conception. None of these folklore beliefs have any validity in science or medicine.

The evidence for the effects of caffeine is actually quite mixed.

Once a couple has achieved pregnancy, of course, they want to have the healthiest pregnancy possible. This is another source of many beliefs about pregnancy. A healthful diet for the mother is definitely healthy for the baby. Let me go over some nutritional details that are legitimate. You may have heard that fish is brain food and therefore is good for mothers to eat while they're pregnant. This is true, but seafood may also contain mercury. While fish is a good source of certain nutrients during pregnancy, pregnant women should avoid swordfish, shark, and white tuna and should eat no more than 12 ounces of fish per week.

In order to have a healthy pregnancy, there are certain foods that should be avoided. These include unpasteurized milk; soft cheeses such as feta, Brie, or Roquefort unless the label says it's made with pasteurized milk; refrigerated meat spreads or pâtés; and hot dogs and deli meats, unless they are very thoroughly steamed.

What about alcohol? We cannot say, based on the evidence, what a safe level of alcohol is during pregnancy. Therefore, it's best to just avoid it completely.

What about caffeine in pregnancy? The evidence for the effects of caffeine is actually quite mixed. In order to be conservative, it is recommended that pregnant women take less than 200 milligrams of caffeine per day, which is about the amount of caffeine you would get in a 12-ounce coffee.

What about other exposures during pregnancy? Accutane, which is a drug commonly used to treat acne, increases the number of birth defects. Therefore, Accutane should not be used during pregnancy or even while trying to become pregnant. Another thing that women should avoid is nail polish. Nail polish contains phthalates, which are endocrine disruptors and may interfere with certain hormones. What about using a hair dryer? That is safe, as is hair dye.

There have been some concerns raised about pregnant women sitting in front of a computer monitor for hours at a time. There is no evidence or theoretical basis for any health concerns from using computers. However, pregnant women are at higher risk of developing carpal tunnel syndrome. This is because their tissues tend to retain more fluid.

What about air travel—should pregnant women restrict their air travel? The increased exposure to radiation is minimal and of no health concern. But there are legitimate health concerns from long flights. One is to make sure that you keep well hydrated. Also, you should get up and walk around the cabin as often as possible to prevent the occurrence of blood clots in your legs from stasis.

Another genuine risk to pregnancy is smoking. Smoking inputs toxins into the body and can be associated with decreased fetal weight and premature birth. These factors are in turn associated with learning disabilities, increased risk of cerebral palsy, and lifelong problems. ∎

Suggested Reading

Bouchez, "Separating Pregnancy Myths and Facts."

Harms and Mayo Clinic, *Mayo Clinic Guide to a Healthy Pregnancy.*

Stone and Eddleman, *The Pregnancy Bible.*

1. What are the ways you can predict or determine the sex of a child before it is born?

2. What do you really need to know to have a safe pregnancy?

Myths about Pregnancy
Lecture 22—Transcript

Pregnancy is a powerfully emotional event in our lives, especially for the women who become pregnant, but also for every family member. It seems that, at every stage of life, pregnancy is important to someone that we're close to—whether it's our own mother, perhaps ourselves, our spouse, our brothers and sisters, our cousins, or when we get older, our children, and our grandchildren. At every stage of life, pregnancy is important to someone close to us. It's no surprise that when pregnancy or the question of pregnancy comes up, friends and relatives come out of the woodwork with medical advice trying to be helpful.

But, is this advice really true or is much of it myths? That's what we're going to explore in this lecture—pregnancy myths and beliefs. Many of these beliefs and advice center around how to get pregnant in the first place. For some basic review, in terms of how to get pregnant, timing is everything. The egg and the sperm have to be in the same place at the same time. If timing is optimal—if you achieve the sperm and the egg getting in the same place at the time—fertilization occurs with a 30 percent success rate.

In order to make this happen, sperm survive three to four days while the egg survives for one day. The timing has to work out so that living sperm are there when the egg is dropped and still alive. Ovulation occurs 14 days prior to onset of menses, regardless of the duration of the menstrual cycle. Therefore, it is best to have intercourse in the two to three days prior to ovulation, during ovulation, and for one day following ovulation.

There are some other variables, however, that people consider in how to increase the odds of getting pregnant. For example, position—does position matter? The bottom line is no, at least not to the probability of getting pregnant. Should you save up the sperm? If you need the sperm to be maximal at the time of ovulation, should you save up so that you have this maximum sperm count when it counts? It turns out that maximum sperm counts occur at about 48 hours, so there is no point in saving up beyond a 48-hour time period. In fact, this led to the belief that having intercourse about every other day or every 48 hours around the time of ovulation was the optimal strategy. Those were the recommendations. However, recent evidence shows that having intercourse every 24 hours around ovulation has a slightly higher chance of conception than every 48 hours. Therefore, those are now the current recommendations.

What other variables are there? If using a lubricant, make sure that it is non-toxic and that it is not a spermicide, which means that you have to read the label very carefully. Yes, this does really happen. I'll never forget a lecture I had in medical school by a fertility expert. He related the story of counseling couples in all the various ways in which they ran into trouble trying to conceive. He told the story of a couple that could not conceive. It was discovered that they were using a lubricant that was a spermicide and just were not aware of it.

There's no evidence that moving around after sex reduces the chances of conception. Also, heat does reduce the sperm count slightly. You may have heard that if you sit in a hot bath or a hot tub, that that will reduce the chance of getting pregnant or conception for the male. That is true. If a man sits in a hot tub for greater than 30 minutes, it will slightly decrease their chances of getting pregnant.

While some people may be trying to conceive, other people may be trying to avoid getting pregnant or avoid conception. There are perhaps more myths about how to avoid pregnancy than how to become pregnant. For example, let's go back to the hot tub myth that I just discussed. While sitting in a hot tub or a hot bath will slightly reduce the sperm count, this certainly is not enough of an effect or a reliable enough effect in order to prevent pregnancy entirely. Thus, you can't rely upon this hot tub effect.

Likewise, having sex in water at all does not prevent or even reduce the chances of conception. In fact, if you're relying upon the use of a condom as a method of contraception while having intercourse in water, the heat of the water or maybe some chemicals in that water may break down the condom and cause it to fail—or the water itself can get in and cause the condom to slip off. Again, it's another way to result in contraceptive failure.

It is true that anyone can get pregnant, any female that is, and any male can cause pregnancy the first time. It is a myth that for first timers, there's no risk for pregnancy. How about early withdrawal? This certainly decreases significantly the probability of resulting in conception. However, it is not an absolute protection, even if done correctly. The reason for this is that there is a small amount of sperm in the lubricant that males excrete during sex. In some cases, this small amount of sperm is enough to cause conception.

What about standing up or jumping around on the part of the female after intercourse? This has no effect on the prevention of pregnancy and is not a reliable method of contraction. Sperm have evolved to be really good swimmers upstream. Jumping around just doesn't help.

There are also methods called calendar methods or more popularly known as the rhythm method or rhythm methods. This basically involves restricting intercourse to times of the month when there is no ovulation. I mentioned previously that if you're trying to maximize your chances of conception, you'll want to have intercourse just before, during, and just after the probable time of ovulation. If you're trying to avoid pregnancy, then you can avoid having sex at those same times. This does result in a dramatic decrease in the probability of conception. However, there is a particularly high failure rate from relying upon this method.

What are those failure rates? Let's just look at some recent surveys examining the failure rates of the various methods of what are called reversible contraception—not surgery to make somebody permanently infertile, but just reversible or short-term methods. For example, taking the contraceptive pill has a 7 percent failure rate. I want to emphasize this is a failure rate from all causes, not necessarily a failure rate from the medicine itself. It's mainly from women forgetting to take the pill for two or more days. There is a 9 percent failure rate when using a male condom. There is an 8 percent failure rate for a diaphragm and a 20 percent failure rate for periodic abstinence or the calendar or rhythm methods. There's also a 15 percent failure rate for spermicides. The calendar method is one of the most unreliable methods of contraception.

Once a woman is pregnant, they often want to predict the gender of the child that they're going to have. There are scientific ways to do this, for example with ultrasound. Ultrasound uses harmless sound waves that bounce off the fetus. It gives a pretty good image of the fetus, enough to see enough anatomy that you can sex children with about a 93 percent accuracy.

At 12 to 14 weeks, the orientation of what's called the genital tubercle— upwards equals a boy and down or parallel equals a girl—is 93 percent accurate in predicting the gender of the child at birth. In the second trimester, there's an even more accurate method, but it still relies upon ultrasound. Here, basically if a penis is present or visible, it's a boy. If a penis is not visible, then it's a girl. In the second trimester, this method—although it may seem very straightforward—is 99 percent accurate.

Other than ultrasound, you can rely on amniocentesis or chorionic villus sampling. In amniocentesis, some of the amniotic fluid is removed from the mother. This is then looked at for chromosomes. The DNA determines whether a child is a male or a female. In mammals, the XX chromosomes equal a girl and XY equals a boy. This method is essentially 100 percent accurate in determining the gender of a child.

But, there is a lot of folklore that pretends to be able to determine or predict what the gender of the child will be. For example, carrying low is supposed to equal being a boy and carrying high is supposed to predict a girl. Actually, whether or not a woman carries high or carries low is determined by muscle tone and baby position and has nothing to do with the gender of the fetus. This dates back to England. This is Old English lore. It was based upon the notion that boys need to be out in front and independent, while girls need to be close and protected. It is somewhat based on the sexist notions of the time.

What about the activity of the unborn child? If the fetal heart rate is greater than 140, there are those who claim that that predicts a boy while less than 140 predicts a girl. This has actually been studied in scientific experiments. It has been shown to be completely false. The heart rate has nothing to do with whether or not the child is a girl or a boy. Another method is fetal activity rather than heart rate. Fetal activity is how much the child is moving around. If it's greater, that is supposed to predict a boy and if it's less, that would predict a girl. This, again, is based upon sex stereotypes—the notion that boys are more aggressive and more active than girls. But, this has no relationship in the perceived activity level and gender. Again, it's been studied and this one is simply false.

What about urine testing? There is a myth that if a pregnant woman mixes her urine with Drano, the change in color will determine the gender. There is no one accepted scheme for what color change equally which sex. However, there is no validity to it either so it doesn't matter that there isn't a consensus.

Here's another myth. If the mother is craving sweets, then they will have a girl. If they are craving salty foods, they will have a boy. Whether or not cravings and aversions actually occur in pregnancy is a little bit controversial. But, it is somewhat accepted that pregnant women will have cravings. Most pregnant women do report that they do have that. This is due, when it occurs, to altered taste and smell. But, there may be other factors like nutritional needs, although that is not completely clear in the research. However, these cravings bear no relationship to the gender of the child.

There are many gastrointestinal and weight related myths for pregnancy. If the husband puts on weight, it's supposed to predict that his wife is going to have a girl. That one is pure folklore. It has no relationship or even plausibility in biology. If the mother has a round or full face, that is alleged to predict that she will be having a girl. Again, it's pure folklore. The more severe the nausea and vomiting—that is also supposed to predict a girl. There have been only a couple of studies looking at that and there is no consistent or clear relationship.

Some methods for predicting gender in pregnancy are little more than just dowsing. For example, if you take your wedding ring and suspend it over the belly of the pregnant woman, it is alleged that it will swing in a circle is she is carrying a girl. It will swing back and forth if she is carrying a boy. This is just a form of dowsing, which is nothing more than the ideomotor effect. Small and unconscious movements in the hand can cause a dangling object to either move in a circle or move back and forth. There is no plausible scientific mechanism for how that can work. There is no evidence to show that dowsing can predict the gender of a child or anything else.

There is something called the Chinese conception chart. This is meant to predict gender based upon the time of conception. It is based upon the age of the mother and the time of the month or the month in which the conception occurred. Belief in this is actually fairly strong in China. There have been studies of whether or not the timing of conception does alter the chances of having either a boy or a girl, but studies have failed to validate any legitimacy to this Chinese conception chart.

The bottom line here is that you have about a 50/50 chance of predicting the gender of a fetus with any of these folklore methods. However, scientific methods that have been developed are very accurate. As I said, using ultrasound is 93 percent accurate or more as the child ages—as you get into your second trimester, for example. Amniocentesis is 99 percent accurate. If you really must know the gender of your child before birth, I suggest using one of those methods and not relying upon any folklore.

What about choosing the gender? Some couples may not want to just predict what gender of child they're going to have. They may want to actually determine whether or not they have a boy or a girl. As I said, sex is determined entirely by the sperm from the male because the males in mammals carry an XY combination of chromosomes, one X chromosome and one Y chromosome. Females carry an XX. The mother can only contribute an X to their child. The male—the father—can contribute either an X or a Y. It is that X or Y which determines at least the genetic gender of that child.

But, of course—you saw this coming—there are many folklore beliefs about choosing gender. Many of them involve timing, whether or not conception occurs during the day or at night. Sometimes there are myths about conceiving during a full moon or at other times of the month. Many of these folklores involve position. Some involve foods that the mother eats at the time of conception or around that time. All of these folklore beliefs about influencing gender have no validity in science or medicine. They are mostly superstitions.

There are some methods, though, that people have been trying to develop for influencing the gender of a child rather than just leaving it up to a 50/50 or close to 50/50 chance. There is one method called the Ericsson method. This has been used since the 1970s. Even though that was many decades ago, there are still few studies to support its validity. The Ericsson method alleges to enrich sperm with either Y or X chromosomes. Therefore, this enriched sperm—more X or more Y—can be used in insemination and thereby affect the chances of conceiving a boy or a girl.

There is one Hong Kong study that showed an 83 percent success rate of, producing a male baby using the Ericsson method. But, it failed to enrich the sperm that was used with Y chromosome. That is a contradiction. If it was really working, the only real plausible method by which it could work was that it enriched the sperm with a greater proportion of Y chromosomes. It's hard to explain how it worked in that study, but failed to enrich the sperm with Y chromosomes.

There is speculation that the Ericsson method may preferentially inactivate X sperm. Even though there were the same number of X and Y in the sperm, the X carrying sperm were preferentially inactivated. Therefore, a Y sperm had a greater chance of leading to conception and therefore, a greater chance of being a boy. However, this is mainly speculative and there is no empirical data at this time to support that mechanism.

Some couples rely upon a technique called in vitro fertilization. In vitro means "in glass" or outside of the body, for practical purposes. The sperm and the egg are collected separately. They are fertilized in vitro—this is the so-called test tube baby approach—and then implanted in the womb of the mother. This provides an opportunity for sex selection simply by doing chromosomal analysis prior to implantation.

Once you have fertilized the eggs in the Petri dish or in the test tube, you can then examine them and see whether or not they are carrying an XX or an XY. You can then implant only the desired sex or gender into the womb. This also allows for the opportunity for methods of sorting sperm. You don't have to use all of the sperm in order to do the fertilization in the test tube.

You can use one method or another to separate X and Y sperm. You can then use just the X or the Y that's desired in order to achieve conception or fertilization. There is what is called cytometric methods of separating, which have been shown to be 80 percent effective in separating X and Y sperm.

Once a couple has achieved pregnancy, of course everyone wants to have most healthy pregnancy possible. This is another source of many beliefs about pregnancy. A healthy or healthful diet for the mother is definitely healthy for the baby. Let me go over some nutritional details that are actually legitimate. You may have heard that fish is brain food and therefore is good for mothers to eat while they're pregnant. This is true.

However, seafood may also contain mercury. While seafood and fish in particular is a good source of certain nutrients during pregnancy, pregnant women should avoid swordfish, shark, and white tuna. It is recommended that they should eat no more than 12 ounces of these fish per week. However, eating some fish is beneficial because, as I said, fish is brain food. It contains essential fatty acids. There was a Harvard study that showed that eating fish in the second trimester correlated with increased IQ at six months of age.

There are also infections that are more likely or are more dangerous during pregnancy. In order to have a healthy pregnancy, there are certain foods that should be avoided. The FDA in the United States has a list of foods that pregnant women should avoid. These include unpasteurized milk; soft cheeses such as feta, Brie, or Roquefort unless the label says "made with pasteurized milk;" refrigerated meat spreads or pâtés; refrigerated smoked seafood, unless it is cooked afterwards in a casserole or other dish as the cooking kills the bacteria and reduces the chance of infection; and hot dogs and deli meats, unless they are very thoroughly steamed, should also be avoided.

What about weight gain? Of course, it's expected that mothers who are pregnant will gain weight from the pregnancy itself. But, how much weight gain is okay? It's not necessary actually for a woman to significantly increase her intake of food. An additional 300 calories per day is the average need of a pregnant woman in order to get all the nutrition that she needs. However, this is highly individualized. It is based primarily on the weight of the mother at the time of becoming pregnant. Women who are overweight when they become pregnant may in fact not need to increase their caloric intake at all. They may gain very little or no weight overall during the pregnancy.

What about alcohol? Alcohol should be entirely avoided during pregnancy. This data is mostly correlational because it's just not ethical to do experimental studies on potentially toxic effects in pregnancy. You can't randomize pregnant women to take something that you're trying to figure out whether or not it's going to damage them or their child. But, we can ask women about their behaviors both during and after pregnancy and then try to correlate that with outcomes. Therefore we cannot say, based upon the evidence, what a safe level of alcohol is during pregnancy. Therefore, it's best to just avoid it completely.

Specifically, there's something known as the Fetal Alcohol Syndrome. This may be associated with either binge drinking or multiple episodes of heavy drinking during pregnancy. This causes multiple congenital abnormalities in the child including mental retardation.

What about caffeine in pregnancy? Most pregnant women are told that they should restrict their caffeine intake while pregnant. Sources of caffeine include coffee, tea, cola, and chocolate. The evidence for the effects of caffeine in scientific studies is actually quite mixed. In order to be conservative, it is recommended that pregnant women take less than 200 milligrams of caffeine per day which is about the amount of caffeine you would get in a 12 ounce coffee. A 2008 study from the *American Journal of Obstetrics and Gynecology* found that drinking 200 milligrams or more per day doubled the risk of miscarriage. Therefore, there is the recommendation of less than 200 milligrams per day. Some institutions have lowered that recommendation just to have an increased buffer of safety.

What about other exposures, other things that pregnant women might be likely to be exposed to during pregnancy? What should they avoid? Should mothers, for example, avoid getting close to or using a microwave oven? Other than the general safety recommendations of not standing right next to an operating microwave for any prolonged period of time, there does not appear to be any special risk to pregnant women or to the pregnancy from microwaves. You can use microwaves and eat food that has been cooked in microwaves safely.

Accutane, which is a drug commonly used to treat acne, increases the number of birth defects. Therefore, Accutane and no product with Accutane should be used during pregnancy or even if you are trying to become pregnant. That is an important point to emphasize because if you're trying to become pregnant, then you will be pregnant for four to six weeks before you realize you're pregnant. Most of the really important development occurs during that first six weeks or so. Therefore, most of the risk from these kinds of environmental exposures will have already occurred.

If you're trying to become pregnant, you should be engaged in all of the healthy activities that you should do while you are pregnant. Another thing that women should avoid is nail polish. Nail polish contains phthalates. These are also found in hairsprays and deodorants. These are what we call endocrine disruptors. They may interfere with the effect of certain hormones. A small 2005 study found an association with genital problems in boys whose mothers were exposed to phthalates. While this is preliminary evidence, it is reasonable to avoid things that are optional in any case—like products like nail polish—that contains these compounds.

What about using a hair dryer? Can you dry your hair with either a portable or a full hair dryer? That is safe. Other hair products are as well, like hair dye. There's no evidence to suggest that dye in hair contains anything unsafe for a mother. There have been some concerns raised about using computers, sitting in front of a computer monitor for hours at a time for pregnant women. But, there is no evidence or theoretical basis for any health concerns from using computers in pregnant women. However, pregnant women are at higher risk of developing carpal tunnel syndrome. This is because their tissues tend to retain more fluid and using a keyboard may also contribute to carpal tunnel syndrome. But, that is not a risk to the child itself.

What about air travel? Should pregnant women restrict their air travel? The concern here is increased exposure to radiation. As you rise in the protective blanket of the earth's atmosphere, you get exposed to more and more cosmic rays. This is because less of those cosmic rays are being filtered out by bombardment with the atmosphere. However, this amount of radiation that you get from taking even a long jet flight is minimal and of no health concern.

There are legitimate health concerns from long flights if you are pregnant. One concern is that you need to make sure that you keep well hydrated. Pregnant women may have increased needs for hydration so carry plenty of water with you. Also, you should get up and walk around the cabin as often as possible while on a plane in order to prevent the occurrence of blood clots in your legs from stasis and from sitting around for hours at a time.

There is one parasite called toxoplasma, which is of specific concern in pregnant women. You may have heard to avoid exposure to cats while pregnant. This is true—specifically cat fecal matter, which can contain the toxoplasma parasite. Many people are walking around with some antibodies or even a little bit of toxoplasma in them, so it is actually a fairly common thing to be exposed to probably because many people are exposed to cats and kitty litter.

However, this infection can be extremely serious in pregnant women and therefore, any chance of contracting toxoplasmosis should be minimized. Therefore, the standard recommendation is for women who are pregnant to avoid kitty litter. You can also get toxoplasma from the soil. If a pregnant woman is going to do any gardening, they should wear protective gloves. Also, all food should be thoroughly cooked.

Another very genuine risk to pregnancy is smoking. Smoking inputs toxins into the body. It can be associated with decreased fetal weight and premature birth. While you shouldn't smoke anyway because smoking has many health risks, it has additional health risks for the child in pregnant women. These premature births and decreased fetal weight are in turn associated with learning disabilities, increased risk of cerebral palsy, and lifelong problems. They are significant.

There are a number of myths surrounding the notion of certain activities or positions that women who are pregnant should avoid. I'm just going to list a number of these myths. An example is sleeping on one's back. Pregnant women are told that while pregnant, they shouldn't sleep on their back. However, this is safe. The belief is that it may compromise blood flow to the placenta or the fetus. But, this is simply not true. If it's comfortable, feel free to sleep on your back.

What about raising your arms over your head? Will it cause the umbilical cord to twist up? This one is pure folklore. Raising your arms in any position won't affect the umbilical cord position. There is another myth that you should not start any new exercise, any exercise that you haven't engaged in prior to the pregnancy. This one is a myth because starting a new form of exercise does not pose any special risk to the pregnancy. However, like anyone starting a new form of exercise, there is a risk of injury if you overdo it and are not used to it.

Women do not need to avoid swimming or bathing while pregnant. This poses no risk. Nor do you need to avoid bumpy car rides. The false belief here is that it may induce a premature labor. This has actually been studied and has been found to have no risk.

There is a tremendous amount of misinformation and myths surrounding pregnancy. When a woman becomes pregnant, there are many people in their lives that are certain to make an effort to bring that misinformation and myths to them. It's understandable, however, that there will be so much concern surrounding pregnancy. It is an incredibly important event in all of our lives. I'm going to end with a quote from George Bernard Shaw who wrote, "Life is a flame that is always burning itself out, but it catches fire again every time a child is born."

Medical Myths from around the World
Lecture 23

There are many claims that bee pollen is a superfood, an especially nutritious food. It is a really good food for the bees, and it does contain many useful nutrients. But years of research have not found any specific health benefits for humans.

Taking a broad cultural view might help put beliefs and myths into a broader perspective. Are there some common themes, or is it true that medical myths are specific to individual cultures? We're going to take a look at some medical myths from around the world to try to put this all into a broader perspective.

Let's start with the Korean fan death myth. There is a belief, unique to South Korea, that sleeping with an electric fan running overnight can result in death. Fans in South Korea, in fact, are made with a timer switch so that they will automatically shut themselves off in order to avoid this feared calamity. But is there any plausibility to this belief?

There are several putative causes for what might cause harm or death from sleeping with a running fan. One is hypothermia—that the fan will cause someone to lose too much body heat, their body temperature will drop to dangerous levels, and their heart will stop. Another is that the fan will cause suffocation; it will interfere with the person's ability to breathe.

Is there any real risk from using a fan? In a very hot environment, relying entirely upon a fan may be insufficient. It can lead to hyperthermia and dehydration, which can be dangerous. While fans themselves do not present any risk, relying on a fan under the false assumption that it's cooling a dangerously hot environment may pose some risk.

Now we turn to Africa, where there are many human immunodeficiency virus (HIV) myths. HIV is at epidemic proportions in Africa, with an estimated 22.4 million infected people. Efforts to stem this epidemic rely heavily on the population having accurate information. HIV myths in Africa are therefore especially pernicious and are hampering attempts at controlling this dangerous epidemic.

One horrible myth surrounding HIV in Africa is that it can be cured by having sex with a virgin. This has led to much child rape and the spreading of HIV to children. It also may lead to the false belief that one has been cured, therefore leading to the further spread of HIV.

There's also a belief called HIV denial. This is the denial of scientific evidence establishing that HIV is the cause of the clinical syndrome known as acquired immunodeficiency syndrome (AIDS). This myth is largely based on conspiracy theories—that there is a conspiracy among governments and pharmaceutical companies to sell medications or to decrease unwanted populations.

HIV denial, while somewhat of a worldwide phenomenon, is especially harmful in Africa. Some of these HIV fears were tied to vaccines. There was specifically the myth that HIV was being spread by the West deliberately in the polio vaccine. This crippled vaccine efforts, especially in Nigeria. This decreased compliance with the polio vaccine led to the return of almost epidemic polio in Nigeria, which then spread to other countries, setting back eradication efforts by years, if not decades.

To wrap up our world tour of medical myths, let's look at one that originated entirely in the United States. Many people think that the caduceus is the symbol of the medical profession. The caduceus is essentially a staff with wings at the top that has 2 snakes winding around it. The caduceus is actually the wand of Hermes and has nothing in Greek mythology—or in any other mythology—to do with medicine or the healing arts.

The actual symbol of the medical profession is the staff of Aesculapius. Aesculapius is a Greek god and the son of Apollo. He was the god of medicine. His staff is a staff with no wings and a single snake wrapping around it. That staff is the symbol of medicine and was thought to be a healing staff. The mistake of confusing the caduceus for the staff of Aesculapius was first made by the U.S. Army Medical Corps in the late 19th century. Its spread from there led to medical institutions and hospitals using the caduceus for decades, thinking that it was an appropriate symbol of medicine.

In the middle of the 20th century, the knowledge that the staff of Aesculapius was more appropriate began to take hold. The American Medical Association (AMA) now uses the staff of Aesculapius, and you may notice it painted on the back of ambulances. Even though this story isn't really a health myth, it shows how one authoritative source can be responsible for the spread of misinformation. The spread of this misinformation to other sources like hospitals and the AMA lent it the further appearance of authority. This reinforces the notion that you need to question everything, even if it seems to be coming from a reliable source.

Medical myths from around the world tend to have some similar themes.

Taking a look at these various myths, we see that cultures do vary, but people are fundamentally the same. Medical myths from around the world tend to have some similar themes. These themes include a desire for control, a desire to understand our health, and a desire to have a simple system by which we can understand and improve our health. Another common theme is that people who are ill may become desperate and seek out things to help their problems. I think that by looking at the various myths from around the world, we see that people are the same no matter where you go. ■

Suggested Reading

Brenneman, *Deadly Blessings*.
Epstein, *The Invisible Cure*.

Questions to Consider

1. To what extent are medical myths the same or unique in various cultures?

2. Where in the world is HIV denial most prevalent and pernicious?

3. Why is the caduceus believed to be the symbol of the medical and healing professions?

Medical Myths from around the World
Lecture 23—Transcript

Taking a broad cultural view might help put beliefs and myths into a broader perspective. For example, do various cultures tend to harbor the same misconceptions? Are there some common themes or is it true that medical myths are just a matter of culture and therefore specific to individual cultures or language? We're going to take a look at some medical myths from around the world to try to put this all into a broader perspective.

Let's start in Korea with the Korean fan death myth. There is a belief, actually unique to South Korea only, that sleeping with an electric fan running overnight can result in death. Fans in South Korea, in fact, are made with a timer switch so that they will automatically shut themselves off in order to avoid this feared calamity. But, is there even any plausibility to this belief? Can there be any risk from sleeping in a room with a running fan?

There are several putative causes for what might cause harm or death from sleeping with a running fan. One is hypothermia—that the fan will essentially cause someone to lose too much body heat and their body temperature will cool down to dangerous levels and their heart will stop. Another one is that the fan will cause suffocation. It will interfere with the person's ability to breathe.

Related to that is that it might cause depletion or decrease in the amount of oxygen in the air in the room. There are thoughts that it may do this in a couple of ways. One is that it may chop up the O_2 air molecules—oxygen molecules—in the air. If O_2 is chopped up into just elemental oxygen, it won't be in the air in a form that can be breathed, go into the blood, and do its job. There are beliefs that maybe it sucks the oxygen out of the room. Either way, with decreasing levels of oxygen, that's what causes the death.

Others believe maybe it's not sucking air out of the room, but it might be sucking the breath out of the lungs of the sleeping person. Still others believe that it may keep the skin itself from breathing, which itself is a little bit of a minor myth. The skin doesn't need to necessarily breathe in order for someone to stay healthy. All of these beliefs are medically wrong. They are pure urban legend.

But, can there be any real risk from using a fan? It is true that fans do not decrease air temperature in a room. They move the air around and make you feel cooler by causing evaporation of sweat on your skin. They cause evaporative cooling, but they don't reduce the air temperature. In fact, if anything, they may slightly increase the air temperature due to the heat produced by the motor in the fan. However, this increase in air temperature is insignificant and not worth worrying about.

The real point here is that, in a very hot environment, relying entirely upon a fan may be insufficient. It can lead to hyperthermia and dehydration. Once dehydration occurs, a person's sweating will decrease. That will reduce and maybe even eliminate the evaporative cooling causing hyperthermia, which can be dangerous. While fans do not present any risk, relying upon a fan under the false assumption that it's cooling the environment in a dangerously hot or warm environment may pose some risk.

Let's turn to another Asian myth, that of Koro. Koro is the name given to a believed disease or disorder in which the male penis can shrink up entirely and retract inside the body. Fears that this dreaded disease was spreading spread in waves of mass delusion. However, there are also isolated cases. This is actually a real disorder in that belief that Koro exists is a delusion. It's a specific type of delusion called body dysmorphic delusion where people have a fixed false belief about something about their body.

Another example of this would be anorexia nervosa. This is people who believe that they are overweight or obese even while they are dangerously underweight. Anorexics can look in the mirror and look at skin over bones and emaciated form, and in their minds, they see somebody who is overweight. That's a body dysmorphic delusion.

Koro is similar in that people who fear that they are suffering from that believe that their penis is actually shriveling up or being retracted inside the body. When there are news reports or stories about a case of Koro cropping up, in the cultural setting of belief that this is a real disorder, fear often spreads. This becomes what we call a mass delusion or a community panic, which has been described in the psychological literature and can occur for other types of belief as well.

Those who believe that Koro is a real biological disorder have thought of several possible causes for it. There, of course, is no genuine scientific cause. Some believe that it is due to an imbalance of yin and yang, the two types or sides of chi, the Asian name for a vitalistic life energy. Some people say that perhaps it's caused by excessive masturbation or by sex with someone other than your wife. Perhaps there are many women in the culture who specifically spread that belief. Some think it can be spread through food or contact like a contagion. It is in fact a contagion; it's just a mental contagion, not a biological contagion. There is a West African version of this Koro belief. However, in the West African version, penis theft is thought due to black magic rather than due to some medical disorder.

Turning to Africa, there are many HIV or human immunodeficiency virus false myths in Africa. HIV is at epidemic proportions in Africa. There are an estimated 22.4 million people living with HIV in the Africa. That's two-thirds of all people living with HIV in the world. In 2008, 1.4 million people died of AIDS in sub-Saharan Africa. It is a full-fledged epidemic that, if anything, is getting worse. Therefore, efforts to stem this epidemic are important. They rely heavily on the population having accurate information. HIV myths in Africa are therefore especially pernicious and are hampering attempts at controlling this very dangerous epidemic.

One of the most horrible myths surrounding HIV in Africa is that it can be cured by having sex with a virgin. This, of course, may lead to the false belief that one has been cured and therefore leads to further spread of HIV. But, it's also responsible for much child rape in Africa in addition to spreading HIV to children through that rape.

There's also a belief called HIV denial. This is the denial of scientific evidence establishing that the human immunodeficiency virus is the cause of the clinical syndrome known as AIDS or the acquired immunodeficiency syndrome. This was first promoted by a German physician Peter Duesberg, so belief in HIV denial is not isolated to Africa. But, once this belief got out into the general public, a subculture of belief based upon this notion that HIV does not cause AIDS began to spread.

It is largely based on the notion of conspiracy theories—that there is a conspiracy to spread the lie that HIV causes AIDS. Sometimes that conspiracy is framed as one among governments and pharmaceutical companies to sell medications to treat HIV. It may be a conspiracy to literally decrease unwanted or unpopular populations. It is embedded largely in distrust of any authority.

Those who believe in this notion of HIV denial claim that HIV does not cause AIDS. However, they do not really have a coherent or cogent alternative theory for which there is any evidence. Usually, those who believe that HIV doesn't cause AIDS replace it with some vague claims about toxins in the environment. They may also in fact blame it on HIV medications themselves.

HIV denial, while somewhat of a worldwide phenomenon—we have it in Europe and we certainly have it here in the United States—it is especially harmful in Africa. Belief in HIV denial has waxed and waned over the years. It was noted that it did decrease somewhat in the wake of effective HAART medication. By HAART, I mean highly active antiretroviral therapy. The human immunodeficiency virus is a retrovirus. It works by inserting its DNA into the DNA of the host.

Medications that target this process and prevent it from occurring have successfully interfered with the life cycle of HIV. They have extended the life expectancy of people living with HIV by decades, almost to the point where they have a normal life expectancy. When these medications in the 1990s really started to take hold and people with HIV were living longer and longer, that took a lot of steam away from the HIV denial movement. But, it didn't go away entirely. It is still around and if anything, may be coming back with more vigor.

However, it also took hold firmly in Africa, especially in the country of South Africa. South African President Thabo Mbeki bought into the whole notion of HIV denial, making statements essentially echoing those of prominent HIV deniers. He crippled his country's HIV efforts for many years. However, now South Africa is trying to get back on track with HIV control. There is no longer any official governmental belief in HIV denial and hopefully, they'll be able to get back on track.

Some of these HIV fears were tied to vaccines. There was specifically the myth that HIV was being spread by the West deliberately in the polio vaccine. This crippled vaccine efforts, especially in the country of Nigeria. This foiled attempts at eradicating polio worldwide. In fact, the World Health Organization estimated that we were on the brink, just maybe a couple of years away from worldwide eradication of polio. It would have been the second eradication, following smallpox.

However, fears were being spread in Nigeria, one of the last countries to still have endemic polio virus. The fear was that the polio vaccine was being used to deliberately spread HIV—and also infertility drugs—to the population. This led to decreased compliance with the polio vaccine and the return of almost epidemic polio in Nigeria, which then spread to other countries, setting back the eradication efforts by years if not decades. However, these false beliefs have been largely put in check. The World Health Organization efforts are now back on track, but we are still years away from achieving this goal.

Let's turn now to India in which something called urine therapy remains popular. There's a religious Sanskrit text called the *Damar Tantra* which contains 107 stanzas on the benefits of "pure water, or drinking one's own urine." Urine therapy is referred to as *Sivambu Kalpa*, also part of what is known as Ayurvedic medicine or the Ayurvedic tradition. Urine therapy itself may be called *amaroli*. It is often taken orally or it may be rubbed on the skin. There are claims that drinking urine is beneficial for many aspects of health, most specifically that it can fight off cancer. This has led to other kinds of claims about the cancer fighting activities of constituents of urine.

In 1978, the former Prime Minister of India, a longtime practitioner, spoke to Dan Rather on *60 Minutes* about the benefits of urine therapy. This largely increased its popularity in the West and elsewhere. Claims for the cancer fighting ability of urea—one of the main constituents of urine—and also alleged cancer fighting proteins excreted in urine are that they stimulate the immune system against cancer. That's the core of the claims that are being made. There is no evidence for this premise or for the efficacy of urine therapy. In fact, urine therapy has been condemned by the National Cancer Institute and other organizations.

It's important to recognize that urine is waste. Urine is our body's attempt, through the kidneys, to eliminate harmful toxins and waste from our body. The kidneys filter out our blood and take out as much as possible things like urea and other toxins in order to get them out of the body. If your kidneys fail, if you have kidney failure, then things like creatine and blood urea nitrogen will increase to dangerous levels causing organs to fail, brain dysfunction, and eventually death. Therefore, urine is not something that you want to be putting back into your body.

But, ideas tend to spread around the world. While I may be talking about ideas that are originating in one country, it is true that we live with an increasing global network of information. While urine therapy may have originated in Indian beliefs, it has spread to the United States and elsewhere where urine therapy cancer cures have cropped up. In Japan, for example, Dr. Hasumi claims to cure cancer with a vaccine made from a patient's own urine.

In the United States, most notoriously, a doctor by the name of Stanislaw Burzynski, claims that he has purified what he calls antineoplastons from the urine. He claims that he's isolated several of these antineoplastons. It turns out that antineoplastons do not exist. He has merely identified previously recognized proteins in urine. These proteins don't have any particular anti-cancer fighting or antineoplastic activity. Therefore, they are completely useless in treating cancer.

In Japan, there are many mythological beliefs about blood type. In fact, blood type or blood typing is a form of astrology in Japan. It is believed that personality profile can be determined simply by knowing one's blood type. Compatibility and other things depend on whether or not you are a type A, B, AB, or O—what we call the ABO blood type system. Companies hire based upon blood type. There are politicians who feel obliged to publicly disclose their own blood type as part of their campaign. It is thought that maybe they're hiding something if they won't make their blood type disclosed publicly.

It's hypothesized that belief in this blood type personality profile, in a country like Japan, may provide some level of difference or differentiation in what is otherwise a very homogenous culture. Although, that kind of psychological explanation about the popularity of these blood typing myths is mainly speculation.

What are the blood type personalities, in case you want to know? A type A blood type is supposed to be earnest, creative, sensible, and fastidious. A type B blood type is supposed to be wild, active, selfish, and irresponsible, while AB is rational, cool, critical, but may be indecisive. Type O is agreeable, social, optimistic, vain, and rude. If these descriptions sound like astrological horoscopes, it's because essentially that's what they are.

Other beliefs have emerged out of the notion of different biological factors from blood type and have spread to other countries. For example, one is the Blood-Type Diet, which was developed by naturopath James D'Adamo. He claimed that different blood type proteins affect blood chemistry and determine both what your optimal diet would be and your optimal activities for health. Therefore, if you have a type B blood type, then your health would be optimized by eating certain kinds of food and engaging in certain kinds of exercise. This is not based upon any evidence or even any plausible underlying theory.

We may understand this better by understanding what blood type actually is. The ABO blood type system is based upon specific proteins, what we call antigens on red blood cells. Antigens are something that interact with or activate the immune system. If A antigens are present on the red blood cells, then that person will make antibodies against B proteins. They'll have anti-B antibodies. This is because your immune system, in development, is prevented from making antibodies against your body's own natural proteins. If you have A type proteins, your immune system's production of anti-A antibodies is suppressed. If you don't have the B type on your red blood cells, then your immune system is free to make anti-B antibodies.

However, the ABO antigen blood typing system is only 1 of 30 blood group systems. There are in fact many different antigen systems that we have identified and that we look at on blood. This is very important for transfusion and transplant. In order, for example, to have a successful kidney or other organ transplant and minimize the effect of rejection, at the very least, the donor and the recipient must be compatible in terms of their ABO blood type. This is because it is most significant blood type antigen. But, it's important to have compatibility also with as many as possible of the other 29 blood group systems. The more similar all of these blood types are, then the fewer antibodies the recipient will make against the host's organ because these antigens not only occur in the blood, but also occur on other tissues as well.

No one, except for an identical twin, would be a perfect match. There are so many different antigens that there are far more permutations than there are people on the people. Therefore, you never get a perfect match from this extensive typing unless you are a genetically identical twin. However, all of this complex biochemistry, while it affects immune activity against blood and tissues, it does not affect other aspects of biochemistry or physiology. It has no plausible effect on your personality, certainly on how you digest food, on your nutrient needs, or on how you would respond to various types of exercise.

In Europe, there is a very popular belief for many benefits from the various bee products. Again, this is a belief that has become truly international, but it is extremely popular in Europe. The notion that what bees produce may be beneficial for human health is somewhat understandable in that honey bees, for example, produce a lot of useful things for humanity. As a poet once said, they produce both sweetness and light. They give us honey and they give us wax for candles.

But, bees make things other than wax and honey. For example, they collect bee pollen. There are many claims that bee pollen is a superfood, an especially nutritious food. It is a really good food for the bees, and it does contain many useful nutrients. But, years of research have not found any specific health benefits for humans.

Also, there are serious concerns about allergies. Bee proteins do have a tendency to cause human allergies. In fact, allergic reactions to bee stings is the number one animal death in the world, more than other things that you may worry about like sharks and snakes. More people who die from animals die from bee stings than anything else. Any bee products always come with the caution that it may cause an allergic reaction in people who have a sensitivity.

Also, bee pollen is not considered safe for pregnancy as it might have some uterine stimulant effects. Therefore, there is the concern that it may promote a premature contraction or premature labor. There isn't a lot of evidence for this so that's more on just the cautious concern level than a proven risk.

Another bee product is called royal jelly. This is a milky substance made by worker bees containing water, sugars, fats, and proteins. This is food intended for the queen and for the queen's larva. Again, it contains many nutritious things that they need. However, there are claims that are made that this royal jelly can be used to treat arthritis, high cholesterol, baldness, and many other disparate health conditions. There is no evidence, especially reliable clinical evidence in humans, to back up any of these claims. There is some interesting research in animals showing some effects and royal jelly may have some application for animals. But, right now there are no science-based indications for people.

One other bee product that you may be surprised to hear is offered as a therapeutic agent is bee venom. There are people who actually let themselves be stung repeatedly by different honey bees, a process which is called apitherapy or therapy from bees. It is believed that the bee venom is a powerful natural agent that can have some properties that can be exploited. Specifically, it's claimed that bee venom is a powerful anti-inflammatory.

It is true that there are anti-inflammatory chemicals in bee venom. Bee venom is actually quite a powerful cocktail of chemicals, but there is no clinical evidence to support any specific health claims. The disease that has been most studied with bee venom is a neurological disorder that I'm very familiar with called Multiple Sclerosis. There are people who suffer from multiple sclerosis or MS who treat themselves with bee venom therapy in the hopes that it will reduce the severity of their disease. There have actually been some preliminary studies looking at bee venom therapy in MS. They show, unfortunately, at this point in time, no significant or measurable benefit.

However, it may be true that we can identify and isolate useful compounds or chemicals in bee venom that may one day lead to effective treatments, but this has not occurred yet. It also needs to be emphasized that bee venom contains a very high risk of allergic reaction. Therefore, this should not be done by anyone who has a bee venom allergy and certainly unless you're pretty sure that you don't have an allergy.

For me, the most surprising bee product for which there are health claims is something called propolis. Propolis is a substance used by bees to build their hives. It also has some pesticide activity for the bee hives. It reduces the population of mites and other pests. Propolis is a sticky material—literally a building material—mostly harvested from tree sap and resins. It contains many volatile oils and terpenes. But, also in our modern world, bees collect caulking, tar, and things that contain lead like paint and other contaminants. Therefore, propolis, in addition to being fairly inedible tree sap, also may contain some harmful contaminants.

It is claimed, however, as a medicinal agent and that it has antibacterial activity. There is documented antibacterial activity in some of the things in propolis, but it's not significant. It hasn't been shown to be safe and effective when used by people. There is also a recognized significant risk of what's called an allergic dermatitis from propolis, from being exposed to propolis. Essentially, it can cause a bad rash. Therefore, it should be used only with caution.

Let's turn now to the Philippines and psychic surgery. In 1984, actor Andy Kaufman went to the Philippines to receive psychic surgery for a rare form of lung cancer. Psychic surgery has been popular in the Philippines and in Brazil since the mid 20th century. It is born out of the spiritualist movement in those countries. Practitioners claim to reach inside the body of their client psychically and pull out diseased or malignant tissue. However, there is no evidence to suggest that they're actually reaching inside the body.

Investigative teams have shown that psychic surgeons are merely palming chicken parts and pretending to pull it out of their clients' bodies. It is a bit of prestidigitation and misdirection—nothing else. Many magicians have delighted in reproducing the effects of psychic surgeons and showing how convincing the illusion can be.

Another myth in Asia—this one originating in China, but common in other countries as well—is the notion that cold liquids should not be drunk during meals because they will increase the risk of cancer. The belief is that the cold fluid will solidify fats, causing them to clog up the intestines. This, in fact, increases the risk of cancer. It is therefore advocated to drink hot liquids, like hot tea, with meals. It's not clear if the tradition of drinking hot tea with meals came before or after this myth about the risks of cold liquids, but this one also is not true.

To wrap up my around the world tour of medical myths, I'm going to return home to one that originated entirely in the United States. Many people think that the caduceus is the symbol of the medical profession. The caduceus is essentially a staff with two snakes winding around it and with wings at the top of the staff. The caduceus is actually the wand of Hermes and if anything, is a symbol of commerce. It has nothing in Greek mythology—or in any other mythology—to do with medicine or the healing arts.

The actual symbol of the medical profession is the staff of Aesculapius. Aesculapius is a Greek god and the son of Apollo. He was the god of medicine. His staff is a staff with a single snake wrapping around it and no wings. You could see how the confusion can be made. That staff is the symbol of medicine and was thought to be a healing staff. This mistake was first made by the U.S. Army Medical Corp in the late 19th century—confusing the caduceus for the staff of Aesculapius. It spread from there and included medical institutions and hospitals using the caduceus for decades, thinking that it was an appropriate or proper symbol of medicine.

However, in the middle of the 20th century, the belief or the knowledge that the staff of Aesculapius was more appropriate began to take hold. The AMA now uses the staff of Aesculapius. If you get behind an ambulance, for example, you may notice that the medical symbol on the back of that ambulance is a staff with a single snake, not a caduceus.

This is interesting, this story, even though it's not really a health myth because it shows how one authoritative source can be responsible for the spread of pure misinformation—the misinformation about the caduceus. In addition, this source spread this misinformation, this myth, to many other sources like hospitals and the AMA. This lent the further appearance of authority to this false belief. This reinforces the notion that you need to question everything, even if it seems to be coming from a reliable source. You should question whether or not the source is just copying it as a secondary source or if this really is a primary and reliable source of information.

Taking a look at these various myths, we see that cultures do vary, but people are fundamentally the same. The same kind of medical myths from around the world tend to have some similar themes. These themes include a desire for control, a desire to understand our health, and a desire maybe to have a simple system by which we can both understand our health and also improve our health. Another common theme is that people who are sick or ill may become desperate and seek out things to help their problems. People are perhaps easy to frighten with medical myths. I think that, by looking at the various myths from around the world, we see that people are the same no matter what culture you go to.

Roundup—Decluttering Our Mental Closet
Lecture 24

> What about the notion that if you die in your dreams, then you will die in real life? ... This is contradicted by reported experiences where people actually do die in their dreams and then live to tell the tale. There is also no theoretical reason why we would expect that dying in one's dream would cause someone to die in reality.

We've taken a look at many medical myths over this course, some serious, others less so—hopefully all interesting. Some myths have a false reliance on authority. Others have a kernel of truth to them that is often misinterpreted or exaggerated. There are also some themes that seem to have been around forever and just won't die; perhaps they appeal to something that's fundamental about human psychology. In this last lecture, we make roundup of many medical myths.

The first myth is that you lose most of your body's heat through your head. This notion is based on a 1970 U.S. Army survival manual claiming that 40% to 45% of body heat is lost from the head. However, this study looked at soldiers who were wearing heavy coats and thermal gear everywhere except for their head. Where does heat loss actually occur? There are several mechanisms of heat loss in your body: One is the evaporation of sweat on your skin. We also radiate body heat away from us.

We lose heat primarily through the entire surface area of our skin, but there are some places on the body where we lose more heat than others. These mainly include those parts of the body that stick out, like our hands, feet, nose, chin, and ears—but not especially our scalp or our heads. The bottom line is that it simply is a myth that you lose most of your heat through your head. You don't even lose more heat through your head than through other parts of the body.

Let's look at another simple myth you may have heard. Does cracking your knuckles cause arthritis or otherwise damage your joints? First, what causes the cracking sound? You are stretching the ligaments that hold your joints together. The joints are filled with fluid called synovial fluid, which expands when you stretch the joint and ligaments. An expanding liquid has less pressure, which causes gases that are dissolved in the synovial fluid to come out and form bubbles. When these large bubbles pop, they form the cracking noise.

There actually has been only one published study looking at the health effects of frequently cracking one's knuckles. The study examined 300 people who were frequent knuckle crackers. It found no increased risk of arthritis, but there was an interesting finding. People who frequently cracked their knuckles did have loose ligaments and grip weakness, probably caused by repeatedly stretching those ligaments.

Rather than seeing it as an unpleasant experience to be told that I am wrong, I've come to appreciate and even enjoy having my own myths corrected.

Here's another quick one: Does hair continue to grow after we die? The answer to this is a simple no. Neither hair nor nails continue to grow after we die. This observation may stem from the fact that after death the skin becomes desiccated, or dehydrated. The skin retracts, giving the false impression of the hair or nails being more prominent.

It may interest you, or perhaps concern you, to learn that even physicians harbor myths. While medical school makes an effort to eliminate any lingering myths from physicians' thinking, this is not a 100% effective process. Even physicians in practice may still have lingering myths that they simply have not had illuminated during their education or careers.

A recent survey of pediatricians, for example, asked many questions about pediatric medicine, focusing on those beliefs known to be common myths. It turns out that 2% to 10% of pediatricians surveyed still believed many false things. Here are some examples: Some pediatricians believe that ice baths can be used to treat a high fever. In fact, you shouldn't give somebody an ice bath to treat a high fever; it's not necessary or safe. Some believe that chicken pox is not contagious before the rash appears. This is also false.

Is it safe to put infants to sleep on their side? It is, though 32% of pediatricians still harbored an older false belief that it wasn't safe to do so. Small percentages of pediatricians think that drinking milk can cause an increase in phlegm, which is not true. Twelve percent still believe in the Mozart effect—the notion that listening to Mozart will make babies smarter—though that has been entirely debunked.

Having our false beliefs challenged is often not a pleasant experience. I understand that I have popped a lot of balloons in the course of these lectures. Perhaps I've even challenged some beliefs that were comforting and that you were relying on for a sense of control. I long ago accepted the fact that my head is filled with misinformation; that's an inevitable consequence of living in our information society. We are constantly surrounded by information, and much of it is not true.

Therefore I have tried to flip my relationship with the notion that I harbor myths and misinformation. Rather than seeing it as an unpleasant experience to be told that I am wrong, I've come to appreciate and even enjoy having my own myths corrected. It is an empowering experience to have this intellectual clutter removed from our mental closet, as it were.

I don't want you to treat me as a definitive authority. I'm just one physician trying to understand the evidence and the literature as I see it. I hope that I have given you a lot to think about and challenged many of your beliefs. Most of all, I hope that I have taught you that you can't assume that what you've always heard must be true simply because many other people believe it and spread it around. You should challenge all of your beliefs. Whenever possible, try to rely on a consensus of authority or, even better, primary sources to verify what you think you know to be true. ■

Suggested Reading

Barrett, "Questionable Cancer Therapies."

Jenicek and Hitchcock, *Evidence-Based Practice.*

Shermer, *Why People Believe Weird Things.*

1. What would you say about the idea that the medical establishment is hiding a cure for cancer?

2. Are there some types of medical myths that doctors themselves are more likely to believe?

3. What false beliefs might you be harboring, and how is it best to deal with them?

Roundup—Decluttering Our Mental Closet
Lecture 24—Transcript

We've taken a look at many medical myths over this course and these lectures, some serious, others less so, hopefully all interesting. It is especially interesting, however, to take a step back and get the broader view about common themes of myths and common origins. Some myths, for example, have a false reliance on authority. Others have a kernel of truth to them although that kernel of truth is often misinterpreted or grossly exaggerated. There are also some themes that seem to have been around forever and just won't die. Perhaps they appeal to something that's fundamental about human psychology.

Some things that you may think are myths may actually be true. In this last lecture, I'm going to take a look at some smaller myths and quickly run through a roundup of these many medical myths. We'll touch on all of these themes and then come back to this broader view at the end.

The first one is that you lose most of your heat through your head. This is actually based upon the false notion that heat rises. You may have read that heat rises in your high school science textbook. This is an example of an authority, an apparent authority that frequently gets it wrong. It turns out that heat itself has no inherent tendency to rise, sink, or move in any particular direction. But, what is true and what is misinterpreted is that often, hotter fluids or gases—like air and water—will rise above relatively cooler fluids. Warm air rises above cooler air. But, the heat itself does not rise or go in any particular direction.

The notion that you lose most of the heat through your head specifically is based upon a 1970 U.S. Army survival manual claiming that 40 to 45 percent of body heat is lost from the head. However, this study looked at soldiers who were wearing heavy coats and thermal gear everywhere except for their head. Therefore, it really wasn't a fair comparison. But, again, that lead to this false authority leading to a common belief and myth.

Where does heat loss occur? First of all there, are several mechanisms of heat loss in your body. One is evaporation. You sweat and that fluid on your skin then evaporates. The evaporating sweat carries away heat with it. There is also radiation. Human bodies glow in the infrared. You may have seen on a movie or maybe even had access to infrared goggles yourself, where you can see a red outline or somebody glowing in infrared. That infrared glow is body heat. We are always radiating this body heat away from us, from every part of our skin.

There's also convection. Air and water next to our skin will be warmed up and will carry away some of that heat. There's also just breathing. If the air you exhale is warmer than the air you inhale, that is also a loss of heat.

We lose heat primarily through the surface area of our body, the entire surface area of our skin—not just one place and certainly not just our heads. But, there are some places on the body where we will lose more heat than others. These mainly include those parts of the body that stick out, like our hands, feet, nose, chin, and ears—but not especially our scalp or our heads. These parts of the body have particular regulation of the blood flow.

In all parts of our body we regulate the blood flow to our skin in order to regulate heat loss when it's very hot out or we have a lot of heat in our body. Let's say you've just exercised and you've built up body heat. Your body will increase the blood flow to the skin, particularly in the hands, feet, and parts of the face and ears—again, the things that stick out. That blood will bring more heat to the surface and cause an increased amount of heat to be lost through evaporation, convection, and radiation. When it's very cold, the opposite happens. Your body will clamp down on those blood vessels, reducing the amount of blood flow to the skin in order to conserve heat. If that's taken to an extreme, you can get what's called frostbite because your limbs will not be getting enough blood flow to keep them alive.

The regulation of blood flow to the hands, feet, and parts of the face are exquisite so you get more blood flow there and therefore more loss of heat from those parts of the body. Your scalp is particularly vascular, but not as much and certainly not as closely tied to heat loss as these other parts that I mentioned. The bottom line is that it simply is a myth that you lose most of your heat through your head. You don't even especially lose more heat through your head than through other parts of the body.

Let's also take a very simple myth, one that I hear quite a bit. People ask me about this because they think I know these things because I'm a physician. Cracking your knuckles—does it really cause arthritis? Is it bad for your joints? First, what causes the cracking when you stretch your knuckles? What happens is that you are stretching the ligaments that hold your joints together. The joints themselves are filled with fluid called synovial fluid. When you stretch the joint and ligaments, that causes this liquid to expand. An expanding liquid has less pressure. Therefore, that causes gases that are dissolved in the synovial fluid to come out and form bubbles. They come out and are actually gases rather than being dissolved in the fluid itself.

These large bubbles form and when these large bubbles pop, they form the cracking noise of cracking your knuckles. They burst into a bunch of smaller bubbles. You can then continue to pop or crack your knuckles; however, you will deplete the gas in the synovial fluid. You will no longer be able to crack your joints until the little bubbles re-dissolve back into the synovial fluid.

There actually has been only one study looking at the health effects of frequently cracking one's knuckles. This was done by a man named Raymond Brodeur. He published the study in the *Journal of Manipulative and Physiological Therapeutics*. He examined 300 people who were frequent knuckle crackers. He found that they had no increased risk of arthritis. However, he did make an interesting finding. They did have lax or loose ligaments and grip weakness, probably caused by repeatedly stretching those ligaments. While frequent knuckle cracking does not cause arthritis, there is a kernel of truth to this myth in that it's not good for you. It could cause your ligaments to become loose and actually compromise your joint function and grip strength.

What about the notion that teething is a frequent cause of fever in infants? Babies often begin drooling and chewing on their fingers at around 3 to 4 months of age. This is often interpreted as teething and as dealing with the fact that their teeth are starting to come in. But in fact, this is just normal behavior for that developmental age. True teething does not start until the teeth start to actually come in. You will see swollen gums and you may even see teeth breaking through the gums.

Some of the symptoms of teething include a decreased appetite for solid foods, biting, ear or gum rubbing, irritability, a rash on your child's face, sucking, or waking up at night. It does not, however, cause diarrhea, cough, or high fever. Those symptoms should not be attributed to teething. It is somewhat controversial whether or not it can cause a low grade fever, but it definitely cannot cause a high fever, say a fever over 102. Therefore, don't assume that a high fever is due to teething.

A lot of people will claim that turkey makes you sleepy. They often offer as evidence their own anecdotal experience of feeling especially sleepy after a large Thanksgiving dinner. Often it is argued that the reason why turkey, a large meal of turkey, will make you sleepy is that turkey is a good source of L-tryptophan. This is an essential amino acid that is metabolized into serotonin and melatonin. Serotonin and melatonin are indeed sleep inducing hormones in the body or chemicals in the body. However, there are many sources of tryptophan in a typical dinner. Turkey is not really special in this regard at all.

In fact, eating turkey or other sources of L-tryptophan do not necessarily increase tryptophan in your blood and therefore serotonin and melatonin. This is especially true when other amino acids, which are the components of protein, are also present in the food. This is the case with protein meals like turkey. Also, it should be considered that there are other components of a large holiday meal that are more likely to contribute to a little bit of sleepiness or lethargy. This includes the large meal itself and some people may consume alcohol during these holiday meals. Those are much more likely to cause lethargy than any amino acids from the turkey itself.

Here's a big question that I get often. There's actually a few myths with respect to the notion of cancer as a disease and if it's curable. One myth right off the bat is that cancer is not a single disease. It's actually a category of diseases. It's many, many individual diseases that share a common pathophysiology. This means that the same kind of thing is happening in the body, but they are different enough that you really can't ask questions about whether or not they can be cured, treated, and what their prognosis is—until you describe very specific types of cancer.

A type of cancer might, for example, be lung cancer, breast cancer, or brain cancer. What part of the body are they affecting? In addition, there are different cell types, so different things can happen to the lungs. There are different types of lung cancer. There are also grades of cancer or how aggressive it is. There are also stages of cancer—how far advanced it is, and whether it's spread locally or remotely, far from its origin. All of these things—every type, grade, and stage of cancer—needs to be pointed out specifically before you can start asking or answering questions about treatment, prognosis, and curability.

It turns out that many types of cancer are in fact largely curable. One very prominent example is leukemia, which is a form of blood cancer. Leukemia has a very high cure rate. By cure, we mean a chance of becoming cancer-free without any recurrence and with a normal life expectancy. However, there are other cancers that are indeed incurable. Pancreatic cancer is a very prominent one for example. Treatments for pancreatic cancer, even given the best current technology, only lead to a modest extension of life expectancy. It is as close to completely incurable as we get in the category of cancer.

A related question is whether or not medical science or advances in medicine are winning the war on cancer. Are we making any progress in the treatment for cancer? Some people think that because cancer still has not yet been cured—which as I just pointed out is a bit of a problematic premise—that therefore we're not making progress. It turns out that cancer survival for different types of cancer—all the different types that I discussed—as well as different age groups is followed very carefully. They have been followed for decades so could make very meaningful comparisons about cancer survival in the 21st century compared to earlier decades.

It turns out that there has been a slow and steady increase in survival with cancer in every single age group. This represents curing cancer, you might say, through a thousand baby steps. We still have a lot of baby steps to go. But, we have made many of them so far. Some people claim that this increase in survival is due only to earlier detection, what we call increased lead time. If you diagnose the cancer earlier, then of course people will seem as if they are living longer even though they're dying when they would have anyway despite treatment. But, this is something that cancer researchers are well aware of. It's taken into consideration in looking at cancer survival statistics.

Even if you adjust for the advanced lead time of early detection of cancers, people are surviving longer with their cancers. Again, we are making slow and steady progress. This also, however, gets to the myth or the notion that there is one day going to be a cure for cancer. This is something that I don't think is really quite reasonable. As I said, cancer is many diseases, not one disease. There's not likely therefore to be one cure. It is probably always or at least for the foreseeable future going to require many different treatment approaches.

A very closely related myth is the notion that there is a hidden cure, that "they" have already cured cancer. But, they are hiding it from the public for some nefarious purpose, perhaps to protect the profits that are being made off of treating cancer with current technology. However, this is definitely a myth. No one is hiding a proven cure for cancer. There are far too many players involved for this to be an effective conspiracy of silence, for example. People often think that "they" is one cohesive monolithic agency or institution, but no such thing exists in medicine. There are, for example, academics and academic institutions, patient groups, government funding and regulatory agencies, professional organizations, and competing private interests. There isn't even one private industry. There are multiple companies that are competing against each other. There are multiple nations that are competing against each other. It simply wouldn't be possible or very plausible to bring all of these disparate institutions together for one grand conspiracy to hide such a profound truth from the public.

In addition, any one entity or person who actually had knowledge of a cure for cancer would only stand to gain by making that knowledge public. The benefits and rewards would far outweigh any perceived short-term loss or profits from other means. Imagine being the person who found a significant cure, a contribution to the cure for cancer—or the company that did it, or the academic institution. This would bring prestige, money, fame, and career advancement that would far outweigh any perceived loss of revenue.

Further, because there are so many types of cancer, it would take years of research for any new treatment—even a significant breakthrough—to be tested with every different type and stage of cancer. This would generate a tremendous amount of new research. Success in treating and curing cancer would lead to more research and profits for everybody. It wouldn't be a detriment or something to be hidden.

What about the notion that if you die in your dreams then you will die in real life? This is one that I've heard multiple times myself. This is contradicted by reported experiences where people actually do die in their dreams and then live to tell the tale. There is also no theoretical reason why we would expect that dying in one's dream would cause someone to die in reality.

The purported reason is that the stress of experiencing one's death, even in a dream-like state, is so significant that it would cause someone to die from that stress, from a heart attack, for example. But, the stress of something occurring in a dream like that is not necessarily sufficient to cause death, especially in a healthy individual. Also, you have to ask yourself the question, if someone did die due to dreaming that they died, how would we ever know? They would never survive to tell us what they were dreaming.

As a neurologist, I'm frequently asked about whether or not the left brain/right brain thing is true. Are people really left-brained with a certain personality and right-brained with a distinct personality and set of capabilities? There is a kernel of truth to this in that the mammalian cortex, the thinking part of the brain, is divided between two independent hemispheres—the right and left hemispheres. These hemispheres can function completely independently as their own brain. In fact, you only need one of these hemispheres, as I said in the lecture on coma, in order to be awake and conscious.

Moreover, it is also true that cognitive functions are lateralized, or many of them are. This means that they exist only in one hemisphere or the other. For example, in the dominant hemisphere are centers for language and mathematics. In the non-dominant hemisphere, there are centers for visuospatial relationship. Some of your strength, therefore, in terms of different abilities may reside more in one hemisphere than the other.

To contrast this, however, there are massive connections and communications between the two hemispheres. This is mainly through a structure called the corpus collosum. It's like a broadband cable connecting the two hemispheres. There's also the anterior and posterior commisures, which are smaller cables going between the hemispheres. Therefore, there is massive real-time communication that allows the two hemispheres to function seamlessly as if they were one entity, one mind.

It also should be noted that there are neural networks. There are connections between different parts of the brain that are involved in specific tasks. These neural networks involve structures in both hemispheres. Both hemispheres are involved in many of the things that we do.

Another weakness of this notion of right brain versus left brain is that the largest part of our cortex, the frontal lobes, are largely not lateralized with respect to things like personality and cognitive ability. The largest part of our personality is what we call bilaterally redundant. This means that either side of the frontal lobes can function and produce the things that make up our personality, like our ability to inhibit our own desires or tendencies, for example. That's another strong argument against personality being located in one hemisphere or the other and us being dominant for one or the other. The bottom line is that people are not left-brained or right-brained. We have one whole cohesive brain.

Here's a quick one. Does hair continue to grow after we die? The answer to this is a simple no. Neither hair nor nails continue to grow after we die. This observation may stem from the fact that after death, the skin will become desiccated or dehydrated. It will retract or it will pull back. This can give the false impression of the hair or nail being more prominent and therefore, appear as if they had grown. But, in order to grow hair or nails, you need living cells. Once the biological death occurs and the organs shut down, the cells in various parts of the body will also begin to die. It may take hours for all cells to completely die, but then all cells in the body are dead including those that cause the hair or the nails to grow. Therefore, they don't continue to grow.

An unrelated myth—but also a hair myth—is the question of whether or not your hair will grow back faster or thicker after you shave it. That is also a myth. The thickness and growth of hair is determined by the hair follicles. These are not affected simply by shaving.

It may interest you or perhaps concern you to learn that even physicians harbor myths. I remember going into medical school. Although I thought I was interested in medical information and had learned quite a bit even before I got to medical school, my head was filled with a ton of misinformation and myths about biology and medicine. During the course of my medical education, these were systematically removed. However, there's a lot of information that we pick up during the course of our lives. While medical school certainly makes an effort to eliminate any lingering myths from physicians' thinking, this is not a 100 percent sure process. Therefore, even physicians in practice may still have some lingering myths that they simply have not picked up or encountered during their education or their careers.

There is a recent survey looking at pediatricians, for example. It asked many questions about pediatric medicine and focused on those beliefs which are known to be common myths. It turns out that even pediatricians—between 2 and 10 percent of pediatricians surveyed—for most of these myths, they still believed many false things. I'm going to run through a few quite quickly.

The notion that honey can be given safely to babies under six months old is a myth. The notion that aspirin may be used to treat fever in children above the age of 5 years old—in fact, you need to wait longer, more like 8 to 10 years, before you can safely give aspirin to children. Teething can sometimes cause high fevers—a myth that I just discussed. Again, a small percentage of pediatricians still believe these things despite the fact that those statements are all myths.

Some pediatricians—again, still in small numbers, about 2 to 10 percent—believe that ice baths can be used to treat a high fever. You shouldn't give somebody an ice bath to treat a high fever; it's not necessary or safe. Chicken pox is not contagious before the rash appears—also false. Chicken pox is contagious. You are shedding virus even before there is a visible rash. Also, since colds are respiratory viruses, they are not often spread by physical contact. This also is a myth. You can spread the cold virus from physically touching somebody without breathing, sneezing, or coughing on them.

Is it safe to put an infant to sleep on their side? It is safe, although 32 percent of pediatricians still harbored an older false belief that it wasn't safe to do so. If a child has a seizure, do not place any objects in their mouth, like a spoon or your finger. You should not do that, although about 5 percent of pediatricians still thought that it was safe and appropriate to do so.

How about the notion that to prevent ear wax build-up, you should clean the ear canals with a cotton swab after a bath when the ear wax is softest? It turns out that you shouldn't clean ear wax out of an ear by putting a cotton swab or anything inside the ear. You should only use things like tissues on the outside of the ear canal. Never stick anything inside the ear canal because of the risk that you may damage or rupture the eardrum.

The notion that rubbing alcohol is not absorbed through a baby's skin as also false, and yet 31 percent of pediatricians thought that that one was true. Also, the best way to stop a bloody nose is to tilt the head back. That too is a myth. Tilting the head back doesn't stop a bloody nose. It just causes the blood to run down the back of your throat. You should, in fact, pinch the nose in order to staunch the flow of blood.

Over 8 percent of pediatricians still think that sugar causes hyperactivity. We learned in this course that there is no correlation between eating sugar and hyperactivity. Reading in the dark causes visual problems—in fact, reading in the dark does not harm the eyes in any way. A small percentage thought that eating chocolate causes acne when there is no correlation between eating chocolate and acne. Also, 15 percent thought that you should wait 30 minutes after eating before swimming. As we learned in the first lecture, there is no particular reason to wait any specific length of time after eating before swimming.

Still, small percentages of pediatricians thought that drinking milk can cause an increase in phlegm when that is not true. They thought that carrots can improve vision. Carrots, as we learned, do contain beta carotene which is a vitamin that is important for vision. But, that doesn't mean that carrots improve vision. They may be useful in treating a vitamin A deficiency, but if you're not deficient, there's no effect on vision. Will wounds heal quicker when exposed to air? Thirty-three percent of pediatricians thought so, but that one is also a myth. Will vitamin C help ward off colds? Seventeen percent of pediatricians thought that one was true but, we learned that that also is a myth and is not backed up by evidence.

Have you heard of the Mozart effect? It's the notion that listening to Mozart will make babies smarter. Twelve percent of pediatricians believe that when, in fact, that one has been entirely debunked. There is no effect on baby intelligence or anyone's intelligence from listening to Mozart. Will sitting too close to a TV damage your vision? No, it won't. Will sleeping with a night light cause nearsightedness? That won't bother you either. Neither will caffeine stunt growth, although a minority of pediatricians still thinks that those things are true.

To summarize the entire course if you will, I've long noticed that having false beliefs challenged is not often a pleasant experience. I understand that I have popped a lot of balloons in the course of these lectures. Perhaps I've even challenged some beliefs that were comforting and that you were relying upon for a sense of control, for example. I long ago accepted the fact that my head is filled with misinformation. That's an inevitable consequence of living in our information society. We are constantly surrounded by information; much of it is not true. A lot of that information just comes from the culture. It spreads very quickly, especially now with the Internet and the global information network that we live in.

Therefore, I have tried to flip my relationship with the notion that I harbor myths and misinformation. Rather than seeing it as an unpleasant experience to be told that I am wrong or that I was mistaken about something, I've come to appreciate and even enjoy having my own myths corrected. It is in fact an empowering experience to have this intellectual clutter removed from our closet as it were.

Why are there so many false beliefs out there? There may be some lessons to learn about this from the myths that I covered during this course. For example, we talked about the placebo effect. It has a very powerful psychological effect to convince people that an intervention or a treatment is working or is having an effect, even when it is worthless or even harmful. There are many historical examples to back that up.

There is, for example, the historical example of the Abrams Dynamizer where millions of people and thousands of clinicians were convinced of the extreme effectiveness of this radio emitter that was diagnosing and treating people allegedly. Then it turns out that the device was completely worthless. It wasn't even producing the radio waves that were claimed for it.

It's interesting how quickly this lesson was forgotten from our culture. Most people I speak with have never heard of an Abrams Dynamizer. Therefore, they continue the false belief or myth that, if millions of people think that something is working, there must be something to it. They aren't aware of the fact of how easy we can fool ourselves and the powerful effect of things like confirmation bias and the placebo effect—when the historical lessons are right there for us to see, like with the Abrams Dynamizer.

We also found that there are many different types of myths. There are beliefs that have no validity at all on any level like homeopathy, for example. There are some beliefs that never seem to die. They have been with us for centuries, perhaps because they appeal to some fundamental notion in human psychology. For example, there's the concept that things that are natural are more healthful than things that are synthetic. This is one that's always there to some degree. It seems to peak, come and go, and wax and wane over the decades, but it's always there to some degree, however. There's also the notion that cutting-edge scientific ideas are going to help all of our problems or cure all of our ills. Things like magnetism seem to have an ageless appeal although they to seem to come and go over time.

It's almost as if there is a tag team of different mythological notions being natural or cutting-edge science, for example, that come and goes in the public consciousness. There's always some myth there to take its place when it becomes less popular over time. There are some ideas that are part myth, but part true, like hypnosis. It's not what you think it is, but it's actually an important neuroscientific interventions. There are some genuine health modalities but with exaggerated claims, like vitamins and nutrition. They're very important for our health, but there are a lot of notions that go well beyond the science and evidence.

There are also effective therapies that suffer from false fears and rumors, like vaccines. There are also many sources to these myths, such as marketing hype, wishful thinking, human psychology, and investing an inappropriate level of authority in an individual or in people who can be wrong. It's reasonable to rely upon appropriate authority figures and the consensus of scientific opinion should be taken seriously. But, anyone or any source can make a mistake and we have seen that in multiple instances throughout this lecture.

In fact, I don't want you to treat me as an end-all, definitive authority. I'm just one physician trying to understand the evidence and understand the literature as I see it. I hope that I have given you a lot to think about and challenged many of your beliefs. But, most of all, I hope that I have taught you that you can't assume that what you've always heard must be true simply because many other people believe it and spread it around. You should challenge all of your beliefs. Also, whenever possible, try to rely upon a consensus of authority or, even better, primary sources in order to check out everything that you think you know to be true.

Glossary

Myths sometimes stick in the mind even after more accurate information has been presented. For that reason, this glossary focuses on currently accurate medical information pertaining to myths discussed in the course. Each entry also mentions specific lectures where relevant information is discussed or mentioned. As always, for specific medical advice or treatment, consult a physician.

acupuncture: Acupuncture originated from multiple prescientific belief systems, including blood-letting, and its current practice lacks both the long tradition and evidence of efficacy that is widely presumed. There are currently no proven indications for acupuncture. Published scientific evidence shows that acupuncture points have no basis in anatomy or physiology, that needle placement does not relate to effectiveness, that needle penetration through the skin is not necessary, and that the training or experience of the acupuncturist does not affect outcome. What does impact outcome is the compassion and interaction of the acupuncturist. All of this suggests that acupuncture has no specific biological effect but is essentially a ritualized placebo intervention (Lecture 17).

amnesia: Amnesia is a loss of memory, which can be either temporary or permanent. Amnesia for events occurring prior to an injury or other cause is called retrograde amnesia; for events after an injury, it is called anterograde amnesia. Amnesia never causes one to forget one's name or identity—such a state is a psychiatric condition known as a fugue state (Lecture 20).

animal magnetism: Animal magnetism is a term invented by Franz Anton Mesmer in the 18th century, which he used to refer to a hypothetical magnetic fluid that he claimed existed within living creatures. He claimed to manipulate this force of nature in order to effect cures of his clients. Mesmer was eventually exposed as a fraud, and the notion of animal magnetism never caught on as a scientific concept. However, the term survives with a very different colloquial meaning (Lecture 18).

antibiotics: Antibiotics are specific to bacteria and do not work against colds (Lecture 9), other viruses, or other types of germs. Use in animals is not directly dangerous to people, although may hasten resistance (Lecture 5). They may reduce the normal bacterial flora, especially broad-spectrum antibiotics (Lecture 6). Overuse of antibacterial products can cause bacteria, not people, to become resistant to an antibiotic (Lecture 12).

antimicrobials: Antimicrobials are drugs that are used to treat infecting organisms, such as viruses, bacteria, fungus, or protozoans (Lecture 12).

antioxidants: Antioxidants are a class of chemicals that react with oxygen-free-radicals and stop them from reacting with and damaging components of cells. They occur naturally in living organisms (such as vitamins C and E and enzymes such as superoxide dismutase). Claims for antioxidant supplements have generally not been supported by clinical evidence. For example, the evidence does not support claims that antioxidants reduce cancer risk or prolong longevity (Lecture 8).

antivirals: Antivirals are a class of drugs that inhibit reproduction of viruses but do not kill viruses. They are useful in a subset of specific viral infections (Lecture 12).

applied kinesiology: Applied kinesiology (not to be confused with simply "kinesiology," which is the study of human movement) is the technique of using muscle strength testing to diagnose a host of diseases and ailments, including allergies. It is used mainly by chiropractors, but has been adopted by other practitioners as well. Published research, however, shows that applied kinesiology is not reproducible under blinded conditions, and is likely nothing but self-delusion and what is called the "ideomotor effect"—subconscious muscle movements based on expectation (Lecture 15).

attention deficit hyperactivity disorder (ADHD): ADHD is a genuine neuropsychological disorder that is currently considered to be a deficit of executive function and correlates with reduced activity in the frontal lobes. Recommended treatments include prescribed central nervous system stimulants and behavioral management using clear routines, boundaries, and positive reinforcement (Lecture 7).

autism: (Now considered part of autism spectrum disorder.) Autism is a neurodevelopmental disorder characterized by a deficit of social development. While the precise cause is unknown, current evidence strongly suggests autism is largely a genetic disorder affecting brain development. There is no scientific evidence linking autism to a significant environmental factor, including parenting style, specific foods (such as dairy products) or toxins (Lecture 7). Despite some credulous media coverage, multiple studies have failed to show any correlation between vaccines and autism. Also, despite claims by a few, mercury toxicity is a distinct neurological condition that does not resemble autism (Lecture 11).

bacteria: Bacteria are the most populous kingdom of life on earth. Most bacteria do not cause disease or have any implications for human health (Lecture 6). Some bacterial species are actually necessary for health, as they colonize our skin, bowels, and other mucous membranes. Only a small percentage of bacterial species are infectious to humans and can cause illness. Illnesses such as flus and colds are not caused by bacteria, but rather by viruses (Lecture 9). There are vaccines available for certain common and serious bacterial infections. Attenuated bacteria are used in typhoid and tuberculosis (TBG) vaccines, while killed bacteria are used in typhoid, cholera, plague, and pertussis vaccines (Lecture 10). *See also* **probiotics**.

bee venom therapy: Bee venom therapy involves allowing honey bees to sting and inject their venom, which is believed to have anti-inflammatory properties. While bee venom contains many interesting biologically active chemicals, there is currently no evidence supporting the safety and effectiveness for bee venom for any specific disease. Bee stings also come with the risk of serious allergic reactions (Lecture 23).

biofeedback: Biofeedback is a technique of using monitoring of biological functions, such as heart rate or electrical brain activity, in order to achieve a state of maximal relaxation. This can be a useful technique, but there is no evidence for medical benefits beyond that of relaxation (Lecture 19).

blood type diet: Blood type refers to various protein antigens that are found on blood cells and that are reactive to the immune system. The most commonly known (but not only) system is the A-B-O blood type. Individuals will make

Glossary

antibodies against whatever antigen they do not possess themselves, so those with blood type B will make antibodies against type A. Therefore blood typing is essential for matching blood donors, or for any organ transplant.

However, there is no theoretical reason or evidence to suggest that blood type has any other biological significance. There are popular claims that different blood types require different dietary needs for optimal health, but this is not based on any science or evidence (Lecture 23).

bottled water: Bottled water has become a popular product, and many people purchase bottled water for the convenience. However, bottled water varies in quality as much as tap water, and there is no consistent advantage to taste, purity, or healthfulness to bottled water over tap water (Lecture 2).

brain death: Brain death is defined as a complete lack of brain activity, which must be documented to strict criteria either by neurological exam, electroencephalography, or other diagnostic testing. In many states and countries brain death meets the legal definition of death (Lecture 20).

brain usage: Anatomical and functional studies show that humans use their entire brains. Despite the popular myth, we do not use only 10% of our brains and, in fact, it is not possible to be conscious using just 10% of the brain. The source of this myth is not clear, but it is not based on any scientific belief or evidence (Lecture 20).

caduceus: The winged staff of Hermes (with two snakes) is not the official symbol of medicine. This was a simple mistake made by the US Army Medical Corp in the late 19th century and was then perpetuated. The Staff of Asclepius (with one snake) is the actual symbol preferred by medical professionals and now recognized by the AMA (Lecture 23).

caffeine: Caffeine is a widely consumed drug with multiple biological effects. It acts as a mild diuretic, but you can still rehydrate with fluids that contain caffeine. Regular caffeine drinkers become tolerant to the diuretic effect (Lecture 2). While caffeine is a stimulant and can interfere with sleep, its use has not been linked to hyperactivity (Lecture 7).

calories: A calorie is a standard measure of energy. The term "Calorie" (sometimes designated with a capital "C") is also used to refer to a kilocalorie of energy in food (so 1 food Calorie = 1000 calories of energy). And 3500 Calories translates to one pound of fat, which is the body's way of storing energy. Weight control is about the proper balance of total calories consumed versus total calories expended. Overeating by 50 calories per day can mean gaining 5 pounds per year. It does not matter when you eat the calories; late-night eating does not necessarily affect weight (though it can cause problems with reflux; Lecture 4).

cancer prevention: Cancer is not one disease but a category of diseases (also called neoplasms). Therefore there are different methods for preventing and treating different kinds of cancer. Cancer prevention is largely accomplished through lifestyle choices, such as avoiding smoking. The relationship between diet and risk of cancer is complex and still the focus of ongoing research, but in general a diet rich in fruits and vegetables may be of benefit (Lecture 23).

cell phones: Cell phones are a source of nonionizing radiation. This has caused some popular concern about their potential health risks. However, nonionizing radiation (electromagnetic radiation of near-ultraviolet or longer wavelength) is too low energy to break chemical bonds, and therefore cause any direct damage to DNA or other cell molecules (Lecture 18).

chewing gum: Chewing gum is made of indigestible gum resin, but normally passes through the gastrointestinal tract without getting stuck. Not recommended for children under 5 years due to choking hazard (Lecture 1).

chiropractic: Chiropractic is a system of practice originating with D. D. Palmer in 1890s based on notions of life energy. Some chiropractic continues to follow Palmer's unscientific ideas, while others more closely resemble contemporary physical therapy and sports medicine (Lecture 18). Chiropractic generally continues to focus on manipulation of the back to affect the alignment of the vertebra. Chiropractic remains controversial due to the lack of a scientific basis for many of its practices.

cholesterol: Cholesterol is a waxy steroid-like molecule used as a structural component in living cells. It is also a building block of other important substances, and is essential for life. It is transported in various forms in the blood and can build up on the inside of blood vessel walls, eventually leading to plaques and blockages. To minimize cholesterol buildup, it is optimal to keep total cholesterol levels relatively low and to maintain a relatively high ratio of HDL (so-called good cholesterol derived from plants) to LDL (so-called bad cholesterol derived from animal fat; Lecture 4). *See also* **fats**.

chronic fatigue syndrome: This is a controversial disorder characterized by a state of chronic fatigue without any identifiable causes. In a minority of patients with chronic fatigue a chronic infection with the Ebstein-Barr virus (EBV) has been identified and is considered a plausible cause. However, many people without chronic fatigue are EBV positive, and many people with chronic fatigue are EBV negative. Therefore there may be other unrecognized causes. In addition, patients with chronic fatigue may simply have a known but currently undiagnosed condition to explain their fatigue (Lecture 13).

chronic Lyme disease: The term "chronic Lyme" can refer to chronic symptoms following an acute infection with the bacterial spirochete *Borrelia burgdorferi*. However, there are patients and practitioners who believe that it is possible to have a chronic active infection with *B. burgdorferi* that survives even thorough antibiotic treatment. This claim remains controversial and without empirical evidence (Lecture 13).

coma: Coma is a term used to define a disorder of consciousness caused by damage to or physiological impairment of the brain. For nonreversible causes of coma, patients rarely "wake up" without neurological impairments. Conscious processing (seeing/hearing) is unlikely in persistent vegetative state (PVS) but may occur in a minimally conscious state (MCS)—although currently there is little difference in prognosis between PVS and MCS (Lecture 20).

common cold: The common cold is an upper respiratory infection caused by many different viruses. Cold weather does not cause colds; it is possible to catch a cold in the summer. Vitamin C, Echinacea, and supplements like Airborne will not prevent or treat a cold. There is nothing special about chicken soup, although hot liquids may provide some symptom relief (Lecture 9).

copper: Copper is a nonferromagnetic base metal (it cannot contain a magnetic field). There is no evidence of benefits for pain or other indications from copper jewelry (Lecture 18).

dehydration: Dehydration defines a relative lack of water in the body. Most people in most situations can maintain proper hydration simply by drinking when thirsty. Drinks with caffeine do not worsen dehydration (Lecture 2). In extremely hot or dry environments, at high altitudes, and with extreme physical exertion special effort may be required to stay hydrated. Looking at the color of your urine is one way to quickly assess your level of hydration. *See also* **water**.

detoxing: The human body's inherent ability to remove toxins is often sufficient (kidneys, skin, and breath). Drinking lots of water does not "flush out" the system. Although this is a common claim, there are no diets or supplements which have been shown to aid dotoxifying the body (Lecture 16).

diabetes mellitus (DM): Diabetes mellitus is a group of disorders of glucose metabolism. Adult onset DM is often due to a combination of genetic predisposition and being overweight or obese. Diet is also important, specifically avoiding foods with a high glycemic index (GI), meaning that they are rapidly converted into glucose (Lecture 4).

dieting: Special diets are sometimes required for specific health conditions, like diabetes and heart disease. However, for weight control and overall health it is recommended to adopt healthy eating habits and lifestyle for life, rather than going on a restrictive or crash fad diet. Fasting is also of no long-term benefit. Diet pills do not aid in long-term weight control and may be harmful (Lecture 4). *See also* **calories**.

disorder: A condition characterized by the lack or impairment of a function usually possessed by healthy individuals and resulting in demonstrable harm. A disorder is distinguished from a disease, which has a specific demonstrable pathology (Lecture 13).

dying in dreams: Although there is a common belief that dying in one's dream will cause one to die in real life, there is no evidence to support this. Dreaming of dying is not uncommon, and if someone did in fact die from a dream they would not live to tell about it. Even if later revived, they would likely not remember the event, given that the process of dying and being resuscitated would likely lead to brain anoxia and therefore lack of memory of the event (Lecture 24).

facilitated communication (FC): FC is a disproven technique developed in the 1980s involving a facilitator who will aid a client who is not able to communicate on their own by "helping" them move their hand across a keyboard or other pointing device. Early popularity among therapists gave way to carefully controlled scientific studies that clearly indicated that the facilitator was doing all the communication, not the client. FC is now known as an example of the ideomotor effect in which a person makes small subconscious muscle movements, such as during the operation of a ouija board. Despite scientific evidence that FC does not work and is a deception, it remains in use by fringe practitioners (Lecture 20).

fats: Fats, or lipids, are one of the macronutrients from which we derive much of our calories (energy) and are also essential building blocks for life. However, too much of the wrong kinds of fats can increase disease risk, especially vascular risk. So-called "good" fats are monounsaturated and polyunsaturated fats that increase high-density lipoprotein (HDL) levels. The term HDL refers to the size of fat globules in the blood, and they are "good" because they shuttle fat and cholesterol from the lining of blood vessels to the liver. "Bad" fats are saturated fats and trans-fats which increase low-density lipoprotein (LDL) levels. LDL contributes to fat and cholesterol deposition in the blood vessels (Lecture 4).

fever: A fever is an abnormal increase in body temperature. 98.6° F is not the normal temperature for everyone; that number is based merely on an average computed in the 19th century. There is a range of normal body temperature, and the cutoff for a fever is a temperature over 100 degrees F. Most fevers do not pose any health risk (unless they are very high, 107 degree F or greater), and therefore the only need to treat them is for comfort (Lecture 9).

flu vaccine: The flu is a severe upper respiratory infection caused by various strains of influenza virus. Vaccines made from either attenuated or inactivated versions of flu viruses have been shown to be effective in reducing the risk of getting the flu and morbidity from the flu. Despite some claims, flu vaccines do not contain aborted fetal cells (Lecture 10).

genetically modified (GM) food: Genetically modified food refers to cultivars of edible plant and animal species that are the result of direct genetic manipulation. This involves either inserting a gene from another variety, or even species, or modifying existing genes. Critics claim that GM foods are inherently risky and have not been adequately safety tested. Supporters point out that all foods consumed by humans have been substantially modified over centuries and millennia with breeding and cultivation, and GM simply speeds up this process (Lecture 5).

hangover: Hangover refers to a set of symptoms, including headache, dehydration, and nausea, caused by the after effects of alcohol toxicity, and is the target of many popular, but untrue, preventions and remedies (Lecture 1).

head injury: A head injury serious enough to cause unconsciousness is also likely to cause long term or even permanent brain injury (called traumatic brain injury). Unlike in the movies, someone suffering a blow to the head that causes unconsciousness does not simply revive minutes or hours later with no long-term impairment (Lecture 20).

heat loss through head: This notion is inaccurately based on the idea that heat rises (heat has no tendency to rise, although some hotter fluids, like air, will rise above relatively cooler fluids). Heat is lost through entire surface area of skin through radiation and evaporation, and is affected by various factors, including blood perfusion and exposure (Lecture 24).

herbal treatments: Herbs have been used for millennia as drugs and remedies, and are an important source of modern drug development (pharmacognasy). However, while they are used for their pharmacological effects, they are often poorly regulated as dietary supplements (Lecture 14).

hiccups: A hiccup is an involuntary contraction of the diaphragm resulting in a sharp intake of air followed by a glottal stop. There are countless folk remedies, none of which work but may appear effective because most hiccups stop even without intervention (Lecture 1).

HIV and **HIV prevention**: The human immunodeficiency virus (HIV) is the virus which causes the acquired immunodeficiency syndrome (AIDS). Preventing the spread of HIV is a major goal of the world's health organizations. Their efforts are sometimes hampered by myths about HIV and prevention, including the myth that HIV is not the true cause of AIDS (Lecture 23).

homeopathic products: Homeopathy is a prescientific medical philosophy dating from the late 18th century. Its premises or "laws" are fanciful and not supported by modern science. They include using substances diluted to the point where not even a single molecule remains. Claims for homeopathic products have been shown in clinical trials to be no different from placebos. Homeopathy does not refer to herbal or natural remedies (Lecture 15).

honey: Honey is highly concentrated flower nectar made by honeybees. Its extremely low moisture content makes it an effective antiseptic for wounds (Lecture 12).

hormones in meat and dairy: Natural and synthetic hormones are used to increase growth and production. Small amounts can be found in beef, slightly more in eggs and dairy, but overall levels of added hormones are much less than naturally occurring hormones in people and animals. There is no current evidence for adverse health effects (Lecture 5). *See also* **antibiotics**.

hyperactivity: Although normal in children to some extent, increased hyperactivity is considered a disorder and may occur with or without attention deficit. Hyperactivity is often erroneously linked to food as the cause, particularly sugar, caffeine, or preservatives but scientific studies do not support a causal link (Lecture 7).

hypnosis: Hypnosis is not a trance but rather a state of heightened alertness and suggestibility. People are capable of lying when hypnotized. Hypnosis does not grant access to otherwise forgotten memories and, in fact, may result in the formation of false memories. There is evidence to support medical use of hypnosis for pain, blood pressure, stress management, and muscle relaxation—essentially using hypnosis as a form of relaxation (Lecture 19).

infrared lasers: Infrared lasers refer to coherent light in the infrared spectrum, which is efficient at transferring heat. They are legitimately used to relax muscles, which is a response to the heating effect (Lecture 18).

ionized water: All water contains ions of H+ and OH- in a steady state. The balance of these ions in water determine the water's pH. Technically pH is a logarithmic scale of the H+ concentration in water, with a pH of 7 being neutral, less than 7 being acidic, and greater than 7 being alkaline or basic. So called "ionized" water has no health benefit over nonionized water. The term "ionized water" is not an accepted scientific term but rather is used in marketing. Pure water always has a pH of 7 and cannot be "ionized." Water may contain ions of other substances, and it is they that make water acidic or alkaline. There is no health benefit to consuming "ionized" or alkaline water, as is sometimes claimed (Lecture 2).

iridology: Iridology is a form of diagnosis based on the false notion that the colors and flecks in the iris of the eye are connected to all parts of the body and reflect the health or disease state of the body. Practitioners therefore claim to infer a person's state of health by looking at the iris. This idea, however, is not based on any known anatomy or physiology, nor is there any evidence for its claims (Lecture 19).

irradiated foods: Irradiated foods are those that have been treated by passing radiation through them in order to kill any bacteria or other organisms. The food is therefore sterilized, which greatly reduces spoilage and extends safe shelf-life. Irradiated foods are not radioactive (Lecture 5).

kidney stones: Kidney stones are formed from solid concretions or small crystals forming from substances dissolved in urine. Some individuals are predisposed to kidney stones due to genetics or certain medications or chronic medical conditions. Drinking enough fluid helps keep the urine dilute and washes out any small crystals or concretions before they form into stone (Lecture 2).

knuckle cracking: Knuckle cracking is the process of making a popping sound by stretching the joints, thereby expanding the synovial fluid which forms bubbles that then "pop." This activity has not been linked to arthritis; but in one study was shown to be associated with some loss of strength in the hands, perhaps due to lax ligaments (Lecture 24).

locked-in syndrome: Locked-in syndrome is a syndrome in which a person is mostly paralyzed but still fully conscious. This may result, for example, from a brainstem stroke or other injury that causes a person to be paralyzed everywhere except for some remaining eye movement. Some patients who are locked in may communicate by blinking their eyes or by computer tracking of their gaze (Lecture 20).

low fat versus low carb: *See* **dieting.**

magnets: Most magnets are permanent magnets, which are made by ferromagnetic material, like iron, being exposed to a magnetic field while being stroked or struck. Static magnets, like refrigerator magnets, have a static (unchanging) magnetic field. There is no demonstrated biological effect or medical benefit for static magnets, despite centuries of products with such claims. Dynamic magnets, however (such as electromagnets with an alternating magnetic field), do have biological effects and may have potential benefit for migraine and other indications (Lecture 18). *See also* **cell phones** and **copper.**

meditation: Meditation is a self-induced state of relaxation. This may be achieved through self-reflection, rhythmic chanting, or "mental silence." There is no consensus on a more specific neurological definition. Meditation is useful medically to achieve relaxation, reduce pain, and lower blood pressure or stress, but evidence is lacking for applications not related to relaxation (Lecture 19).

microwaving: Microwave ovens use microwave frequency electromagnetic fields to heat water molecules inside food. This has the same overall effect on food as other forms of cooking. Using microwave-safe plastic containers does not release cancer-causing toxins, although not all plastic is safe to microwave (some are too thin and might melt; Lecture 16). Microwave ovens are shielded, but to minimize potential risk do not stand directly in front of microwaves for extended periods. Liquids may become superheated in a microwave causing rapid boiling and pose a burn risk (Lecture 18).

migraines: Migraines are a chronic neurological disorder characterized by recurrent headaches, often associated with nausea and sensitivity to bright lights and noise (Lecture 2). Many migraine sufferers require medications to prevent and treat headaches. Several nutritional supplements, such as Vitamin B2 and magnesium, may aid in prevention (Lecture 3).

minerals: Minerals are required, often in trace amounts, for normal health. Plants require minerals also, and humans derive much of their minerals from plants in the diet. Reports of mineral depletion in soil are often misinterpreted. Soil is tested and minerals are added during farming, and mineral content in food is generally adequate (Lecture 3). *See also* **vitamins.**

minimally conscious state (MCS): MCS is a type of coma characterized by severe decrease in consciousness with only minimal signs of any interaction with the environment. MCS is the result of severe brain injury and has a very poor prognosis but slightly better than persistent vegetative state (Lecture 19). *See also* **coma** and **persistent vegetative state**.

morbidity: The term morbidity refers to disease, injury, illness and other biological adverse conditions, events, and effects. The term "mortality" specifically refers to death, and therefore "morbidity" is often used in medicine to refer to all diseases and adverse consequences short of death.

natural: The term "natural" refers to substances that occur in nature, but in terms of food and products the definition is often vaguely applied and not carefully regulated. "Natural" is used more as a marketing term than for any meaningful scientific definition (Lecture 5).

neti pot: A container used to flush the sinuses with warm water or saline (salt water). While use may improve an acute sinus infection by helping to remove mucous, there is no evidence for benefit from routine preventive use, and in fact frequent use may lead to sinus infections.

organic foods: The term "organic" refers to a collection of farming practices that avoids the use of synthetic fertilizers and pesticides and the use of other techniques such as irradiation and genetic modification. The regulation of the organic label refers to the process of farming and production, and does not necessarily say anything about the final product. Proponents argue that organic farming methods are more sustainable and better for the environment, while others argue that sustainable farming methods should be supported whether or not they meet the definition of "organic." Some may prefer organic produce because they wish to support local farms, although much organic farming is conducted by large agricultural companies as well. Claims for nutritional or health benefits of organic produce remain somewhat controversial. After 50 years of research there is no evidence of a specific health benefit to consuming organic food. Organic produce does contain fewer synthetic pesticides, but the health implications of this are unclear as pesticide levels are generally low (and can be reduced further by thorough washing) and organic farming often uses nonsynthetic pesticides. (*See also* **hormones**.) There are only slight nutritional differences in organic versus conventional produce, with unclear impact on nutrition and health. An additional concern for organic meat, eggs, and dairy is the humane treatment of the animals in question (Lecture 3).

persistent vegetative state (PVS): A type of coma defined by a complete lack of any interaction with the environment. People in a PVS can have sleep-wake cycles, and display eye movement, facial grimacing, and other movements but have no discernable conscious awareness. PVS is usually the result of severe permanent injury to the brain (Lecture 20). *See also* **coma** and **minimally conscious state**.

pharmacognasy: The study and development of medicinals from natural substances, such as plants and animals products. This has been and remains an important part of modern drug development (Lecture 14).

placebo effect: There are many types of placebo effects which cause the impression or illusion of a health benefit from an inactive intervention. These effects include psychological effects, nonspecific benefits surrounding the ritual and attention of treatment, biases of observation, and statistical effects (like regression to the mean; Lecture 21).

prebiotics: Prebiotics are foods that contain nondigestible components that are meant to be food for intestinal bacteria in order to support the intestinal ecosystem. While theoretically plausible, there is currently no evidence to support specific health benefits (Lecture 6).

pregnancy, conception: Conception is the result of the union of male and female gametes. There are many myths and beliefs surrounding this event— most involving methods of preventing, ensuring, or controlling conception so as to determine gender (Lecture 22).

pregnancy, determining gender: The two scientifically established methods of determining the gender of a child prior to birth are through examination of the anatomy by ultrasound or examination of the genetics through amniocentesis (Lecture 22).

pregnancy, labor: Having a safe and healthy pregnancy and delivery is important, but many myths as to how to achieve this may cause unnecessary fear. It is best to listen to expert advice. For example, it is safe to sleep on one's back while pregnant. Raising arms will not twist the umbilical cord; moderate exercise is okay; bumpy roads will not induce labor; and it is safe to use microwave ovens (though don't stand close for long periods while they're operating; Lecture 22).

prepared foods: In terms of nutritional content, food choice is overall more important than food preparation. Excessive cooking can reduce the nutritional content of food, but normal cooking will have a negligible effect. Fresh fruits and vegetables will often have the most nutrients, but frozen may in fact be better as frozen produce is often picked at peak ripeness, while canned has slightly less (Lecture 3).

probiotics: Probiotics are products that contain live bacteria, intended to improve the helpful bacterial flora of the body, mainly in the intestines. Existing products, however, have not been shown to significantly alter the complex bacteria ecosystem of the body, with either short-term or long-term use (Lecture 6).

raw foods: Raw foods refers to food that has not been cooked or treated in a way that would alter its composition. Despite claims, raw foods are not nutritionally superior to cooked foods. Normal cooking only has a minor effect on some nutrients, while actually making some foods more digestible and therefore more nutritious. Raw milk has no more nutritional value than pasteurized and carries an increased risk of contamination and infection (Lecture 5).

sneezing: A sneeze is an involuntary reflex that results in the explosive expulsion of air from the lugs through the nose and mouth. It is possible to voluntarily suppress a sneeze. Despite common belief, this is not dangerous. However violent sneezing itself does have some rare risks, including muscle strain, arterial dissection, and venous thrombosis (Lecture 1).

sweating: Sweating is the secretion of water through sweat glands in the skin. Its primary function is to cool the body through evaporation. If one becomes dehydrated the ability to sweat will be diminished, which can lead to overheating (Lecture 2).

swimming: Swimming is a physical exercise like any other. There is no special reason to wait an hour after eating before swimming, although any physical exertion on a full stomach may be uncomfortable (Lecture 1).

syndrome: A syndrome is a constellation of symptoms and signs that tend to occur together and display a characteristic natural history, prognosis, and response to treatment. Syndromes can be described and named even in the absence of knowledge of their underlying cause, and in fact may have many possible underlying causes (Lecture 13).

teething: Teething is the process of infant teeth emerging through the gums. Infants may often become fussy from the discomfort. However, there is no evidence to support an association between teething and diarrhea, cough, or high fever (Lecture 24).

turkey: Turkey meat is a source of protein, including the amino acid L-tryptophan. It is a popular belief that tryptophan contributes to the sleepiness attributed to a large turkey meal, however tryptophan from turkey alone does not cause sleepiness (Lecture 24).

urine therapy: Urine therapy (or urotherapy) is the practice, dating back to many ancient cultures, of drinking one's own urine as a remedy or health tonic. It is based on the false belief that vital nutrients or therapeutic proteins are expelled in the urine and drinking them can cure many diseases or ailments. However, this is superstition and not science. Urine is waste and is used to remove toxins and waste from the body as well as to regulate electrolytes and hydration (Lecture 23).

vaccination: Vaccination is the medical intervention of stimulating the immune system with a component of an infectious agent in order to provoke long term immunity to the infection. Vaccines use either live attenuated (not harmful) versions of bacteria or viruses, or killed organisms, or sometimes just proteins from the organisms. In this way vaccines strengthen the immune system and allow it to mount a much more vigorous response when the recipient is exposed to the infecting agent the next time (Lectures 10 and 11). *See also* **flu vaccine** and **autism.**

vitalism: Vitalism is an ancient belief, common in almost every culture, that living things are animated by a life energy. In Chinese culture the vitalistic force is referred to as chi (or qi), in India it is called prana, while in the West it was referred to as spiritus and in modern manifestations it has been called "innate" (by chiropractors) and the "human energy field" (by practitioners of therapeutic touch). The vitalistic force was used to explain aspects of biology that were not yet understood scientifically, but by the middle of the 19th century the notion of a vital force was abandoned by science, essentially because there was nothing left for it to do (biological processes had been adequately explained scientifically to make it superfluous). Further, there is no scientific evidence for a special life energy or any claims based on its manipulation (Lectures 15 and 17).

vitamins: Nutritional substances essential to health in tiny amounts that an organism cannot manufacture in sufficient quantities, and therefore must be obtained from the diet. There are deficiency syndromes associated with each vitamin, which can be treated by supplementation. Overdoses of specific vitamins are also possible. A balanced diet can be sufficient for most people to provide enough vitamins without the need for supplements. Women who are pregnant or may become pregnant should be taking a prenatal vitamin, especially folic acid. Other specific medical conditions may also benefit from specific vitamin supplements (Lecture 3).

water: Water is the most fundamental component of life, and also a target of much misinformation. All life requires water to live, and the average person could only survive a few days without access to water. However, 8 ounces of water 8 times per day is not a rule based on any evidence. For most people in most situations thirst is an adequate guide to hydration (Lecture 2). *See also* **dehydration**.

Bibliography

Allen, Arthur. *Vaccine*. New York: W. W. Norton, 2008. Everything you ever wanted to know about the history of vaccines.

Australian Skeptics. "Debunking the Detox Myth." http://skepticzone. wordpress.com/2009/01/15/debunking-the-detox-myth. This article contains information on detox scams.

Barbour, Alan G. *Lyme Disease: The Cause, the Cure, the Controversy*. Baltimore, MD: Johns Hopkins University Press, 1996. The author does a good job of presenting the controversy surrounding chronic Lyme disease and putting it into cultural and scientific perspective.

Barrett, Stephen. "Homeopathy: Is It Medicine?" Chapter 13 in *The Health Robbers*. Buffalo, NY: Prometheus Books, 1993. An excellent, brief overview of homeopathy and why it is pseudoscience.

———. "Questionable Cancer Therapies." This is an excellent and well-referenced discussion of the most popular dubious treatments for cancer. http://www.quackwatch.org/01QuackeryRelatedTopics/cancer.html.

Bauby, Jean-Dominique. *The Diving Bell and the Butterfly: A Memoir of Life in Death*. New York: Knopf, 1997. This book tells the personal story of Jean-Dominique Bauby, who suffered a stroke that left him locked-in. He wrote the book by blinking his eyes to indicate each letter to an assistant. This is a compelling story that gives insight into this tragic condition.

Bausell, R. Barker. *Snake Oil Science: The Truth about Complementary and Alternative Medicine*. New York: Oxford University Press, 2007. Bausell does an excellent job of reviewing medical research methodology as a way of determining which treatments are safe and effective. He also reviews the research for many controversial and fringe health claims.

Benedetti, Fabrizio. *Placebo Effects: Understanding the Mechanisms in Health and Disease.* New York: Oxford University Press, 2009. This book reviews the history of our understanding of placebos and how it was shaped by research.

Bouchez, Colette. "Separating Pregnancy Myths and Facts." WebMD. This is a fun review of common pregnancy myths. http://www.webmd.com/baby/guide/separating-pregnancy-myths-and-facts.

Brenneman, Richard J. *Deadly Blessings: Faith Healing on Trial.* Buffalo: Prometheus Books, 1990. The author gives an excellent exposé of frauds passing themselves off as faith healers, exploiting the sick and desperate.

Brown, Kevin. *Penicillin Man: Alexander Fleming and the Antibiotic Revolution.* Gloucestershire, UK: Sutton, 2004. The story of Fleming is one of the most fascinating in the history of medicine, and Brown tells it well. The past, present, and future of antibiotics are also discussed.

Centers for Disease Control. http://www.cdc.gov. The CDC site does not cover all medical topics, but it is a comprehensive resource on everything to do with infectious diseases and public health, including vaccines. It is also an excellent source for statistics. The site can be a bit clunky, but once you get used to the interface, it becomes easier to find the exact information you need.

Crislip, Mark. "Probiotics." http://www.sciencebasedmedicine.org/?p=344. This is a primer on probiotics from an evidence-based critical perspective by an infectious disease specialist. The author's style is also a pleasure to read.

Denisov, Evgeny T., and Igor B. Afanas'ev. *Oxidation and Antioxidants in Organic Chemistry and Biology.* Boca Raton, FL: CRC Press, 2005. This reference is a bit technical but contains detailed information on antioxidants for those who want to delve deeply into the science.

Eades, Mary Dan. *The Doctor's Complete Guide to Vitamins and Minerals.* New York: Dell, 2000. This reference of individual vitamins and minerals contains exhaustive information.

Eccles, Ronald, and Olaf Weber, eds. *Common Cold.* http://www.springerlink. com/content/g5tt72/?p=33f33dadb341480d8a14979d37492c2b&pi=0. This is a collection of essays on the history and science of the common cold and other respiratory infections. Many of the essays are dry and technical, but others are very readable for the layperson.

Eckman, Peter. *In the Footsteps of the Yellow Emperor: Tracing the History of Traditional Acupuncture.* Rev. ed. San Francisco: Long River Press, 2007. This is a good source for the cultural history of acupuncture but is not a critical scientific resource.

Epstein, Helen. *The Invisible Cure: Why We Are Losing the Fight against AIDS in Africa.* New York: Picador, 2008. This book tells the tale of how myths and superstition about HIV and AIDS are impairing public health measures to fight one of the most serious epidemics of modern times.

Ernst, Edzard, ed. *Homeopathy: A Critical Appraisal.* Oxford: Butterworth-Heinemann, 1998. This is designed to be a reference for professionals, but it is very accessible. While it is not as critical of the theoretical basis of homeopathy as I would like, it does provide an excellent review of the published evidence.

Ernst, Edzard, and Simon Singh. *Trick or Treatment: The Undeniable Facts about Alternative Medicine.* New York: W. W. Norton, 2009. Ernst and Sigh review the scientific method in the opening chapters and then apply that method to a variety of medical practices. They give excellent examples of good science, and not-so-good science, in medicine.

Fallacy Files. "Appeal to Nature." http://www.fallacyfiles.org/adnature.html. This is a brief description of the naturalistic fallacy and gives examples.

Flamm, Bruce. "Magnet Therapy: A Billion Dollar Boondoggle." *Skeptical Inquirer* 30 (2006). http://www.csicop.org/si/show/magnet_therapy_a_ billion-dollar_boondoggle. This is a quick overview of the modern marketing of dubious magnetic devices.

Floch, Martin, and Adam Kim. *Probiotics: A Clinical Guide.* Thorofare, NJ: SLACK, 2010. This is a clinical reference to the history, principles, and research involving probiotics. Overall a good reference, but a bit more positive than I think is deserved by the current research.

Gardner, Martin. *Fads and Fallacies in the Name of Science.* Mineola, NY: Dover, 1957. Gardner is a giant in science education—and one of the original intellectuals of modern skepticism. *Fads and Fallacies* is a classic in the genre of the promotion of science and logic, and despite the fact that it was written half a century ago, the topics and underlying principles are timeless and relevant.

Hallowell, Edward, and John Ratey. *Driven to Distraction: Recognizing and Coping with Attention Deficit Disorder from Childhood through Adulthood.* New York: Touchstone, 1995. This is an excellent reference on ADHD for the layperson.

Harms, Roger and Mayo Clinic. *Mayo Clinic Guide to a Healthy Pregnancy.* New York: HarperResource, 2004. This is a review intended for the average reader. It is a good primer but lacks depth in areas.

Henderson, D. A. *Smallpox: The Death of a Disease.* Amherst, NY: Prometheus Books, 2009. As the title suggests, this book has a narrow focus—on the eradication of smallpox—but it is a fascinating tale about perhaps the single best success of modern medicine.

House of Commons Science and Technology Committee. "Evidence Check 2: Homeopathy." http://www.publications.parliament.uk/pa/cm200910/cmselect/cmsctech/45/45.pdf. This is the comprehensive report of the House of Commons' Science and Technology Committee. You will likely not want to read it from beginning to end, as it is a sprawling treatise, but the conclusions of each section nail the scientific status of homeopathy from the basic science and clinical points of view. It is also thoroughly referenced.

ICON Group International. *Pharmacognosy: Webster's Timeline History, 1832–2007.* San Diego, CA: ICON Group International, 2009. This is a compilation of *Timeline* references dealing with pharmacognosy. You can use it as a reference to read individual articles.

Jamieson, Graham. *Hypnosis and Conscious States: The Cognitive Neuroscience Perspective.* New York: Oxford University Press, 2007. More than just a discussion of hypnosis, this book explores the neuroscience of consciousness itself and the nature of altered states of consciousness. This is a dense book, focusing on basic science, but not overly technical.

Jenicek, Milos, and David L. Hitchcock. *Evidence-Based Practice: Logic and Critical Thinking in Medicine.* Chicago: American Medical Association Press, 2004. The authors provide a thorough discussion of critical thinking in medicine, with plenty of illustrative examples. It is organized like a textbook, and is definitely not casual reading but is an excellent resource for those who wish to delve deeper into clinical thinking.

Karasov, William H., and Carlos Martinez del Rio. *Physiological Ecology: How Animals Process Energy, Nutrients, and Toxins.* Princeton, NJ: Princeton University Press, 2007. This is a technical reference for those interested in the hard science of toxins.

Kavoussi, Ben. "Astrology with Needles." http://www.sciencebasedmedicine. org/?p=583. The author puts astrology into an interesting historical context in this essay.

Lipson, Peter. "Fake Diseases, False Compassion." http://www. sciencebasedmedicine.org/?p=241. An excellent overview of the nature of problematic diagnoses.

Lynn, Steven Jay, and Irving Kirsch. *Essentials of Clinical Hypnosis: An Evidence-Based Approach.* Washington, DC: American Psychological Association, 2005. This book focuses on the clinical applications of hypnosis and reviews the evidence for each. It is reasonably balanced, though perhaps more favorable overall than others might be.

Mayo Clinic Online Reference. http://www.mayoclinic.com. This is an excellent topic-based resource on health information compiled by professionals. When dealing with uncontroversial topics, the Mayo Clinic provides a reliable and up-to-date resource. However, like other all-purpose medical references intended for the public, the site takes a wishy-washy approach at best to controversial topics.

MedlinePlus. "Hyperactivity and Sugar." http://www.nlm.nih.gov/medlineplus/ency/article/002426.htm. This is a quick primer on hyperactivity and sugar, with some useful references.

Mesmer, Franz Anton. *Mesmerism: The Discovery of Animal Magnetism (1779); A New Translation*, edited and translated by Joseph Bouleur. Edmonds, WA: Holmes Publishing Group, 1997. For those who like to read original sources, this is a translation of Mesmer's original work on animal magnetism.

Novella, Steven. "All Natural Arsenic." http://www.theness.com/neurologicablog/?p=231.This essay explores the naturalistic fallacy in detail.

————. "Antioxidant Hype and Reality." *Science-Based Medicine* (blog). http://www.sciencebasedmedicine.org/?p=38. This essay is an overview of the history and science behind the current antioxidant hype.

————. "The Detox Scam." http://www.theness.com/neurologicablog/?p=452. This is an overview of the current hype surrounding detox products.

————. "The Skeptic's Diet." http://www.theness.com/the-skeptics-diet.

This essay is a primer on diet, nutrition, and health. It is periodically updated as significant new research is published.

————, ed. "Vaccines and Autism." *Science-Based Medicine* (blog). This reference page contains a quick overview of topics on vaccines and autism, a list of articles published on the *Science-Based Medicine* blog on the topic, and a fairly complete list of references with a summary of their results. http://sciencebasedmedicine.org/reference/vaccines-and-autism.

Offit, Paul. *Autism's False Prophets*. New York: Columbia University Press, 2010. Dr. Offit has been on the front lines of vaccine education and fighting against antivaccine propaganda for years. Much of the book covers the alleged connection between vaccines and autism, also put in the perspective of the many other false treatments for autism that have cropped up through the years.

Parker, James and Philip Parker, eds. *The Official Patient's Sourcebook on Coma: A Revised and Updated Directory for the Internet Age*. San Diego, CA: ICON Health Publications, 2006. This reference is designed to be updated and accessible and is therefore a good primer on coma.

Posner, Jerome, Clifford B. Saper, Nicholas Schiff, and Fred Plum. *Plum and Posner's Diagnosis of Stupor and Coma*. 4th ed. New York: Oxford University Press, 2007. This book is intended for professionals, but for those with a science background or an interest in being challenged, it is the definitive reference on coma.

Price, Donald D., Damien G. Finniss, and Fabrizio Benedetti. "A Comprehensive Review of the Placebo Effect: Recent Advances and Current Thought." *Annual Review of Psychology* 59 (2008): 565–590. This is an updated review of research into placebo effects.

Rippe, James M. *Weight Watchers Weight Loss That Lasts: Break Through the 10 Big Diet Myths*. Hoboken, NJ: Wiley, 2005. Weight Watchers is the one dieting system that is evidence-based and based on teaching people how to have healthful eating habits (rather than relying on gimmicky diets).

Sagan, Carl. *The Demon-Haunted World*. New York: Ballantine Books, 1997. This book is perhaps *the* best introduction to critical thinking, and probably the first one you should read out of this entire Bibliography. Sagan's style is unmatched.

Sampson, Wallace, and Lewis Vaughn, eds. *Science Meets Alternative Medicine: What the Evidence Says about Unconventional Treatments*. Amherst, NY: Prometheus Books, 2000. This is an eclectic collection of essays by various authors addressing myths, misconceptions, and frauds in medicine.

Samuelsson, Gunnar, and Lars Bohlin. *Drugs of Natural Origin: A Treatise of Pharmacognosy.* 6th ed. Stockholm, Sweden: Swedish Pharmaceutical Press, 2010. Samuelsson and Bohlin review the history of pharmacognosy—the use of natural products as a source for drugs and drug development. They treat pharmacognosy as a mainstream science, which it is.

Science-Based Medicine (blog). http://www.sciencebasedmedicine.org. This is a website dedicated to the discussion and promotion of science in medicine. It contains hundreds of published articles and a reference section for major topics. Dr. Novella is the senior editor of this site.

Science-Based Medicine (blog). Archive for the "Acupuncture" Category. http://www.sciencebasedmedicine.org/?cat=8.

Science-Based Medicine (blog). "Homeopathy." http://sciencebasedmedicine.org/reference/homeopathy. This is a compilation of essays and research on homeopathy.

Scientific American Readers. *Infectious Disease: A Scientific American Reader.* Chicago: University of Chicago Press, 2008. Scientific American is a recognized leader in translating cutting-edge science for the educated layperson, and this reader is no exception.

Segal, Alan. "Body Fluids: Physiology of Salt and Water." Department of Molecular Physics and Biophysics, University of Vermont. http://physioweb.med.uvm.edu/Fluids_1_files/Lecture1.pdf. This reads more like a reference than a good story, but it contains everything you would want to know about how our bodies handle water and electrolytes.

Shermer, Michael. *Why People Believe Weird Things.* Rev. ed. New York: Henry Holt, 2002. The author provides an excellent introduction into logic and critical thinking and then applies it to several popular topics.

Shils, Maurice E., James A. Olson, Moshe Shike, and A. Catherine Ross, eds. *Modern Nutrition in Health and Disease.* 9th ed. Baltimore, MD: Lippincott Williams and Wilkins, 1998. Excellent overview and reference for nutritional information.

Stone, Joanne, and Keith Eddleman. *The Pregnancy Bible: Your Complete Guide to Pregnancy and Early Parenthood.* 2nd ed. Buffalo, NY: Firefly Books, 2008. A comprehensive and easy-to-read guide to the medical and social aspects of pregnancy.

Taub, Arthur. "Acupuncture: Nonsense with Needles." Chapter 18 in *The Health Robbers.* Buffalo, NY: Prometheus Books, 1993. This chapter is a bit out of date, but the basic information is still relevant.

Tyrrell, David, and Michael Fielder. *Cold Wars: The Fight against the Common Cold.* New York: Oxford University Press, 2002. This is a nicely written and illustrated book about the history of the common cold and our efforts to fight it.

Additional references by lecture

Lecture 2

Bae J. S., J. B. Lee, T. Matsumoto, T. Othman, Y. K. Min, and H. M. Yang. "Prolonged Residence of Temperate Natives in the Tropics Produces a Suppression of Sweating." *Pflügers Archiv: European Journal of Physiology,* 453 (2006): 67–72. http://www.ncbi.nlm.nih.gov/pubmed/16736205.

Baker, Arnie. "Sweat Mineral Losses." Arnie Baker Cycling. http://www. arniebakercycling.com/pubs/Free/NS%20Sweat.pdf.

Dartmouth Medical School. "Drink at Least 8 Glasses of Water a Day"—Really? ScienceDaily (2002). http://www.sciencedaily.com/releases/2002/08/020809071640.htm.

Gift Log. "Koala bear facts." http://www.giftlog.com/pictures/koala_fact.htm.

Godek, S. F., A. R. Bartolozzi, and J. J. Godek. "Sweat Rate and Fluid Turnover in American Football Players Compared with Runners in a Hot and Humid Environment." *British Journal of Sports Medicine* 39 (2005): 205–211. http://www.ncbi.nlm.nih.gov/pubmed/15793087.

High Altitude Living. "Dehydration." http://www.highaltitudelife.com/dehydration.htm.

Jegtvig, Shereen. "Which Foods and Drinks Are Good Sources of Water?" http://nutrition.about.com/od/askyournutritionist/f/water.htm.

Mentes, Janet, Kennith Culp, and Bonnie Wakefield. "Use of a Urine Color Chart to Monitor Hydration Status in Nursing Home Residents." Biological Research for Nursing. http://brn.sagepub.com/cgi/content/short/7/3/197.

National Kidney and Urologic Disease Information Clearinghouse (NIH). "Kidney Stones in Adults." http://kidney.niddk.nih.gov/Kudiseases/pubs/stonesadults.

Palmer, Janice. "Armstrong's Study Shows Caffeine Does Not Increase Dehydration." Advance, University of Connecticut. http://advance.uconn.edu/2002/020722/02072207.htm.

Segal, Alan. "Body Fluids: Physiology of Salt and Water." Department of Molecular Physics and Biophysics, University of Vermont. http://physioweb.med.uvm.edu/Fluids_1_files/Lecture1.pdf.

Survival Topics. "How Long Can You Survive Without Water?" http://www.survivaltopics.com/survival/how-long-can-you-survive-without-water.

Utz, Jeffrey. "What Percentage of the Human Body Is Composed of Water?" MadSci Network. http://www.madsci.org/posts/archives/2000–05/958588306.An.r.html.

Wikipedia. "Cabin Pressure." http://en.wikipedia.org/wiki/Cabin_pressurization.

Lecture 3

Allen, E., A. D. Dangour, S. K. Dodhia, A. Hayter, K. Lock, R. Uauy. "Nutritional Quality of Organic Foods: A Systematic Review." *American Journal of Clinical Nutrition* 90 (2009): 680–5. http://www.ncbi.nlm.nih. gov/pubmed/19640946.

Caplan, Gary E. "Vitamin E Deficiency." http://emedicine.medscape.com/article/126187overview.

U.S. Department of Health and Human Services and U.S. Department of Agriculture. "2005 Dietary Guidelines for Americans." http://www. cnpp.usda.gov/Publications/DietaryGuidelines/2005/2005DGPolicy Document.pdf.

Wikipedia. "James Lind." http://en.wikipedia.org/wiki/James_L.

Lecture 4

Akkary, E., T. Cramer, O. Chaar, K. Rajput, S. Yu, J. Dziura, K. Roberts, A. Duffy, and R. Bell. "Survey of the Effective Exercise Habits of the Formerly Obese." *Journal of the Society of Laparoendoscopic Surgeons* 14 (2010): 106–114.

Carels, R. A., K. Konrad, and J. Harper. "Individual Differences in Food Perceptions and Calorie Estimation: An Examination of Dieting Status, Weight, and Gender." *Appetite* 49 (2007): 450–458.

Centers for Disease Control. "Trends in Intake of Energy and Macronutrients—United States, 1971–2000." *Morbidity and Mortality Weekly Report* 53 (2004): 80–82. http://www.cdc.gov/mmwr/preview/mmwrhtml/mm5304a3.htm.

Chambliss, H. O. "Exercise Duration and Intensity in a Weight-Loss Program." *Clinical Journal of Sport Medicine* (2005): 113–115.

Davis, L. M., C. Coleman, J. Kiel, J. Rampolla, T. Hutchisen, L. Ford, W. S. Andersen, and A. Hanlon-Mitola. "Efficacy of a Meal Replacement Diet Plan Compared to a Food-Based Diet Plan after a Period of Weight Loss and Weight Maintenance: A Randomized Controlled Trial." *Nutrition Journal* 11 (2010): 9–11.

Flegal, K. M., M. D. Carroll, C. L. Ogden, and L. R. Curtin. "Prevalence and Trends in Obesity among U.S. Adults, 1999–2008." *Journal of the American Medical Association* 303 (2010): 235–241. doi:10.1001/jama.2009.2014.

Metcalf, B. S., J. Hosking, A. N. Jeffery, L. D. Voss, W. Henley, and T. J. Wilkin. "Fatness Leads to Inactivity, but Inactivity Does Not Lead to Fatness: A Longitudinal Study in Children (EarlyBird 45)." *Archives of Disease in Childhood*, June 23, 2010 (Published online ahead of print).

Mokdad, A. H., E. S. Ford, B. A. Bowman, W. H. Dietz, F. Vinicor, V. Bales, and J. Marks. "Prevalence of Obesity, Diabetes, and Obesity-Related Health Risk Factors, 2001." *Journal of the American Medical Association* 289 (2003): 76–79.

Nordmann, A. J., A. Nordmann, M. Briel, U. Keller, W. S. Yancy Jr., B. J. Brehm, and H. C. Bucher. "Effects of Low-Carbohydrate versus Low-Fat Diets on Weight Loss and Cardiovascular Risk Factors: A Meta-Analysis of Randomized Controlled Trials." *Archives of Internal Medicine* 166 (2006): 285–293.

Vázquez, C., C. Montagna, F. Alcaraz, J. A. Balsa, I. Zamarrón, F. Arrieta, and J. I. Botella-Carretero. "Meal Replacement with a Low-Calorie Diet Formula in Weight Loss Maintenance after Weight Loss Induction with Diet Alone." *European Journal of Clinical Nutrition* 63 (2009): 1226–1232.

Wansink, B., and P. Chandon. "Meal Size, Not Body Size, Explains Errors in Estimating the Calorie Content of Meals." *Annals of Internal Medicine* 145 (2006): 326–332.

Weightloss for All. "Calorie Needs when Losing Weight." http://www. weightlossforall.com/calorie-requirements-daily.htm.

Lecture 5

Allen, E., A.D. Dangour, S.K. Dodhia, A. Hayter, K. Lock, and R. Uauy. "Nutrition-Related Health Effects of Organic Foods: A Systematic Review." *American Journal of Clinical Nutrition* 92 (2010): 203–210. doi:10.3945/ ajcn.2010.29269.

Bahlai, C. A., Y. Xue, C. M. McCreary, A. W. Schaafsma, and R. H. Hallett. "Choosing Organic Pesticides over Synthetic Pesticides May Not Effectively Mitigate Environmental Risk in Soybeans." *PLoS One* 5 (2010): e11250.

Boor, K., S. Murinda, S. Murphy, and S. Oliver. "Food Safety Hazards Associated with Consumption of Raw Milk." *Foodborne Pathogens and Disease* 6 (2009): 793–806.

Kataria, A., and M. B. Chauhan. "Contents and Digestibility of Carbohydrates of Mung Beans (*Vigna radiata* L.) as Affected by Domestic Processing and Cooking." *Plant Foods for Human Nutrition* 38 (1988): 51–59.

McKenzie, A., and M. Whittingham. "Birds Select Conventional over Organic Wheat When Given Free Choice." *Journal of the Science of Food and Agriculture* 90 (2010): 1861–1869.

Novella, Steven. "All Natural Arsenic." *Neurologica* (blog). http://www. theness.com/neurologicablog/?p=231.

Lecture 6

Briand, V., O. Bouchaud, P. Buffet, A. Fontanet, S. Genty, N. Godineau, C. Goujon, K. Lacombe, S. Matheron, P. Ralaimazava, J. Salomon, and E. Vandemelbrouck. "Absence of Efficacy of Nonviable Lactobacillus Acidophilus for the Prevention of Traveler's Diarrhea: A Randomized,

Double-Blind, Controlled Study." *Clinical Infectious Diseases* 43 (2006): 1170–5. http://www.ncbi.nlm.nih.gov/pubmed/17029137.

Dublin, S. and L. V. McFarland. "Meta-Analysis of Probiotics for the Treatment of Irritable Bowel Syndrome." *World Journal of Gastroenterology* 14 (2008): 26506. http://www.ncbi.nlm.nih.gov/pubmed/18461650.

McFarland, L. V. "Meta-Analysis of Probiotics for the Prevention of Antibiotic Associated Diarrhea and the Treatment of Clostridium Difficile Disease." *American Journal of Gastroenterology* 101 (2006): 812–22. http://www.ncbi.nlm.nih.gov/pubmed/16635227.

———. "Meta-Analysis of Probiotics for the Prevention of Traveler's Diarrhea." *Travel Medicine and Infectious Disease* 5 (2007): 971–05. http://www.ncbi.nlm.nih.gov/pubmed/17298915.

Meurman, J. H. and I. Stamatova. "Probiotics: Health Benefits in the Mouth." *American Journal of Dentistry* 22 (2009): 329–38. http://www.ncbi.nlm.nih.gov/pubmed/20178208.

Nelson, R. and A. Pillai. "Probiotics for Treatment of Clostridium Difficile-Associated Colitis in Adults." *Cochrane Database of Systematic Reviews* (2008). http://www.ncbi.nlm.nih.gov/pubmed/18254055.

Lecture 7

Hale, K. L., and J. R. Hughes. "Behavioral Effects of Caffeine and Other Methylxanthines on Children." *Experimental and Clinical Psychopharmacology* 6 (1998): 87–95. http://www.ncbi.nlm.nih.gov/pubmed/9526149.

Sampson, H. A., and S. H. Sicherer. "Food Allergy." *Journal of Allergy and Clinical Immunology* 125 (2010): S116–25. http://www.ncbi.nlm.nih.gov/pubmed/20042231.

Warner, Jennifer. "Can Food Really Affect your Child's Behavior?" Medicine Net. http://www.medicinenet.com/script/main/art.asp?articlekey=52516.

Lecture 8

Argellatia, F., C. Domenicotti, M. Pronzatoa, and R. Ricciarelli. "Vitamin E and Neurodegenerative Diseases." *Molecular Aspects of Medicine* (2007): 5–6.

Bardia, A., J. R. Cerhan, P. J. Erwin, P. J. Limburg, V. M. Montori, A. K. Sood, and I. M. Tleyjeh. "Efficacy of Antioxidant Supplementation in Reducing Primary Cancer Incidence and Mortality: Systematic Review and Meta-Analysis." *Mayo Clinic Proceedings* 83 (2008): 23–34. http://www.ncbi.nlm.nih.gov/pubmed/18173999.

Blumberg, Jeffrey. "Unraveling the Conflicting Studies on Vitamin E and Heart Disease." Linus Pauling Institute, Oregon State University. http://lpi.oregonstate.edu/ss02/blumberg.html.

Boothby, L. A., and P. L. Doering. "Vitamin C and Vitamin E for Alzheimer's Disease." *Annals of Pharmacotherapy* 39 (2005): 2073–80. http://www.ncbi.nlm.nih.gov/pubmed/16227450.

Chandrashekhar, D. Kamat, Sunyana Gadal, Kenneth Hensley, Molina Mhatre, Quentin N. Pye, and Kelly S. Williamson. "Antioxidants in Central Nervous System Diseases: Preclinical Promise and Translational Challenges." *Journal of Alzheimer's Disease* 15 (2008): 473–493. http://iospress.metapress.com/content/0385r5h41k2022w7.

Cleveland Clinic. "Antioxidants, Vitamin E, Beta Carotene, and Cardiovascular Disease." Cleveland Clinic. http://my.clevelandclinic.org/heart/disorders/cad/vitamin_e.aspx.

"High Doses of Antioxidant Supplements Induce Stem Cell Genetic Abnormalities" e! Science News.

Bibliography

http://esciencenews.com/articles/2010/05/04/high.doses.antioxidant.
supplements.induce.stem.cell.genetic.abnormalities.

Lecture 9

Arroll, B., and T. Kenealy. "Antibiotics for the Common Cold." *Cochrane Database of Systematic Reviews* (2002). Update in *Cochrane Database of Systematic Reviews* (2005). http://www.ncbi.nlm.nih.gov/pubmed/12137610.

Chalker, E., R. M. Douglas, H. Hemilä, B. Treacy. "Vitamin C for Preventing and Treating the Common Cold." *Cochrane Database of Systematic Reviews* (2004). http://www.ncbi.nlm.nih.gov/pubmed/17636648.

Chang, Y. J., H. M. Cho , Y. W. Hwang , S. Y. Kim, and Y. S. Moon. "Non-Steroidal Anti-Inflammatory Drugs for the Common Cold." *Cochrane Database of Systematic Reviews* (2009). http://www.ncbi.nlm.nih.gov/pubmed/19588387.

Lecture 10

Centers for Disease Control and Prevention. "Vaccine Excipient & Media Summary."   http://www.cdc.gov/vaccines/pubs/pinkbook/downloads/appendices/B/excipient-table-1.pdf.

Lecture 11

Centers for Disease Control and Prevention. "Vaccine Excipient & Media Summary."   http://www.cdc.gov/vaccines/pubs/pinkbook/downloads/appendices/B/excipient-table-1.pdf.

Gellin, Bruce G., Michael A. Gerber, Charles J. Hackett, Tobias R. Kollman, Sarah Landry, Edgar K. Marcuse, Paul A. Offit, and Jessica Quarles. "Addressing Parents' Concerns: Do Multiple Vaccines Overwhelm or Weaken the Infant's Immune System?" *Pediatrics* 109 (2002): 124–129. http://pediatrics.aappublications.org/cgi/content/full/109/1/124.

Mayo Clinic. "Autism Symptoms." http://www.mayoclinic.com/health/autism/DS00348/DSECTION=symptoms.

Lecture 12

Aiello, A. E., E. L. Larson, and S. B. Levy. "Consumer Antibacterial Soaps: Effective or Just Risky?" *Clinical Infectious Diseases* 45 (2007) Suppl 2:S137–S147.

Holton, R. H., M. A. Huber, and G. T. Terezhalmy. "Antimicrobial Efficacy of Soap and Water Hand Washing versus an Alcohol-Based Hand Cleanser." *Texas Dental Journal* 126 (2009): 1175–1180.

Ledder, R. G., P. Gilbert, C. Willis, and A. J. McBain. "Effects of Chronic Triclosan Exposure upon the Antimicrobial Susceptibility of 40 Ex-Situ Environmental and Human Isolates." *Journal of Applied Microbiology* 100 (2006): 1132–1140.

Liu, A. H. "Hygiene Theory and Allergy and Asthma Prevention." *Paediatric and Perinatal Epidemiology* 21 (2007) Suppl 3:2–7.

Trampuz, A., and A. F. Widmer. "Hand Hygiene: A Frequently Missed Lifesaving Opportunity during Patient Care." *Mayo Clinic Proceedings* 79 (2004): 109–116.

Lecture 13

Baker, P. J. "Perspectives on Chronic Lyme Disease." *American Journal of Medicine* 121 (2008): 562–564.

Knoop, H., J. B. Prins, R. Moss-Morris, and G. Bleijenberg. "The Central Role of Cognitive Processes in the Perpetuation of Chronic Fatigue Syndrome." *Journal of Psychosomatic Research* 68 (2010): 489–494.

Marques, A. "Chronic Lyme Disease: A Review." *Infectious Disease Clinics of North America* 22 (2008): 341–360, vii–viii.

Lecture 14

Botanical Gardens Conservation International. "Plant Species Numbers." http://www.bgci.org/ourwork/1521.

Davis, Roger B., Stefanos N. Kales, Nadia Khouri, Janet Paquin, Russell S. Phillips, Robert B. Saper, Anusha Sehgal, and Venkatesh Thuppil. "Lead, Mercury, and Arsenic in U.S.- and Indian-Manufactured Ayurvedic Medicines Sold via the Internet." *Journal of the American Medical Association* 300 (2008): 915–923. http://ihealthbulletin.com/blog/2008/08/27/ayurvedic-herbs-may-be-contain-toxic-heavy-metals.

Dekosky, et al. "*Ginkgo biloba* for Prevention of Dementia: A Randomized Controlled Trial." *Journal of the American Medical Association* 300 (2008): 2253–2262.

Izzo, A. A., and E. Ernst. "Interactions between Herbal Medicines and Prescribed Drugs: An Updated Systematic Review." *Drugs* 69 (2009): 1777–1798.

National Center for Complementary and Alternative Medicine. National Institutes of Health. "Echinacea for the Prevention and Treatment of Colds in Adults: Research Results and Implications for Future Studies." http://nccam.nih.gov/research/results/echinacea_rr.htm.

Palacio, C., G. Masri, and A. D. Mooradian. "Black Cohosh for the Management of Menopausal Symptoms: A Systematic Review of Clinical Trials." *Drugs & Aging* 26 (2009): 23–36. doi: 10.2165/0002512-200926010-00002.

Shelton, R. C. "St John's Wort (*Hypericum perforatum*) in Major Depression." *Journal of Clinical Psychiatry* 70 (2009): Suppl 5:23–27.

Tacklind, J., R. MacDonald, I. Rutks, and T. J. Wilt. "Serenoa Repens for Benign Prostatic Hyperplasia." *Cochrane Database of Systematic Reviews* 15 (2009): CD001423.

Web MD. "FDA: Chinese Herb Causes Kidney Failure, Cancer." http://www.webmd.com/news/20010416/fda-chinese-herb-causes-kidney-failure-cancer.

Lecture 15

Altunç, U., M. H. Pittler, and E. Ernst. "Homeopathy for Childhood and Adolescence Ailments: Systematic Review of Randomized Clinical Trials." *Mayo Clinic Proceedings* 82 (2007): 69–75.

Ernst, E. "Homeopathy: What Does the "Best" Evidence Tell Us?" *Medical Journal of Australia* 192 (2010): 458–460.

House of Commons Science and Technology Committee. "Evidence Check 2: Homeopathy." United Kingdom Parliament. http://www.publications.parliament.uk/pa/cm200910/cmselect/cmsctech/45/45.pdf.

Science-Based Medicine (blog). "Homeopathy." http://sciencebasedmedicine.org/reference/homeopathy.

Lecture 16

Australian Skeptics. "Debunking the Detox Myth." *Skeptic Zone* (blog). http://skepticzone.wordpress.com/2009/01/15/debunking-the-detox-myth.

Lee, C. J. "Coffee Enema Induced Acute Colitis." *Korean Journal of Gastroenterology* 52 (2008): 251–254.

Roazen, L. "Why Ear Candling Is Not a Good Idea." Quackwatch. http://www.quackwatch.org/01QuackeryRelatedTopics/candling.html.

Sashiyama, H. "Rectal Burn Caused by Hot-Water Coffee Enema." *Gastrointestinal Endoscopy* 68 (2008): 1008; discussion 1009.

Seely, D. R., S. M. Quigley, and A. W. Langman. "Ear Candles—Efficacy and Safety." *Laryngoscope* 106 (1996): 1226–1229.

Lecture 17

Derry, C. J., S. Derry, H. J. McQuay, and R. A. Moore. "Systematic Review of Systematic Reviews of Acupuncture Published 1996–2005." *Clinical Medicine* 6 (2006): 381–386.

El-Toukhy, T., S. K. Sunkara, M. Khairy, R. Dyer, Y. Khalaf, and A. Coomarasamy. "A Systematic Review and Meta-Analysis of Acupuncture in In Vitro Fertilisation." *BJOG* 115 (2008): 1203–1213.

Haake, M., et al. "German Acupuncture Trials (GERAC) for Chronic Low Back Pain: Randomized, Multicenter, Blinded, Parallel-Group Trial with 3 Groups." *Archives of Internal Medicine* 167 (2007): 1892–1898.

Kavoussi, Ben. "Astrology with Needles." *Science-Based Medicine* (blog). http://www.sciencebasedmedicine.org/?p=583.

Ramey, David. "Acupuncture and History: The "Ancient" Therapy That's Been around for Several Decades." *Science-Based Medicine* (blog). http://www.sciencebasedmedicine.org/?cat=8.

Ying Cheong, Luciano G. Nardo, Tony Rutherford, and William Ledger. "Acupuncture and Herbal Medicine in IVF: A Review of the Evidence for Clinical Practice. British Fertility Society, Policy and Practice Guidelines." *Human Fertility* 13 (2010): 3–12.

Lecture 18

Jarvis, William T. "Chiropractic: A Skeptical View." Chirobase. http://www.chirobase.org/01General/skeptic.html.

Macklis, Roger M. "Magnetic Healing, Quackery, and the Debate about the Health Effects of Electromagnetic Fields." *Annals of Internal Medicine* 118 (1993): 376–383.

Miller, William Snow. "Elisha Perkins and His Magnetic Tractors." *Yale Journal of Biology and Medicine* 8 (1935): 41–57. http://www.ncbi.nlm.nih.gov/pmc/articles/PMC2601307/pdf/yjbm00545-0050.pdf.

Museum of Quakery. "Albert Abrams." Museum of Quackery. http://www.museumofquackery.com/amquacks/abrams.htm.

Pittler, M. H., E. M. Brown, and E. Ernst. "Static Magnets for Reducing Pain: Systematic Review and Meta-Analysis of Randomized Trials." *Canadian Medical Association Journal* 177 (2007): 736–742.

Lecture 19

Chadwick, Catherine. "Brain Research on Hypnosis." Suite101. http://hypnotherapy.suite101.com/article.cfm/brain_research_on_hypnosis.

Green, J. P., and S. J. Lynn. "Hypnosis and Suggestion-Based Approaches to Smoking Cessation: An Examination of the Evidence." *International Journal of Clinical Experimental Hypnosis* 48(2000): 195–224.

Patterson, D. R., and M. P. Jensen. "Hypnosis and Clinical Pain." *Psychological Bulletin* 129 (2003): 495–521.

Rogovik, A. L., and R. D. Goldman. "Hypnosis for Treatment of Pain in Children." *Canadian Family Physician* 53 (2007): 823–825.

Lecture 20

Andrews, K., L. Murphy, R. Munday, and C. Littlewood. "Misdiagnosis of the Vegetative State: Retrospective Study in a Rehabilitation Unit." *British Medical Journal* 313 (1996): 13–16. http://bmj.bmjjournals.com/cgi/content/full/313/7048/13. PMID 8664760. PMC 2351462.

Owen, A. M., M. R. Coleman, M. Boly, M. H. Davis, S. Laureys, and J. D. Pickard. "Detecting Awareness in the Vegetative State." *Science* 313 (2006): 1402. doi:10.1126/science.1130197. PMID 16959998.

Bibliography

Whyte, J., and R. Myers. "Incidence of Clinically Significant Responses to Zolpidem among Patients with Disorders of Consciousness: A Preliminary Placebo Controlled Trial." *American Journal of Physical Medicine & Rehabilitation* 88 (2009): 410–418.

Lecture 21

Hróbjartsson, A., and P. C. Gøtzsche. "Placebo Interventions for all Clinical Conditions." *Cochrane Database of Systematic Reviews* 20(2010): CD003974.

Nuhn, Tobias, and Rainer Lüdtke. "Placebo Effect Sizes in Homeopathic Compared to Conventional Drugs—A Systematic Review of Randomised Controlled Trials." *Homeopathy* 99 (2010): 76–82.

Lecture 22

Aberg, M. A., N. Aberg, J. Brisman, R. Sundberg, A. Winkvist, and K. Torén. "Fish Intake of Swedish Male Adolescents Is a Predictor of Cognitive Performance." *Acta Paediatricia* 98 (2009): 555–560.

Barrett, Julia R. "Phthalates and Baby Boys: Potential Disruption of Human Genital Development." *Environmental Health Perspectives* 113: A542. http://www.ehponline.org/docs/2005/113-8/ss.html.

Kost, K., S. Singh, B. Vaughan, J. Trussell, and A. Bankole. "Estimates of Contraceptive Failure from the 2002 National Survey of Family Growth." *Contraception* 77 (2008): 10–21.

Oken, Emily, Jenny S. Radesky, Robert O. Wright, David C. Bellinger, Chitra J. Amarasiriwardena, Ken P. Kleinman, Howard Hu, and Matthew W. Gillman. "Maternal Fish Intake during Pregnancy, Blood Mercury Levels, and Child Cognition at Age 3 Years in a U.S. Cohort." *American Journal of Epidemiology* 167 (2008): 1171–1181. doi:10.1093/aje/kwn034.

Peck, J. D., A. Leviton, and L. D. Cowan. "A Review of the Epidemiologic Evidence Concerning the Reproductive Health Effects of Caffeine Consumption: A 2000–2009 Update." *Food and Chemical Toxicology* 48 (2010): 2549–2576.

Rose, G. A., and A. Wong. "Experiences in Hong Kong with the Theory and Practice of the Albumin Column Method of Sperm Separation for Sex Selection." *Human Reproduction* 13 (1998): 146–149.

Scarpa, B., D. B. Dunson, and E. Giacchi. "Bayesian Selection of Optimal Rules for Timing Intercourse to Conceive by Using Calendar and Mucus." *Fertility and Sterility* 88 (2007): 915–924.

Wilcox, Allen J., Clarice R. Weinberg, and Donna D. Baird. "Timing of Sexual Intercourse in Relation to Ovulation—Effects on the Probability of Conception, Survival of the Pregnancy, and Sex of the Baby." *New England Journal of Medicine* 333 (1995): 1517–1521.

Lecture 23

Chowdhury, A. N. "The Definition and Classification of Koro." *Culture, Medicine and Psychiatry* 20 (1996): 41–65.

"HIV and AIDS in Africa." AVERT. http://www.avert.org/hiv-aids-africa.htm.

Novella, Steven. "Bee Venom Therapy—Grassroots Medicine," *Science-Based Medicine* (blog). http://www.sciencebasedmedicine.org/?p=296.

Stapleton, Paul. "Blood Type and Personality." http://paulstapleton.info/Fact%20Fable%20and%20Fiction/Chapter%201%20Blood%20Typing.htm.

"Urine Therapy." Academic Dictionaries and Encyclopedias. http://en.academic.ru/dic.nsf/enwiki/321591.

Lecture 24

Adesman, A., A. Cohn, N. Kohn, R. Milanaik, H. Papaioannou, and R. Pritzker. "Pediatric Pearls and Perils: Gaps in Basic Knowledge of Pediatricians that Pose Potential Health and Safety Risks to Children." Baby Facts. http://www.babyfacts.com/PDFs/pediatrician_study_results.pdf.

Barrett, Stephen. "Questionable Cancer Therapies." Quackwatch. http://www.quackwatch.org/01QuackeryRelatedTopics/cancer.html.

Brodeur, Raymond. "What Makes the Sound When We Crack Our Knuckles?" *Scientific American*, October 26, 2001.

Feldens, C. A., I. M. Faraco, A. B. Ottoni, E. G. Feldens, and M. R. Vítolo. "Teething Symptoms in the First Year of Life and Associated Factors: A Cohort Study." *Journal of Clinical Pediatric Dentistry* 34 (2010): 201–206.

"Overview of Population-Based Cancer Survival Statistics." National Cancer Institute. http://srab.cancer.gov/survival.

Unger, D. L. "Does Knuckle Cracking Lead to Arthritis of the Fingers?" *Arthritis and Rheumatism* 41 (1998): 949–950.

Notes

Notes

Notes

Notes

Notes

Notes

Notes